People, Cultures and Societies: Exploring and Documenting Diversities

Series Editors

Sunita Reddy, Godavari Hostel, Jawaharlal Nehru University, New Delhi, Delhi, India

Sanghmitra S. Acharya, School of Social Sciences, Jawaharlal Nehru University, New Delhi, Delhi, India

D1799928

The series proposes to capture the diversities in people and their communities in India. It provides a unique and innovative resource for anthropological knowledge, philosophy, methods, and tools to understand, analyse and formulate sustainable, innovative solutions to address socio-cultural issues in India.

India is a repository of varied cultures and diversities. With the globalisation and development process, the cultural fabric is changing. Customs, traditions, beliefs, on one hand, food habits, art and craft, weaving, dyeing, and handloom artefacts, on the other, are undergoing a metamorphosis. It is imperative to explore, understand and document the process of changing diversity and relational inequalities. The series encompasses richness in art, craft, language, dance, music, folklore, food culture and beliefs, traditions and practices. It addresses the issues of development disparities, inequality, and segregation on the axes of caste, class, religion, region, ethnicity, and gender. The series publishes methodologically rigorous and theoretically sound, critical and comparative, empirical research peer-reviewed volumes related to non-codified healing practices, gender-based violence, migration induced vulnerabilities, child abuse, social identity-based work on a national, regional and local level, welcoming case studies, as well as comparative and applied research.

The series is of interest to the academicians and students in the discipline of sociology, anthropology, psychology, social work, history, philosophy, and public health, and to all of those interested in a wide-ranging overview of art, culture, and politics. It accepts monographs, edited volumes, and textbooks.

More information about this series at https://link.springer.com/bookseries/16479

Sanghmitra S. Acharya · Stephen Christopher
Editors

Caste, COVID-19, and Inequalities of Care

Lessons from South Asia

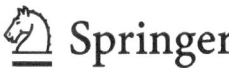 Springer

Editors
Sanghmitra S. Acharya
Centre of Social Medicine and Community
Health, School of Social Sciences
Jawaharlal Nehru University
New Delhi, India

Stephen Christopher
Department of Human and Social Sciences
Tokyo Metropolitan University
Tokyo, Japan

ISSN 2662-6616   ISSN 2662-6624 (electronic)
People, Cultures and Societies: Exploring and Documenting Diversities
ISBN 978-981-16-6919-4   ISBN 978-981-16-6917-0 (eBook)
https://doi.org/10.1007/978-981-16-6917-0

This Springer imprint is published by the registered company Springer Nature Singapore Pte Ltd.
The registered company address is: 152 Beach Road, #21-01/04 Gateway East, Singapore 189721,
Singapore

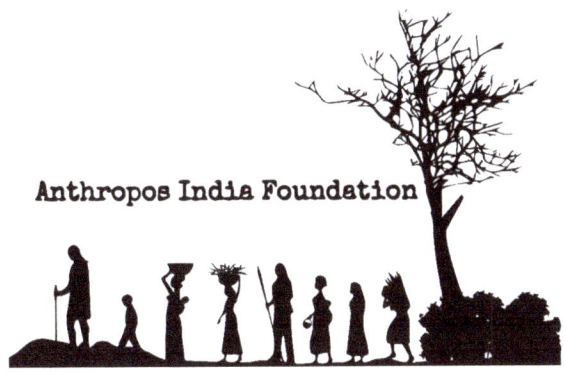

Anthropos India Foundation

Anthropos India Foundation (AIF) is a 2011 registered trust promoting applied anthropology, community-based research and policy recommendations within a South Asian context.

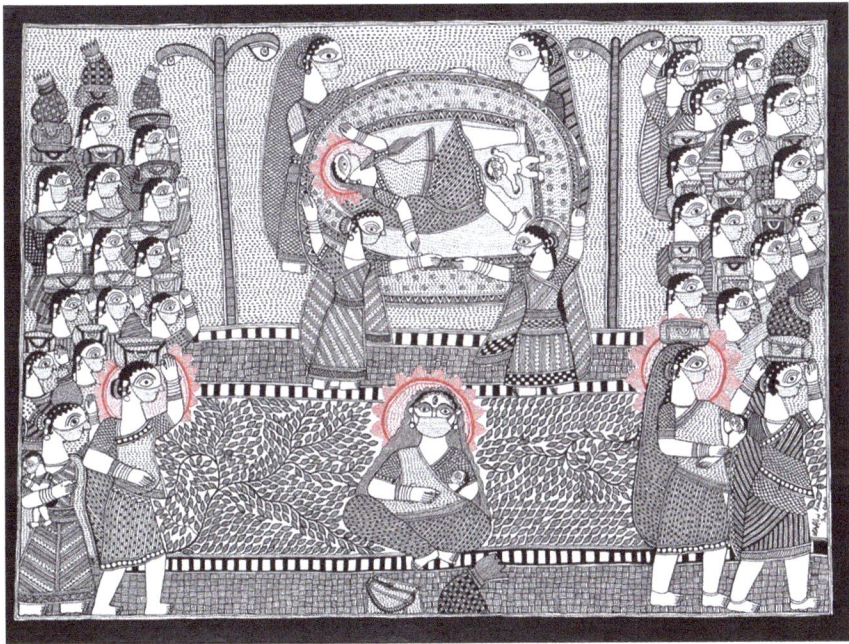

In this painting, the Mithila artist Shalini Karn portrays a real incident that took place during the return home of migrant workers during India's COVID-19 lockdown. Some 60 miles into her 500-mile journey home, Shakuntala gave birth with the help of fellow travelers. Shalini painted this story in black and red, black marking the failure of the government and red the power of women (description by Susan Wadley).

Foreword

At a time of unprecedented global disruption, publishing such a timely edited volume is a noteworthy achievement. The editors and contributing scholars conducted fieldwork, did archival research, collaborated and brought forth this volume during considerable pressures on themselves and their communities. One of the contributors, while researching the COVID-19 response in a Ho tribal village in Jharkhand, had to move his infected father out of Delhi and into a hospital facility in Hapur (UP) to ensure access to oxygen. He described the process as 'honestly speaking one of the scariest moments I've ever come across'. Other contributors lost friends and relatives. Nothing can bring them back, but this volume pays testament to those who lost their lives during COVID-19.

The overarching theme of this book is about how forms of structural inequality shape wellbeing in South Asia. We have come a long way in our analysis, from the days when health was imagined to be purely bio-physical to now, when we recognize the centrality of social determinants of health. This volume analyzes a wide variety of social determinants—from Dalits disenfranchised from Scheduled Caste quotas to the lingering legacy of colonial resource exploitation on tribal communities, from Dalit government hospital employees facing casteist practices to the urban ghettoization of Muslims—and based on these case studies builds upward to theoretical approaches and public health recommendations. Many chapters have critical portrayals of core Indian institutions, such as Reservation and government hospitals. The uneven messaging around COVID-19 lockdowns and the disproportionate impact on minorities paints a critical picture of the federal response.

It is my hope that policymakers will engage with the material in this volume. Each chapter is advocating on behalf of the empowerment of specific groups: tribes, Dalits, Muslims, health care providers and tea plantation workers, among others. The knowledge assembled here, often in dialogue with the aggrieved communities, is meant to be useful and actionable in providing redress and new forms of equity. With inequalities spiking around the world, but especially in India, it is time we take seriously our socialist roots—the founding principles of governance enshrined in the preamble of our Constitution—and implement health care systems that are universally accessible. And it is time we root out systemic discriminations in Indian society to ensure the equal and non-discriminatory wellbeing of all social groups. This volume is immensely useful for crafting policies that address inequalities during this most difficult time in our national history. I thank the many contributors and the two editors—Sanghmitra Acharya and Stephen Christopher—for preparing this volume for public consumption. It will prove useful for reforming public policy and for researchers to advance our future knowledge about these crucial themes.

Sukhadeo Thorat
Professor Emeritus at the Centre for the Study of Regional Development
School of Social Sciences, Jawaharlal Nehru University, New Delhi
Former Distinguished Professor at Savitribai Phule University, Pune
K. R. Narayanan Chair for Human Rights & Social Justice
Mahatma Gandhi University, Kerala (Honorary)
Chairman, Indian Institute of Dalit Studies, New Delhi
Former Chairman of University Grants Commission
Former Chairman of Indian Council of Social Science Research

Contents

Part II   COVID-19 Disparities

Part III   Health Inequalities

Editors and Contributors

About the Editors

Sanghmitra S. Acharya is a Professor in the Centre of Social Medicine and Community Health. Jawaharlal Nehru University, New Delhi. She has been Visiting Faculty at CASS, China; Ball State University, USA; UPPI, Manila; East West Centre, Honolulu; and the University of Botswana. She has received fellowships and grants by UNFPA, Asian Scholarship Foundation, USEFI, ICSSR-CASS and SICI. She works on the issues of health and discrimination and has published in journals of repute, including a book titled 'Social Discrimination in Health Care Access among Dalit Children' (Academic Publications).

Stephen Christopher is a Marie Curie Postdoctoral Fellow at the University of Copenhagen. He is engaged in two interrelated projects: one on casteism within Himalayan tribes and another on the rise of Tibetan Buddhism in East and Southeast Asia. In 2019, he was a JSPS Postdoctoral Fellow at Kyoto University. He serves as the Himalayas editor at the Database of Religious History at the University of British Columbia. Stephen has taught anthropology, South Asian studies and academic writing at Beijing Normal University, Vietnam National University, University of Bremen, Pitt in the Himalayas, Syracuse University, Semester at Sea, Tokyo Metropolitan University and Denki-Tsushin University.

Contributors

Dhananjay W. Bansod is a Professor at the Department of Public Health and Mortality Studies, International Institute for Population Sciences, Mumbai. His research interest includes Population Ageing, Public Health, Large Scale Survey Research, Maternal and Child health and workers' issues in the unorganized sector. He has published several research papers in population ageing, public health and other health-related issues. He has competed many research projects as one of the coordinators like Immunization Coverage Study in Maharashtra (ICM), National Family Health Survey (NFHS)–4 and Building Knowledge Base in Population Ageing in India (BKPAI).

Anwara Begum Ph.D. is a Senior Research Fellow and the Division Chief of the Human Resource Development Division at the Bangladesh Institute of Development Studies. She is Vice President of the Board of Unnayan Shohojogy Team and former Board Member of Campaign for Popular Education and Nari Unnayan Kendra. For the last thirty-two years, her research on development issues have underscored the essence of theoretical frameworks to inform policy and implementation practices. She led the research studies on the Millennium Development Goals Global Report 2003, Poverty Reduction Strategy Papers (PRSP) I and II, several noteworthy Bangladesh Government Reports, UNDP Global Follow-up Report, UNIFEM Female Migration and Education for All Reports. She has extensive experience in international migration research, including Bangladesh, United Kingdom, Ghana and India. She served as the Director of Research at CIRDAP and recently as the Gender and Resettlement Expert, for the International Project titled, DECCMA. Her book *Destination Dhaka* examined the heterogeneity of poor pavement and slum dwellers' migration commitments, and conceptualized a new theoretical framework for migration.

G. Dilip Diwakar teaches in the Department of Social Work, Central University of Kerala. He has more than 15 years of experience in the teaching, research and development sector. Before he joined CUK, he worked with national and international agencies like Indian Institute of Dalit Studies (IIDS), ActionAid, Aide-et-Action and Centre for Equity Studies. He co-authored a book titled *Caste, Discrimination and Exclusion in Modern India* (Sage 2015). He has published research articles in both national, international peer-reviewed journals and chapters in books. He has completed 11 research projects for the government and various funding agencies. He has done his M.Phil. and Ph.D. in Public Health from Jawaharlal Nehru University, New Delhi and MSW for Loyola College, Chennai. His research areas are food security, child nutrition, public health issues and urban poor. He is interested in studying intersectionality and marginalization across class, caste, gender and religion.

Sobin George is with the Institute for Social and Economic Change, Bangalore. His areas of research and writings cover the social gradient of health, critical studies on medical innovation, marginalities and labour rights. He is the author of several books, including: *Medical innovation and disease burden: conflicting priorities and the social divide in India* (2021), *Caste Embededdness of Rural Public Health Services* (2018) and *Work and health in informal economy* (2016). He has edited three books and published several research articles in national and international journals and edited books.

Payal Hathi is a Ph.D. student in Demography and Sociology at the University of California, Berkeley, and a Research Fellow at r.i.c.e. Her research interests centre on social inequality and health. Her current work focuses on the poor measurement of stillbirth as a form of mortality in India and other low and middle-income countries. She has also written on issues of gender, caste, and religion and health in India, including on the cultural reasons why open defecation persists in rural India, the relationship between casteist attitudes and hygiene in public hospitals, and the experiences of discrimination faced by Dalits and Muslims.Originally from southern California, Payal holds a BA in Economics from UC Berkeley and an MPA from Princeton University.

Suresh Jungari is an Assistant Professor in the Department of Public Health & Mortality Studies, International Institute for Population Sciences, Mumbai. His areas of research interest are maternal health, public health, gender issues in reproductive health, violence during pregnancy, health inequities and maternal mental health. He teaches subject of population and health, Gender issues in reproductive health, health economics and social concept in health. He is currently exploring the various dimensions of maternal mental health issues affecting reproductive age women in India. He has published several articles in national and international peer-reviewed scientific journals.

Smritima Diksha Lama completed her doctoral degree at Centre for Social Medicine and Community Health (CSMCH), Jawaharlal Nehru University (JNU), New Delhi. Her research interests include, but are not limited to, public health issues and policy, labour studies and social justice market mechanisms (fair trade) related to the tea plantations. She is currently working in the areas of adolescent health, mental health and impact of COVID-19 in association with the Health Promotion Division at Public Health Foundation of India (PHFI), Gurgaon.

Chandani Liyanage is a Professor at the Department of Sociology at the University of Colombo in Sri Lanka. She was a visiting faculty member at Ljubljana University in Slovenia and a visiting scholar at the Delhi School of Economics. She has received a Fulbright Advanced Research and Lecturing Award, was affiliated with the Centre for South Asian Studies at Syracuse University, and received a fellowship for Professionals-on Demand for Disability Rights in the USA. She works on issues of health, illness, disability and traditional medicine. She has published journal articles and book chapters, recently 'Socio-cultural construction of disability' in *Inclusion, Disability and Culture*(Springer International) and 'A Paradigm for Well-Being: Social Construction of Health' in *Health, Illness and Medicine* (Orient Blackswan).

Nilika Mehrotra is a social anthropologist teaching at the Centre for the Study of Social Systems, at Jawahar Lal Nehru University. She is editor of the journal Indian Anthropologist. She was a Fulbright Senior Researcher at the University of California at Berkeley (2013–2014). She edited the book *Disability Studies in India: Interdisciplinary Perspectives*(Springer, 2020) and has contributed numerous research publications in the areas of gender, disability and development.

Trisha Mukhopadhyay completed a postgraduate Diploma in Public Health Management from the Indian Institute of Public Health in Delhi in 2020. She also holds a Master's Degree in Geography (specialization in Social Geography) from

Jawaharlal Nehru University, batch of 2017–2019. Her area of interest lies in social determinants of health, gender and health, disparities in health, urban health, maternal health and geriatric health.

Prajwal Nagesh is a doctoral researcher with the Department of Human Geography and Planning, Utrecht University, the Netherlands and the Centre for Study of Social Change and Development (CSSCD) at the Institute for Social and Economic Change (ISEC), India. His doctoral research focuses on access inequities in transport for older adults in urban India. Some of his previously researched topics include urban migration, caste-based inequalities and inter-caste marriages.

Mahima Nayar is an independent researcher working in areas of disability, women, children and families. She was previously an Assistant Professor at the Tata Institute of Social Sciences, Mumbai. She has worked extensively with survivors of trafficking (women and children), women facing domestic violence and survivors of sexual assault, and persons with psychosocial disabilities and their families. She is the author of the book *Against All Odds: Psychosocial Distress and Healing among Women*(Sage-Yoda, 2018) and has co-edited *Contemporary Indian Family: Transitions and Diversity* (Routledge, 2020).

Aditi Paranjpe is a Public Health specialist with a background in Microbiology and nutrition. Her areas of interest are Public Health, infectious diseases, nutrition and the social determinants of health. She is currently a Senior Research Fellow at the Institute of Social and Economic Change (ISEC) in Bengaluru.

Sunita Reddy is an Associate Professor at the Centre of Social Medicine and Community Health, Jawaharlal Nehru University. She has twenty years of teaching and research experience. She has a Ph.D. in Medical Anthropology and research on a wide range of issues; disasters, mother-child health, child rights, tribal health, indigenous medicine, migrant workers, medical tourism and surrogacy. She has published three books and few papers in peer-reviewed journals. She has reviewed manuscripts for Springer and Sage. She is founder chair of a trust '*Anthropos India Foundation*(AIF)' which does visual and action research. AIF has signed a book series with Springer '*People, Societies and Cultures: Exploring and Documenting Diversities*'. She is also rooted to a community-based organization 'Satat' to reach out to the rural and urban slums. She was a core member to set up the Special Center for Disaster Studies (SCDR) in JNU. She participated in national debates on surrogacy in national TV channels. She has many awards in sports and co-curricular activities and recently received '*Women Empowerment Award- 2021*' on the International Women's Day by DELSA and Bhagidari Jan Sahyog Samiti.

Firdaus Fatima Rizvi is an Assistant Professor (Senior Scale) in the Department of Development Studies, Central University of South Bihar, Gaya. She holds LLB and Ph.D. (Economics) from University of Allahabad. Her research interests include labour markets, housing, affirmative action and agricultural development. She has published several research articles in reputed journals.

Arindam Roy is currently an Associate professor of Political Science at the University of Burdwan, West Bengal, India. His publications include 'Medical Pluralism and Myopic Public Health: A Study of Memari Block', 'Empowerment Beyond Rhetoric: Intersectionality Perspective to Gender Inequality in Health', 'Making Sense of Multiculturalism'. The latest being 'Privatizing the Pandemic-A Neoliberal Remedy'? and the forthcoming 'Pandemic and Administrative Rationality: Understanding Administrative Responses to the Pandemic'. He has published a book entitled *Mapping Administrative Theories: Problems and Prospects (2018)*. His areas of interest include public administration and political theory.

Sumanta Roy is a research scholar at the Centre of Social Medicine and Community Health, Jawaharlal Nehru University, New Delhi. He is also a student reporter with the People's Archive of Rural India. He writes opinion pieces for leading English and Bengali newspapers and portals. His research interests include political economy, workers health and intersectionality.

Pradeep S. Salve is an Assistant Professor at the Population Research Centre (PRC), Dharwad, Karnataka. He has a Ph.D. from the International Institute for Population Sciences (IIPS), Mumbai. He has received fellowship grant from Brown International Advanced Research Institutes (BIARI), at Brown University, USA and also received the best research paper award in the year 2021 by the Ministry of Health and Family Welfare (MoHFW), Government of India. He has been engaged in monitoring and evaluation of the National Health Missions, national health flagship programmes and public health facilities on behalf of the MoHFW, Government of India. He works on the issues of reproductive, maternal and child health, tropical diseases, occupational health risk among marginalized workers, caste and gender in India. He has published several research articles in the reputed international Journals.

Jay Prakash Sharma is a Ph.D. candidate at the Department of Anthropology at Syracuse University. He specializes in sociocultural anthropology, and his research interests include indigenous movements, land displacement and ecological conflicts. His doctoral research—currently funded by an AIIS Junior Fellowship—analyzes a localized movement against mining and land acquisition among the Ho tribal community in Jharkhand. He completed M.Phil. from the Delhi School of Economics.

Nikhil Srivastav is a researcher with the research institute for compassionate economics (r.i.c.e.) and is associated with Research and Action for Health in India (RAAHI) trust. He holds a Bachelor of Arts in Public Administration from Lucknow University, a postgraduate diploma in rural development from Indira Gandhi Open University (IGNOU), and a Masters of Public Affairs from the University of Texas, at Austin. Nikhil's research interests fall at the intersection of health and social equality. He has written on the issues of caste, religion and health in India, including why issues of caste and sanitation should be discussed together, the costs manual scavenging, and the relationship between caste and hygiene within and outside hospitals. His current work focuses on early life and maternal health. With colleagues, Nikhil is working on piloting a programme that intends to promote breastfeeding and care practices for newborn and low birthweight babies in Uttar Pradesh.

Bamdev Subedi is a medical anthropologist with an interest in public health issues. He holds a Master's degree in Anthropology from Tribhuvan University, Kathmandu, and an M.Phil. and Ph.D. in Social Sciences in Health from Jawaharlal Nehru University, New Delhi. He has more than a decade of working experience in health and community development projects in Nepal. His research interests include traditional medicine, medical pluralism and political economy of health. He has published quite a few research papers in edited volumes and journals. Currently he is contributing as co-author for a book, *From Poverty to Prosperity,* and as co-editor for an edited volume, *Ethnomedicine and Tribal Healing Practices: Challenges and Possibilities of Recognition and Integration.*

Nimisha Thakur is a doctoral student specializing in sociocultural anthropology at Syracuse University. She was also a part of the EMPOWER NSF Research Traineeship at the Department of Earth Sciences, where she was supported by a 2019 Syracuse University Water Initiative Fellowship. Her ethnographic project for her Ph.D. Dissertation focuses on the amphibiousness of river island spaces called *chars*, formed by the river Brahmaputra in Assam, inhabited by a riverine community called the Mising. Nimisha aims to understand how life on these *chars* can contribute to understanding the geo-social fluidity of water and its links to Mising community definitions of belonging and intersecting gender roles. She also aims to understand the gaps between these lived experiences of gendered belonging and state definitions that are caught up in colonial racial categorizations of tribal communities and increasingly in Hindu nationalist attempts that seek to equate 'indigeneity' with being Hindu. Nimisha also worked on an independent climate action group focussing on livelihood impacts of climate change in Majuli river island in Assam, India in 2020. She was awarded an AIIS (American Institute of Indian Studies) Junior Fellowship for 2021–2022. Her writing recently appeared in *Anthropology and Humanism* (December 2020) and *SAPIENS* (April 2021).

Visakh Viswambaran is a Ph.D. candidate at the Department of Social Work, Central University of Kerala. His doctoral dissertation is concerned with creating a pedagogy based on theory of intersectionality. The pedagogy enables the learners to understand how different social identities interact to create unique forms social inequalities in Indian scenario.

K. M. Ziyauddin teaches in the Department of Sociology, Maulana Azad National Urdu University at Hyderabad, India. Earlier he taught in Jamia Millia Islamia and Hamdard University in New Delhi before moving to Hyderabad. His upcoming books are *Sociology of Health in a Dalit Community: Axes of Exclusion* (Cambridge Scholars Publishing 2021) and *Reading Minorities in India: Forms and Perspectives* (Rawat 2021). He is currently working on two manuscripts: *Communalism in India: Socio-Historical and Legal Perspectives* (co-authored) and *Illness and Health: Sociological Narratives of Dalits.* His research involves the Sociology of Minorities, Muslims & Dalit Studies, Health & Sanitation and Urban Sociology. He attained initial degrees in Sociology from Jamia Millia Islamia; worked on *Health in a Dalit community in Polluted Occupation* for his M.Phil. (CSMCH) from JNU and has a

Ph.D. in Sociology on 'Perceptions of Illness and Health among the Dalits' from Delhi School of Economics, DU. He attended the US Department of State's International Visitors Leadership Programme in the USA in 2019. He serves as an executive editor for the Journal of Exclusion Studies and national convener of the Research Committee on Minority Studies of the Indian Sociological Society.

Chapter 1
Of Prejudice and Pandemics

Stephen Christopher and Sanghmitra S. Acharya

Social Discrimination and Well-being

Early in the COVID-19 outbreak, global media portrayed the virus as the 'great equalizer' of castes and classes, the rich and poor, the urban and rural. We were told that the virus does not discriminate. Some Indian commentators drew equal comparisons between the health risk of those domiciled in high-rise luxury apartments to those living precariously in slums, resettlements, illegal encroachments and ethnoreligious ghettos or 'red zones'. With the hindsight knowledge of additional research, we now know that these invidious comparisons were misleading in at least two ways. First, social deprivation and other measurements of inequality (irregular employment, low SES, precarious housing and lack of hygienic facilities) are cross-culturally correlated with mortality rates. Second, the socially marginalized face a host of compounding factors that act like comorbidities and intensify the psychosocial damage of the pandemic.

For the global Haves, those with educational and socio-economic advantage, can jump the line to immunity by buying bootlegged vaccines on the digital darknet. Euro-America and East Asia have dosed far more of their populations than comparatively poorer countries in Africa and Southeast Asia (with Japan being the outlier). Within the United States, vaccination rates privilege Democratic affluent states over Republican poorer states. At the same time that the state of Ohio was announcing a lottery with million-dollar giveaways to incentivize getting vaccinated, COVID-19-infected corpses were washing up on the banks of the Ganga, presumably because crematoria

S. Christopher
Department of Cross-Cultural and Regional Studies (ToRS), Center for Contemporary Buddhist Studies (CCBS), University of Copenhagen, Copenhagen, Denmark

S. S. Acharya (✉)
Centre of Social Medicine and Community Health, School of Social Sciences, Jawaharlal Nehru University, New Delhi, India

© The Author(s), under exclusive license to Springer Nature Singapore Pte Ltd. 2022
S. S. Acharya and S. Christopher (eds.), *Caste, COVID-19, and Inequalities of Care*,
People, Cultures and Societies: Exploring and Documenting Diversities,
https://doi.org/10.1007/978-981-16-6917-0_1

were maxed out and family members could not afford the wood for pyres. Using adjusted modelling to estimate COVID-19 mortality, India had about 2.2 million deaths by late May 2021—one of the worst outbreaks in the world (Guilmoto 2021). Mortality rates, vaccination rates and patterns of viral transmission highlight systemic inequalities between people, groups, regions and nations.

Around the world, we have seen the disproportionate impact of COVID-19 on the marginal Have Nots. African Americans, collectively remembering exploitative medical experiments committed by the US government, have 'vaccine hesitancy' and overall distrust of medical expertise (Brandon et al, 2005). Publicly stigmatized Thai sex workers, and especially transgendered people (primarily *kathoey*), are viewed with increased suspicion as transmitters of the virus. Japanese women, suspended in a web of social precarity, informal employment and patriarchal expectations, have experienced increased suicidal ideation during the cascading States of Emergency (Allison, 2014). Violent anti-Asian discrimination is spiking in several countries. Within China, there is widespread stigmatization of people from Wuhan city and Hubei province (He et al., 2020), reminiscent of Japanese 'radiation stigma' of Fukushima residents after the 3/11 disasters (Maeda & Oe, 2017).

In South Asia, the pandemic outbreak has similarly exacerbated the fault lines of social hierarchy that insidiously structure well-being and life chances. While praiseworthy advancements have been made in eliminating overt casteism, several important studies explore the persistence of group inequality (Jodhka, 2018), the intergenerational continuity of caste (Vaid, 2014), and its correlation to class (Kumar et al, 2002). The rise of neoliberal capitalism has led to upward social mobility for some Dalits in the professional sector, although high castes have disproportionately taken such positions (McMillian 2005, 149). The overt prejudices about symbolic and hygienic purity have, to some degree, transformed into more subtle idioms of discrimination: social pressure to maintain caste endogamy, pejorative associations with reservation quotas, violence against Dalit women and inequalities of access to public institutions, just to name a few. While the idioms have changed, casteism continues to influence health disparities and mental well-being in South Asia, with quantitative correlations between caste ranking, socio-economic status and biophysical health.

This book explores how identity-based discriminations contribute to health disparities and impede well-being. In doing so, it both draws from and extends the robust anthropological literature on how social suffering shapes health outcomes (Nguyen & Peschard, 2003), specifically during the COVID-19 pandemic (Nanda, 2020; Ahmed et al, 2020; Kim & Bostwick, 2020). Farmer (2004, 315) described this as the 'indissociable trio of anthropology, history, and biology' that seeks to understand how persistent inequalities are diachronically structured and naturalized: the political economy of AIDS and tuberculosis epidemics in Haiti, the legacy of slavery and multigenerational poverty on black health in the American South, and cardiovascular degermation and musculoskeletal disorders among manual scavengers in South Asia, among many others. Marginalized groups have increased exposure to environmental toxins and climate change disasters by virtue of their occupations and coerced residential districting; they may live in 'food deserts' and lack access to nutritious staple foods; they may be systematically impeded by bureaucrats or police; they may be treated with suspicion in high-status public and commercial spaces. These social subordinations create real psychic harm—and become important intersectional comorbidities when considering the disproportionate fallout of the pandemic. What are essentially socially constructed classifications of caste and race have become biologized through casteism and racism (Gravlee, 2009); we now understand that to inhabit a subordinate social space is to be deprived of nurturance of the body and mind.

In turn, social discriminations manifest as various disease aetiologies and forms of psychological harm: premature birth, hypertension, stress ulcers, alopecia and increased exposure to diseases, both at home and in health care facilities; and personal feelings of worthlessness, depression, anger and hostility. Many marginalized people suffer not only from empirical forms of discrimination but also from their own perceptions of how high-caste people view them. This doubling—not only what high-caste people think about low-caste people but what low-caste people think high-caste people are thinking about them (*pace* Cooley)—is part of everyday experience. In the Western Himalayas, when a ST Gaddi visits a SC Hali home but refuses *chai* and *chaat* on the pretense of fasting, the Hali may experience considerable mental anguish about their refusal, playing out scenarios, sleuthing about their actual piety and wading into an ocean of resentment where subterranean rivulets of casteism and self-doubt intersect with real physical harm. In Indian metropoles, when Dalits are undesired in marriage websites, barred from entering the homes they collect garbage from, or overlooked as potential renters in high-caste colonies, such experiences, whether inspired by caste prejudice or not, can cause considerable harm.

Social marginalization is not only between clearly dominant and subordinate groups; dominant caste ideologies are reproduced among stigmatized groups through marginal caste jockeying, just as SC/STs can be pitted against religious minorities. Compounding these factors, social identities such as caste shape access to health care resources and community knowledge about disease transmission and reproductive health. And human rights violations against the lower rungs of the caste hierarchy further the pathogenic force in creating health disparities.

Indian Inequality in a Global Perspective

Untouchability practices are historically present in West Africa (Tamari, 2005), East Asia (Korean *baekjeong* and Japanese *burakumin*) and arguably in pre-modern Tibet (Fjeld, 2005). Recently, caste has been invoked to analyse racial discrimination in the United States (Wilkerson, 2020), an argument most persuasively articulated decades before by Berremen (1960). Recognizing this does not deter from the fact that South Asian casteism is unparalleled in contemporary scope.

In India, there is generally higher non-literacy, unemployment, land disenfranchisement and poverty among SCs, STs, OBCs, EWS communities, religious minorities and the disabled, compared to high caste Hindus (Sachchidananda, 1974; Sen,

1992; Thorat, 2002; Shah et al., 2006; Kundu, 2008; Thorat & Madheswaran, 2018). These factors intermesh and form intersectional inequalities at multiple levels of analysis. Caste identities are strongly correlated to some being privileged with land ownership while some remaining landless; some lower castes supplying labour while some others demand it; some being able to freely marry while others meet the iron-clad prejudices of caste endogamy; occupations which are permissible and impermissible for lower castes; situations in which food is shared and collectively eaten, and situations when food, as a biomorphic substances, transmits caste and is restricted; sumptuary restrictions on who wears what and which parts of the body must be covered up by whom and who can and cannot wear footwear in certain social contexts.

Language hegemonies hierarchically scale certain dialects and define who can speak and in which register (Sridhar, 1996; Deshpande, 2000a, 2000b Khare, 2002). Class identities shape who receives certain forms of education, develops cosmopolitan competencies and builds up a cache of symbolic capital. Ethic identities shape ideologies around language, food, dress and geographical centre/periphery. Religious identities are inflected with prejudices and stereotypes about which ritualistic and cultural characteristics are celebrated or criticized.

The Indian social system is an overtly discriminatory, exclusivist and inequitable system which contradicts a parallel tradition of equality (Ambedkar, 1948; Das, 1969; Mungekar, 2017). It is a system that assigns stature, control, supremacy and prosperity to some, and toil, subjugation and oppression to others. Social identities are constructed through the complex interweaving of hereditary transmission of privilege, wealth and opportunity to the Haves, and hereditary disempowerment to the Have Nots (Beteille, 1969). While social identities can positively generate group belonging, cultural schemas, shared values and metaphors to orient around, they also unevenly distribute life chances and forms of mobility based on ethnic junctures (Becker, 1971, Darity, 1998), caste and religious differences (Thorat and Madheswaran, 2018). For instance, caste status is correlated to the hierarchical gradation of employment opportunity, with invisible, yet clear borders that few can cross (Thorat and Attewell, 2007; Borooah et al., 2014, 2015).

These barriers are experienced by marginalized groups as humiliations, injustices and evident forms of structural violence. Being on the wrong side of the social identity divide can induce deprivations and discriminations; those who manage to cross over invite the 'justified' condemnation, explicit or tacit, of dominant populations against boundary-transgressing upward social mobility. Subalterns who struggle into elite residential neighbourhoods or administrative jobs are accused of availing 'undue' Reservation benefits. Their achievements are belittled, rationalized away as government munificence, and they sometimes suffer from Imposter Syndrome for a lifetime. Efforts to redistributes status, power or wealth are opposed, cleverly turned into new forms of caste antagonism through the stereotyping of recipients of affirmative action (Still, 2013) or more violently repressed (Deshpande, 2000a, 2000b; Thorat Committee Report, 2007; Sharma, 2013; Senapati, 2014). The enduring power of social discriminations is evidenced by the effectiveness of positive discrimination to ensure a common starting line for the universal race for resources. These positive discriminations strive to ensure parity in access to vital resources like healthcare, civic participation and equal political representation, and reserved educational and government employment. The 2019 addition of Economically Weaker Sections (EWS) to Indian Reservation, and the ongoing ethnopolitical movements for more equitable distribution to Scheduled Tribal Dalits (Christopher, 2020), suggests that affirmative action is not a *fait accompli* but an ideal in need of vigilant revaluation and critical analysis.

As this book highlights again and again, India is one of the most unequal countries in the world in terms of income inequalities and social indices. Income inequality has continuously increased in India since 1990 (Patnaik, 2008). The 2020 Oxfam Inequality Index ranked India 151st among 158 countries based on its efforts to reverse inequality—especially during the pandemic. Notably, India's health budget is the world's fourth-lowest, and only half of the population has access to even the most basic health care services. India's ranking slipped from 141st in 2018 to 151st in 2020, citing dropping labour rights but increasing employment precarity. Common Sense would dictate that with measurable inequalities so high, the government would address it as the overwhelming crisis of our time. Unfortunately, India ranks 129th among 158 countries in the 2020 Commitment to Reducing Inequality Index (CRI) in terms of actionable government policies in shaping equal access to public services such as education, health care, social protection, taxation and workers' rights. Among the SAARC nations, India is dead last. War-torn Afghanistan fares better than the world's largest democracy (see Table 1.1)! India has also consistently ranked low in the Global Hunger Index (GHI) consistently for the past few years. In 2019, India was 102nd out of 117 countries.

Many chapters address how these systemic inequalities shaped pandemic experiences among minorities and underprivileged segments of Indian society. Certainly, not all groups are affected in the same way. Rounds of lockdowns and 'staying home' have caused joblessness, food insecurity and stress, leading to psychological problems across gender and age cohorts. The poor—disproportionately from SC/ST, minority and migrant labour communities—are the most impacted (NCDHR, 2019).

Table 1.1 SAARC nations in commitment to reducing inequality (CRI)

Countries	Ranking			
	public services*	Taxation	Labour	Over all
India	141	19	151	129
Pakistan	148	71	116	128
Bangladesh	142	32	109	113
Nepal	120	16	130	112
Bhutan	124	130	141	146
Afghanistan	153	06	113	102
Sri Lanka	106	91	86	94

* Healthcare, education and social protection. *Source* Oxfam International (2020), Commitment to Reduce Inequality (CRI) 2020, Oxfam International.

The enforcement of 'staying home' needs to be considered in light of the fact that about one-third of the households in India have to accommodate three to four persons per room, automatically defying social distancing guidelines. The situation of vulnerable groups, especially women, elderly, differently abled and hospice workers, has been particularly dire. Women's workload has increased, as has their exposure to domestic violence (Acharya et al., 2020; Deshpande, 2020; Gupta, 2020; Joy, 2020; Natarajan, 2020). The following chapters provide important insights into how Indian institutional responses to the pandemic have furthered social inequalities and resulted in disparate health care access across social groups. While many of the following chapters remain empirically driven and do not posit moral condemnations, the editors are in agreement that the Indian government broadly failed to implement policies that are responsive to the robust data on the intertwining of social inequalities and public health.

These themes are explored in three sections. The first section addresses institutional forms of marginalization and the downstream impact on well-being. Following the call to study the social field of affirmative action politics using critical ethnography (Shah & Shneiderman, 2013), two chapters analyse how Reservation, when inequitably administered, can deepen the grooves of casteism, jeopardize tribal lifeways and ensnare mountain Dalits in demeaning and expensive rounds of administrative limbo. Two chapters converge on a critique of casteism and neoliberalism within public health intuitions. One chapter addresses how falling on the wrong side of the Digital Divide can have deadly consequences, while another highlights how Muslim urban ghettoization is correlated with systemic inequalities. The last chapter places tribal rumours about COVID-19 in the broader context of historical exploitation by the British, mining companies and health care institutions. We see how the pandemic was perceived by marginal communities within specific legacies of institutional exploitation. Taken together, these chapters marshal considerable ethnographic and quantitative data to highlight the embodied nature of marginalization.

References

Acharya, S. S., Mukherjee, M., & Dutta, C. (2020). The shadow pandemic in India: 'staying home' and the safety of women during lockdown gender forum. *A Journal for Gender Studies, 76*, 46–61.

Ahmed, F., Na'eem, A., Christopher, P., & Joseph, S. (2020). *The Lancet Public Health, 5*(5), 240.

Allison, A. (2014). *Precarious Japan.* Duke University Press.

Ambedkar, BR (1948). The Untouchables: Who were they and Why they became Untouchables Dr Bababsaheb Ambedkar. *Writings and speeches Vol 5 compiled by Vasant Moon. Reprint by Dr Ambedkar Foundation, ministry of social justice and empowerment.* Government of India.

Becker, G. S. (1971). *The economics of discrimination.* University of Chicago Press.

Berreman, G. D. (1960). Caste in India and the United States. *American Journal of Sociology, 66*(2), 120–127.

Beteille, A. (1969). *Caste, class and power.* University of California Press.

Borooah, V. K., et al. (2014). Evaluating the social orientation of the integrated child development services programme. *Economic and Political Weekly,* 52–62.

Borooah, V. K., et al. (2015). *Caste, discrimination and exclusion in modern India.* Sage Publications.

Bora, P. (2010). Between the human, the citizen and the tribal: Reading feminist politics in India's Northeast. *International Feminist Journal of Politics, 12,* 341–360.

Brandon, D. T., et al. (2005). The legacy of Tuskegee and trust in medical care: Is Tuskegee responsible for race differences in mistrust of medical care? *Journal of the National Medical Association, 97*(7), 951–956.

Christopher, S. (2020). 'Scheduled Tribal Dalit' and the emergence of a contested intersectional identity. *Journal of Social Inclusion Studies, Indian Institute of Dalit Studies, 6*(1), 1–17.

Darity, W. A. (1998). Evidence on discrimination in employment: Codes of color, codes of gender. PL Mason. *Journal of Economic Perspectives, 12*(2), 63–90.

Das, B. (Ed.). (1969). *Thus spoke Ambedkar: Selected speeches.* (Vol. 1). Bheem Patrika Publications.

Deshpande, A. (2000a). Hindustani in India. *Economic and Political Weekly, 35*(15), 1240–1242.

Deshpande, A. (2000b). Does caste still define disparity? A look at inequality in Kerala, India. *American Economic Review, 90*(2), 322–325.

Deshpande, A. (2020). In locked down India, women fight coronavirus and domestic violence. *Quartz India.*

Farmer, P. (2004). An anthropology of structural violence. *Current Anthropology, 45*(3), 305–325.

Fjeld, H. (2005). *Commoners and nobles: Hereditary divisions in Tibet* (Vol. 96). Nias Press.

Gravlee, C. C. (2009). How race becomes biology: Embodiment of social inequality. *American Journal of Physical Anthropology, 139*(1), 47–57.

Guilmoto, C. Z. (2021). Estimating the death toll of the Covid-19 pandemic in India. *medRxiv* preprint. https://doi.org/10.1101/2021.06.29.21257965.

Gupta, J. (2020). What does coronavirus mean for violence against women? *Women's Media Centre.*

He, J., He, L., Zhou, W., Nie, X., & He, M. (2020). Discrimination and social exclusion in the outbreak of COVID-19. *The International Journal of Environmental Research and Public Health, 17*(2933), 1–4.

Jodhka, S. S. (2018). Inequality, ethnicity, and caste. In G. Antonelli & B. Rehbein (Eds.), *Inequality in economics and sociology: New perspectives* (pp. 131–147). Routledge.

Joy, Shemin (2020). *Coronavirus crisis: No lockdown for domestic violence.* DHNS.

Khare, S. K. (2002). Truth about language in India. *Economic and Political Weekly, 37*(50), 4993–4994.

Kim, S. J., & Bostwick, W. (2020). Social vulnerability and racial inequality in COVID-19 deaths in Chicago. *Health Education and Behavior, 47*(4), 509–513.

Kumar, S., Heath, A., & Heath, O. (2002). Changing patterns of social mobility: Some trends over time. *Economic and Political Weekly, 37*(40), 4091–4096.

Kundu, A. (2008). Report of the expert group on diversity index. Report of the expert group to propose a diversity index and work out the modalities for implementation. *Ministry of minority affairs.* Government of India.

Maeda, M., & Oe, M. (2017). Mental health consequences and social issues after the Fukushima disaster. *Asia Pacific Journal of Public Health, 29*(2), 26–36.

McMillan, A. (2005). *Standing at the margins: Representation and electoral reservation in India.* Oxford University Press.

Mungekar, B. (Ed.). (2017). *The essential Ambedkar.* Rupa Publication.

Nanda, S. (2020). Inequalities and COVID-19. In J. Michael Ryan (Ed.), *COVID-19: Volume I: Global pandemic, societal responses, ideological solutions* (pp. 109–123). Routledge.

Natarajan, J. (2020). Women's safety during lockdown. *The Hindu.*

NCDHR. (2019). NCDHR-Annual-Report.pdf - National Campaign on Dalit Huma Rights. http://www.ncdhr.org.in>uploads>2019/05. Swadhikar NCDHR ANNUAL REPORT.

Nguyen, V.-K., & Peschard, K. (2003). Anthropology, inequality, and disease: A review. *Annual Review of Anthropology, 32,* 447–474.

Oxfam International. (2020). 'The Inequality Virus' Oxfam Report. https://www.oxfam.org/en/press-releases/megarich-recoup-covid-losses-record-time-yet-billions-will-live-poverty-least.

Patnaik, U. (2008). The Republic of Hunger and Other Essays Delhi Collective.

Sachchidananda. (1974). Education among the scheduled castes and scheduled tribes in Bihar. AN Sinha Institute of Social Sciences, Patna.

Sen, A. (1992). *Inequality reexamined*. Harvard University Press.

Senapati, T. K. (2014). Human rights and dalits in India: A sociological analysis. *International Research Journal of Social Sciences, 3*(3), 36–40.

Shah, A., & Shneiderman, S. (2013). The practices, policies and politics of transforming inequality in South Asia: Ethnographies of affirmative action. *Focaal, 65*(12), 3–12.

Shah, G., Mander, H., Thorat, S., Deshpande, S., & Baviskar, A. (2006). *Untouchability in Rural India*. Sage Publications.

Sharma, S. (2013). Hate crimes in India: An economic analysis of violence and atrocities against scheduled castes and scheduled tribes. *Centre for development economics, department of economics*. Delhi School Economics.

Sridhar, K. (1996). Language in education: Minorities and multilingualism in India. *International Review of Education, 42*(4), 327–347.

Still, C. (2013). 'They have it in their stomachs but they can't vomit it up': Dalits, reservations, and 'caste feeling' in rural Andhra Pradesh. *Focaal, 65*(12), 68–79.

Tamari, T. (2005). Kingship and caste in Africa: History, diffusion and evolution. In D. Quigley (Ed.), *The character of kingship* (pp. 141–169). Routledge.

Thorat, S. (2002). Oppression and Denial: Dalit Discrimination in the 1990s. *Economic and Political Weekly, 37*(6), 123–126.

Thorat, S., Madheswaran, S. (2018). Graded caste inequality and poverty: evidence on role of economic discrimination. *Journal of Social Inclusion Studies, 4*(1), 3–29. https://doi.org/10.1177/2394481118775873.

Thorat Committee Report. (2007). *Report of the committee to enquire into the allegation of differential treatment of sc/st students in All India Institute of Medical Sciences*. Government of India.

Vaid, D. (2014). Caste in contemporary India: Flexibility and persistence. *Annual Review of Sociology, 40*, 391–410.

Wilkerson, I. (2020). *Caste: The origins of our discontents*. Random House.

Part I
Institutional Exclusions

The opening chapters address tribal ethnopolitical mobilizations for state recognition. **Stephen Christopher** analyzes the moving goalposts of state recognition among the Gaddis of Himachal Pradesh. His broader agenda is to advocate for scholarly attention to tribal casteism (and its corollary, tribal heterogeneity) and constitutional recognition of the intersectionality of Dalits either within tribes or petitioning for tribal recognition (Christopher 2020). The Gaddi community—geographically split between Chamba and Kangra in Himachal Pradesh and Bhaderwah in Jammu and Kashmir—is also a caste-heterogeneous community, primarily Rajput but including Scheduled Castes and Brahmins. His chapter explores how tribal casteism contributed to Dalit conversions to the Arya Samaj in the mid-twentieth century. Meant to provide Dalit uplift, caste emendations in the Revenue Record have muddied the waters about which caste groups should be given SC and ST benefits. Based on fieldwork among Halis, a diverse Scheduled Caste community with region-specific propinquity to Gaddi tribalness, Christopher demonstrates how state misrecognition has clear, multigenerational impact on marginalized Halis. Centred on the ongoing saga of his research assistant to emend his caste certificate from general caste 'Arya' to Scheduled Caste 'Hali', Christopher pans out to the systemic problems of labyrinthine administration, shrewd lawyers and bribable bureaucrats. This Kafkaesque drama of rural, often non-literate Dalits, facing years of mental anguish, wasted time, and psychological degradation in order to 'prove' their caste subordination to the state, is the concealed underbelly of an affirmative action system that sometimes disadvantages the very people it was designed to help.

In a similar vein, **Nimisha Thakur** refracts the Assamese Mising tribe's petition for constitutional recognition of the Mising Autonomous Council into a broader discussion about hygiene discourses around pig consumption. She argues that medical expertise aligns with high-caste nationalist discourses about purity to unscientifically blame pig consumption on a range of Mising health problems. Compounding these dietary interventions, climatic changes to the riverine landscape and industrial pork production have further alienated Mising from their traditional lifeways. These changes threaten to undermine the collective spiritual practices, migratory histories, and affective ties to ancestors that are expressed in Mising pig rearing and consumption. Granting constitutional status to the Mising Autonomous Council would ensure the safeguarding of Mising lifeways by increasing their power to internally conduct matters pertaining to tribal land, food, and customary practices. Through detailed ethnographic data, Thakur explores pig practices as a Maussian total social fact, a loci of caste discourses and nationalist imaginings for health experts and a repository of collective memory, spirituality, and autonomy for Mising people. These discrete practices, which span politics, culture, psychology, and health, are interwoven into the body of the pig. Consequently, Thakur's analysis, which explores the recursive looping between state recognition and communal well-being, is an important contribution to the critical analysis of Reservation.

Payal Hathi and Nikhil Srivastav investigate how caste ideologies around purity shape a culture of negligence in government hospitals. Extending previous research on North Indian hospital cleaners, they argue that observable caste practices, under-girded by unscientific attitudes about disease transmissibility, increase the likeli-hood of infection. Their work exposes internalized caste hierarchies with regards to cleaning practices, who receives government training, the perceived replace-ability of Dalit labour, and the unequitable distribution of labour. Moreover, casteist notions shape attitudes around glove use, leaving hospital workers open to infec-tion during medical procedures with high rates of disease transmissibility. Their argument for renewed adherence to the basics of germ theory and dispelling caste prejudice within hospital settings both strengthens overall hygienic conditions and specifically addresses the marginalization of Dalit employees. It reinforces previous studies that correlate discrimination against Dalits in hospitals with the overrep-resentation of general caste medical staff and caregivers (George 2015). Ensuring equal representation of medical staff from lower castes might create a cultural change within hospitals that would lead to the more favourable treatment of Dalit cleaners and improve overall hospital hygiene. Although their data was collected before the pandemic outbreak, it has obvious relevance to curbing the spread of COVID-19.

Further addressing the point that the pandemic was not the 'great equaliser', **Sunita Reddy** explores inequalities within India's health care services that partition lower SES people into government hospitals and higher SES people into for-profit private hospitals. She tracks the emergence of the corporate health sector and its lack of regulatory oversight to serve public interests. She chastises corporate hospitals for sticking to a profit-driven model and price gouging during the COVID-19 outbreak, and proposes amendments to the 2005 Disaster Management Act to compel private hospitals to be more humanitarian and less neoliberal during health emergencies. She echoes the argument of many other chapters in this volume that hospitals are geographically embedded and reproduce gendered, casteist, and classist stereotypes and inequalities of representation and access. Many of her specific policy recom-mendations are buttressed by ethnographic evidence from other chapters, such as the need for federal protections of migrant labourers (pace Sharma's analysis of Ho tribal migrants) and weeding out unscientific caste practices in government hospitals (Hathi and Srivastav).

Dilip Diwakar and Visakh Viswambaran extend the concern about institu-tional exclusions to South Asia's formidable Digital Divide. Rural, poor, and low caste students faced disproportionate burdens to adjust to online education during the pandemic outbreak, contributing to increased mental anguish and suicide rates. Moreover, women face higher rates of suicide because of the difficult balancing patriarchal norms with burgeoning educational aspirations. They call for renewed focus on equitable digital infrastructure, sensitivity training for teachers, an overhaul of online education, and increased resources for psychological counselling for marginalized students placed under increased pressure to negotiate the digital access inequalities. Their work is an important reminder that COVID-19 was not the 'great equaliser'—indiscriminately impacting people from all socioeconomic classes and castes. The pandemic exacerbated existing inequalities and created concomitant social pressures; in the case of Indian students adjusting to expectations of digital access, these pressures sometimes led to suicide. This data is congruent with global data on the disproportionate impact of COVID-19; for example, increased suicidal ideation among Japanese women during the pandemic and ensuring States of Emergency due to their irregular employment and overrepresentation in service industries, which were curtailed by social distancing measures (Sakamoto et al, 2021).

K. M. Ziyauddin analyzes densely packed Muslim neighbourhoods (mohalla) in Hyderabad and argues that intermeshing deprivations contribute to the overall deprivation of Muslims vis-à-vis non-Muslim citizens. Similar to the redlining practices targeting nonwhite citizens in North America, Muslims often live in 'red zone' settlements, sometimes called 'negative geographical zones', not approved for house constructions, unable to secure formal bank loans, and prone to extortionist private money lenders. Muslim ghettoization in these settlements means barriers in registering for a voter card, ration card, Aadhar card, and other official paperwork that allow equal participation. By broadly comparing data on Hyderabad's Muslim-dominated Old City with Hyderabad Central (also called the New City and comprising Secunderabad and Ameerpet), he suggests that Muslim enclaves have less facilities, less police stations, less government buildings and more non-literacy rates and density than non-Muslim counterparts. Ziyauddin concludes that criminalizing Muslim slums and terming them as 'red zones' perpetuates Muslim exclusions from various city and federal institutions. The cloud of illegality over these settlements only furthers their spatial marginalization and discursive othering.

Last, **Jay Prakash Sharma** turned his analytic attention to the pandemic response itself. He tracks how COVID-19 impacted the Ho tribal community in Jharkhand, who are long distrustful of outsiders claiming various forms of expertise in order to exploit indigenous resources and subordinate local peoples. Their historical exploitation extends from British colonization to post-Independence and was often couched as bringing civilization to barbaric tribals (Bora 2010). Recent Jharkhandi statehood has not prevented neoliberal policies, buttressed by anti-worker state legislation, to allow mining companies to continue this legacy of resource extraction. These exclusions frame the analysis of Ho pandemic perceptions which, similar to other indigenous communities, exhibit distrust of the very medical establishment which has long exploited them. He sensitively tracks Ho discourses about the pandemic—rumours that it is exaggerated by state actors and industrialists to further their own benefit, misinformation about its spread, gossip about preventive cures, and conspiracy theories about forced institutionalization. Rather than dismiss these perceptions as village ignorance, he frames them as social facts and forms of indigenous resistance, sometimes unconscious and often partially accommodating the social system it seeks to criticize. Sharma's chapter is an invaluable snapshot, playing out in real time, of how legacies of marginalization track across time. Even when these legacies are countered with indigenous forms of agency, they continue to damage collective well-being.

Chapter 2
Exceptional Aryans: State Misrecognition of Himachali Dalits

Stephen Christopher

Abstract This chapter analyses the positionality of Halis—former bonded labourers, ploughers and animal carcass removers—who constitute the most subordinated Scheduled Caste (SC) community within the Gaddi tribal orbit. For many Halis, the struggle for Scheduled Tribe (ST) recognition begins with legally undoing their ancestral conversion to the Ayra Samaj. In the early twentieth century, many Halis officially replaced their caste name with 'Arya' or 'Gaddi Arya' in the Revenue Record in order to combat tribal casteism. For a time, they adopted the purifying techniques and caste-obliterating ideologies of the Arya Samaj. This strategy of upward caste mobility backfired, however, when Arya was classified as a forward caste and converted Halis were denied SC benefits in the initial constitutional scheduling. Their official status as Aryas continues to deprive thousands of Halis of much-needed SC benefits and protections. Through fieldwork data collected between 2014 and 16, I highlight the psychosocial anguish of many Halis as they waste inordinate amounts of time and resources bribing bureaucrats, negotiating with state administrators, excavating the archive for non-existent property documents, and being exploited by lawyers—all in the pursuit of restoring their Hali caste name to qualify for SC benefits. Many Halis—non-literate village scratch farmers—are defeated by feelings of worthlessness and inadequacy. Their struggle is further complicated by a desire to ascend the escalator of state recognition from forward caste Aryas to SC Halis to ST Gaddi Dalits. Based on 16 months of ethnographic fieldwork, I argue that state (mis)recognition can drive marginalization and coarsen psychosocial wellbeing.

Keywords Gaddi · Hali · Arya · Reservation politics · Tribal dalits

S. Christopher (✉)
Department of Cross-Cultural and Regional Studies (ToRS), Center for Contemporary Buddhist Studies (CCBS), University of Copenhagen, Copenhagen, Denmark

Introduction

Gaddis are a Scheduled Tribe (ST) concentrated in the tribal-reserved area of Bharmour in Chamba district, Himachal Pradesh. Affectionately named Gadderan, Bharmour is the notional Gaddi homeland and focal point of transhumant pastoralism, pilgrimage and various Gaddi beliefs and folktales. Another population of Gaddis inhabits the southern spurs of the Dhauladhar Mountains in Kangra district—roughly stretching from Dharamsala to the west, Bir to the east, and Maharana Pratap Sagar and Gaehr to the south. While the Gaddi communities in both Chamba and Kangra remain interconnected through migration histories, communal festivals, intermarriage and shared spiritual practices, they also exhibit significant differences. Kangra Gaddis have culturally integrated into the wider plains culture of Punjab, inflecting Gaddi dialect with Punjabi, popularizing the *mangal sutra*, and affecting ritual practice.

Many Gaddis consider Kangra to be a place of socioeconomic aspiration, with the city of Dharamsala—once a Gaddi pastoral stopover—now the hub of Tibetan diaspora politics, international spiritual tourism and weekend sojourns for Delhiites (Christopher 2020a, 2020b; Bloch, 2018). Dharamsala boasts an Indian Premier League-accredited cricket stadium, hosted the 2019 Global Investors' Meet, and is currently being modernized into a Smart City. In their aspiration to a lifestyle of novelty, which remains unavailable in their remote natal villages, male Gaddi youth increasingly shift to Dharamsala, Bir and other towns in the Kangra region to learn English, acquire cosmopolitan competencies and work in the tourism sector.

While Chamba has also undergone significant transformations due to large-scale hydro projects, the popular perception is that Bharmouri Gaddis follow more traditional tribal lifestyles: living proximate to the Chaurasi Temple complex (the *axis mundi* of Gaddi cosmology); maintaining Gaddi dialect; retaining a greater number of folk bards and family lineage priests; and conserving a village life dependent on small-scale scratch farming and traditional modes of social interdependence.

Politics have also divided Gaddis in Chamba and Kangra. Although Gaddis in Bharmour were granted ST status in the first post-Independence scheduling in 1950, those Gaddis who since the early nineteenth century had migrated into Kangra—to exploit low-lying winter pasturelands and agricultural land grants—were initially considered to belong to general castes and later to Other Backward Classes (OBCs). Kangra Gaddis had fallen into an administrative paradox: while their affines in Bharmour were constitutionally recognized tribal subjects, they themselves were not. This transpired because Kangra officially belonged to Punjab—an area British administrators considered as uninhabited by tribes. In 1966, however, Kangra was redistricted as a part of Himachal Pradesh, and Gaddis began to appeal for ST status to the end of unification, politically and socially, with their relatives in Bharmour. This appeal accelerated as Mandal reforms and political alliances shifted in favour of the Gaddis and, consequently to an ethnological survey of Dharamsala and adjoining areas, high-caste Kangra Gaddis were awarded ST status in 2002. They are now constitutionally guaranteed government entitlements and political protections as a marginalized community.

Since 2011, my research has focussed on how tribal reclassification of Kangra Gaddis has included *solely* high-caste Rajputs and Bhatt Brahmins. It has excluded five Scheduled Castes—Sippi, Badi, Rihare, Dhogri and Hali—which have maintained a contested purchase on Gaddi identity since the earliest colonial documentation of the annexation of Dharamsala. These SC communities comprise the fullest account of Gaddi social stratification; being partially integrated into Gaddi life in hundreds of villages spanning hundreds of kilometres across Kangra and Chamba. While this chapter focuses on the unique predicament of Halis, who are perceived as the lowest status Gaddi group, the issue of tribal Dalit misrecognition extends to other Gaddi-aspiring SC groups and, indeed, is an under-researched and poorly theorized feature of Himalayan tribal life in general.

Halis and Scheduled Caste Gaddis

In similarity with nearly all Gaddis, Halis trace their origins back to Gadderan, the fifth Scheduled Tribal heartland in Bharmour *tehsil*. However, their migration histories differ from those of Gaddis, who were subject to the efforts of colonial administrators to settle semi-nomadic pastoralists in the non-state space of the Punjabi Himalayas, with increasingly restricted access to pasturelands. Rather, Halis were bonded labourers, 'brought' (*leke ānā*) by dominant Gaddis from Bharmour and settled in Gaddi villages on the southern spurs of the Dhauladhar Mountains during the eighteenth and early nineteenth centuries. Newell (1952, 90) describes how this process occurred in the Gaddi village of Goshen, where three Sippi (another SC Gaddi caste) families were 'called' to resettle, to perform caste-specific labour. Further, Halis were not only 'brought', like mobile commodities; along with other Gaddi Dalits, they were 'kept' (*rakh liyā*) by Gaddis as tenants (*pāocārī*) within a flexible patronage system that paralleled *jajmānī* relations among non-Gaddi castes. These landless tenants performed sedentary and stigmatized social roles, such as exorcism, ploughing, animal carcass removal and hide tanning. While some Halis grazed modest flocks locally—an occupation nowadays referred to as 'goat duty' (*bakrī duti*)—they rarely participated in Gaddi transhumance, during which shepherds traversed Chamba and Kangra as mobile six-monthers (*chemahīne*).

Over the centuries, Halis have faced wide-ranging discrimination, including prohibitions on grazing their flocks at sacred highland pastures, barring of access to temples, segregation of water taps and cremation grounds, ghettoized residential patterning on less arable and symbolically polluted land, ritual exclusions, and rejection by Gaddi Bhatt Brahmin lineage priests (*kul purohit*), who preside over important lifecycle events. In a cluster of interconnected villages, elders recalled how everyone wore the off-white Gaddi woollen cloak (*colā*), but Halis were forced to wear a black mark (*kālī tanki*) on their shoulders as a symbol of exclusion.

Casteist attitudes concerning marriage endogamy and commensality continue to this day and, in a shift of caste idiom, historical exclusions are now buoyed by the stereotyping of SC benefits. However, despite the perpetuation of casteism by Gaddi Rajputs (the demographic majority and reference group), Halis are in the midst of an uneven process of tribal integration. Over multiple generations, they have integrated many of the commonalities of Gaddi culture—culture (*sanskriti*); dialect (*bolī*), dress (*beṣ buśa*), cuisine (*khānpān*) and history—that constitute a Herderian notion of shared ethnic identity. But this Gaddi tribalisation among peripheral labouring castes remains unevenly distributed; operating at multiple scales, and shaped by ethnic entrepreneurs and the successes of ethnopolitical mobilizations.

This process has renewed in urgency since 2002 awarding of ST status to only Kangra Gaddi Rajputs and Brahmins; a classification that excluded Gaddi-identifying SC groups such as Halis. Although the stakes have grown in the past two decades—as caste groups vie for state benefits—colonial administrators, followed by post-Independence anthropologists, have actually mulled over the liminal positionality of Halis within the Gaddi tribe for at least 160 years (Barnes, 1862; Newell, 1952; Phillimore, 1982; Wagner, 2013). The multiple and contradictory accounts of Gaddi social organization over time have contributed to the emergence of tribal Dalit identity. Gaddis are variously defined as the inhabitants of Gadderan, as an administrative category not corresponding with tribal social organization, as a nationality of between two and four classes, as synonymous with Gaddi Rajput, and as a generic group inclusive of either solely high castes, or of all castes. Attempts to reconcile early colonial records with post-Independence scholarship provide no unifying consensus on Gaddi identity, but rather establish the archival parameters by which contemporary scholars and local ethnic entrepreneurs shape their arguments.

This chapter does not delve into the archival record to try to adjudicate Gaddi nomenclature and social belonging. I have argued elsewhere for the place of Dalits within the Gaddi tribe, and examined the broader question of tribal caste pluralism. Instead, this chapter addresses the forms of psychic and social harm that have befallen Halis, as a result of their perceived political misrecognition.

There has been multi-generational fallout from Halis whose ancestors, in an attempt to evade casteism, have nominally adopted the tenets of the Arya Samaj and recast (through legal emendation) their caste from stigmatized Hali to purest Arya. This strategy has backfired and, from Independence to the present, their 'recasting' of caste has disqualified uncounted thousands of Halis from SC benefits. Further, emending their caste names back to Hali has proven an administrative nightmare and source of considerable distress.

Before ethnographically unpacking how the caste-obliterating aspirations of Aryan exceptionalism have given rise to generations of social suffering, I will highlight the broader and more systemic forms of misrecognition that impact Halis. Specifically, Kangra Halis are broadly categorized as SCs and are thus ineligible for less competitive ST benefits. The restriction of the ST administrative category to Gaddi Rajputs and Brahmins alone has left Halis and other self-reporting low-caste Gaddi communities—those which are most fragile and in need of state assistance—socially marginalized. This causes tangible forms of harm. Halis are barred from membership of the Gaddi Welfare Board and the HP State Wool Federation—the primary vehicles of influence peddling to allocate funds and pass favourable legislation. Halis cannot stand in local elections reserved for ST candidates and rarely defeat larger SC communities (specifically Chamar, Lohar, Kori and Julaha) in SC-reserved elections. Hali youth are looked over for leadership roles in the student-run Kailash Association—a Gaddi ethnic association with vast membership. Kangra Halis are legally prohibited from purchasing land in the Fifth Scheduled Reserved Area of Bharmour; their ancestral homeland.

Another reality of tribal exclusion is that Halis must compete for the 15 per cent SC quota reservation in Himachal Pradesh—the state with proportionally the second-highest SC population (25.2%) in India. Halis rightly contend that they are systematically outperformed by those other demographically outsized SC communities that dwell in resource-dense urban centres with more entrenched political support. Conversely, Himachal Pradesh has a modest ST population (5.7%), which competes for 7.5% quota reservations. Given state demographics and the concentration of Halis in underdeveloped rural enclaves sustained by scratch farming, mountain foraging and employment schemes such as the Mahatma Gandhi National Rural Employment Guarantee Act (MGNREGA, the creamy layer of competing SC groups is better positioned to negotiate state bureaucracy and benefit from state assistance. These tangible restrictions augment the overall distortion of 'being misrecognised'; proper recognition being the 'vital human need' that underlies our modern sense of human agency (Taylor, 1994, 26). This contemporary state misrecognition is rooted in the evangelizing efforts of the Arya Samaj, towards the beginning of the twentieth century.

Purification Through the Arya Samaj

The Arya Samaj was established in 1877 in Lahore as a pan-regional, proselytizing organization, dedicated to modernizing Hindu practices. The founder, Dayananda Saraswati, castigated the Puranas and later legends as inauthentic add-ons, responsible for legitimizing undesirable social practices such as *varṇāshram*, idolatry and patriarchy. To overcome these social barriers, Dayananda advocated a return to Vedic living, by emphasizing *brahmacharya* and the intrinsic divinity of humans, and denouncing priestly intermediaries, religious dogmatism and individualistic conceptions of *moksha* that were not aimed at universal emancipation. Dayananda's ambitions exemplified the nineteenth century modernist Hindu zeitgeist, aiming to unify a diversity of practices and beliefs into a single textual hermeneutic, stripped of perceived superstitions. Hindu reform and universalist groups such as the Arya Samaj and the Brahmo Samaj, alongside Neo-Vedanta teachers such Aurobindo, Vivekananda and Ramakrishnan, expanded against the backdrop of colonial subjugation. Such movements attempted to place Hinduism on an equal footing with European enlightenment beliefs, while replacing the ideological underpinnings of

British colonialism with indigenous expressions of Hindu rationality (Prakash 2000, 289).

The cornerstone social practice of Hindu modernization was purification (*śuddi*). Rites to remove ritual pollution and expiate sin (*prāścit*) were documented as far back as the Vedas; in the nineteenth century, *śuddi* was often practised by high-caste Hindus who faced ritual pollution during international travel (Hardiman, 2007, 43). From the late nineteenth century, *śuddi* was transformed from a practice of everyday purification into a social movement focused on the re-Hinduisation of Muslims and Christians (Asani, 2011, 104). Although Dayananda Saraswati never formalized specific conversion rites, there were precedents for the reclassification of Christians as 'Aryas' and the endowment of Hindu names upon reconverted Muslims. The *śuddi* movement entwined Vedic principles of ritual purity with broader sociopolitical anxieties, often unfounded, around the perception that increasing Christian and Muslim demographics were due to the conversion of vulnerable Hindus.

Much of the rhetoric of Hindu reclamation was couched in gendered language concerning the colonial neutering of 'traditional' Indian masculinity—epitomized by valorous Rajputs and Marathas—and the need to restore Hindu male virility (Gupta, 2011, 445). Against this backdrop, the *śuddi* ceremony was in 1893 expanded to include 'the ceremony of tonsure, or cutting of hair, the offering of the *Hom*, or fire-sacrifice, investment in a sacred thread, and the learning of the sacred Gayatri *mantra*, explanation of the Ten Principles of the Arya Samaj, and finally distribution of sweets (*sherbet*) by the converts to all the present' (Ghai, 1990, 48–9).

Having transformed the *śuddi* ceremony, it was several decades before the Arya Samaj shifted reconversion efforts from Muslims and Christians to Hindu Dalits. Earlier attempts to perform *śuddi* ceremonies among several Depressed Classes (including the Dumnas, who were located in low-lying Gaddi villages) were condemned by the Shudhi Sabha; and the conversion of Dalit-Bahujans by the Hindu Sudhar Sabha in 1907 was similarly spurned (Prashad, 2000, 80). Targeting Dalits for Arya Samaj conversion, with the promise of social uplift through personal purification, would begin in earnest in the 1920s. Dalit groups such as Halis were singled out by bourgeois Hindu ideologues and implored to seek liberation through the abandonment of 'defiling behaviour'—as defined by B.S. Moonje of the Hindu Mahasabha in 1927 as lack of personal hygiene, consumption of leftover food (*jūṭhan*), meat and alcohol, and over-indulgence during social ceremonies (Prashad, 2000, 82). Although the Arya Samaj blamed the Puranas and their subsequent mythological accretions for the creation of the caste system, their paternalistic correctives to casteism often reproduced Brahminical disdain for the behavioural 'deficiencies' of the oppressed.

In the decades following the death of Swami Dayanand, the Arya Samaj underwent internal processes of institutionalization and theological fragmentation. By 1890, there were 55 Samaj Centres across 31 districts and two princely states (including Chamba), all of which supported the Dayananda Anglo-Vedic College movement (Jones, 1976, 155–57). 'From the original group of Samajes, the movement spread into the southeastern Punjab, from Multan outward, down along the western border tracts, and finally into the Punjab hills' (Jones, 1976, 155). Between the 1920s and Indian Independence, many indigent and socially ostracized Halis performed *śuddi* ceremonies and at least nominally converted to the Arya Samaj. In successive settlement surveys (*bandobast*), some Halis—encouraged by the promise of self-actualisation and caste transcendence—filed caste emendations and re-registered in the Revenue Record under socially aspirational caste names. Those Halis who were partially integrated into Gaddi life coined and registered the caste name Gaddi Arya. In the decades before tribal scheduling, when tribes connoted uncivilized backwardness without offsetting state benefits (Bora, 2010), identifying as Gaddi Arya was both a description of Hali subjectivity and an aspiration for tribal acceptance of Dalits.

Consequently, Halis living in Gadderan and outlying areas throughout Chamba began to adopt the name Arya. Modern-day elders in Arya-converted villages still recall this conversion narrative, as passed down by their forebears. Bavinder, an elder from a village of predominately Gaddi Aryas, who lives below the iconic Chaurasi Mandir in Bharmour, provides a representative oral history:

> Before 1947, a Punjabi Sanskrit professor and Samaji named Ram Sharan Shastri came to Chamba. When he saw the suffering (*duḥkh-dard*) of Halis, he went from house to house and gave us all the Gayatri *mantra* [he laughingly recites the full *mantra*]. If there were any literate people in the village, he gave them a written copy so they would remember it. Ram Sharan said: 'I've now given you a very powerful *mantra*, you must give up drinking alcohol and eating meat. You must live like a Brahmin, wear a *janeū*, bathe properly daily, and with pride say that you are Arya'. So Halis started to say that they are Arya; out of fear and disgust they erased the name Hali in the Revenue Record. They were Arya, only Arya. You can still see that all Halis are Arya on the Churah side, in Salouni and Rajnagar, and mixed into Hali villages in Bharmour itself.

I have been unable to track down archival references to the language professor-turned-social-reformer Ram Sharan Shastri. However, he is a central historical personage, responsible for spreading Arya Samaj ideology across Chamba, and impacting Arya-converted Halis for generations to come. The following is the most official account I could unearth in my research of Ram Sharan Shastri's propagation of the Arya Samaj in Chamba, as vividly recounted by the headmaster of an Arya Samaj school.

> During the time of kings, a guru was brought to Chamba from Lahore, whose name was Ram Sharan Shastri. This was before Partition, when it was part of Punjab. During that time, the headquarters of Chamba were in Gurdaspur, which is now in Punjab. This was approximately 1932–1933. He was a student of Dayanand Saraswati and he heard the principles of the Arya Samaj in Lahore at the Upadeshak Vidyalay. He was a very strict (*kaṭṭar*) follower of Arya Samaj. He got married in Chamba, had three children, two boys and a girl, and all three became doctors—Dr. Bimla, Dr. Jagdish and a third.
>
> He was a Farsi teacher. He came here to help translate the Revenue Records which were written in Farsi and Arabic; languages he knew. He taught the office people how to correctly read the records. When he came to Chamba, he saw the high rate of illiteracy, especially among women. They were not allowed to be taught at all. So, he struggled against this by starting a school for women in Chamba, in Chameshani Muhalla, near Halvai Gali. Even now there is an Arya Samaj there in which the school was started. Among the people who studied there were Halis, Sipis and Soi, who stitched the king's apparel (*cogā*). They were believed to be low people. Some of these people are still alive, like Sita Ram, who is about 90 and got an education there as a girl.

When Ram Sharan established the school, the king got angry with him and banished him to Mangala, across the Ravi River. But after some time, Ram Sharan came back to Chamba and was captured. He explained to the Raja about the work he wanted to do, and he was given permission to teach Farsi and Arabic, and alongside that to teach the lower castes to 4th class. He gave education at first to four children. Two are still alive—Indrajeet, who lives nearby, and another, who shifted to Kangra. When these first students got educated and started to earn money, they changed their castes to Bhardwaj, Chauhan... They remained SC in the Revenue Record, but socially they adopted higher caste names. Soon another Arya Samaj school was opened in Sarol. He also opened an Arya Samaj temple in about 1940.

Ram Sharan Shastri was a Brahmin. He gave to his followers, who were of all castes, the name Arya. Arya recognises that all humans are born with the same capabilities and rationality. We are not born as elephants or snakes; we are born in the highest position as humans, based on the good *karma* we must have done in previous lives. We came here for a reason. So, based on this recognition, SCs all across the region, up to Pongi [and including Bharmour, Salooni, Ghudei, Churah, and then, after migration, down into Kangra], began to follow Ram Sharan. In the beginning, everyone was taking the name Arya and getting an education but then, after a while, society caught up and recognised that Arya, which was a high-caste (*svarṇ jātī*) name, was actually another name for SC. But it is important to emphasise that Arya is not a caste at all.

In Ram Sharan's life, after all this happened, he renounced (*sannayās*) his name and became Shantanand. After 1950, when the government started giving SC benefits, those lower castes who adopted the name Arya tried to re-enter their original caste names as Hali and so on...

The historical particulars of conversion have faded from the memories of contemporary Arya-converted Hali villagers. For example, several villagers reported to me that Ram Sharan Shastri was a Sanskritist, when he was probably a Farsi scholar. However, one germane historical anecdote emerged during my fieldwork, concerning the *jajmānī* patronage that bound Halis in exploitative subservience to Gaddis, and the contestation—be it historically accurate or imaginatively remembered—that accompanied Hali uplift.

Upon becoming Arya, we Halis left the job of picking up carcasses. Ram Sharan had instructed us to purify. When we refused to do Chamar work, it led to a big distress (*tangī*) among Gaddis. There was a huge meeting held in Chaurasi Mandir, and all the Gaddis of the area called the representatives of the Hali community. This was a long time ago. It was presided over by Tani Ram, a famous Gaddi *lambredār* who is even sung about in songs. He publicly asked us Halis: 'Brothers (*bhaiyon*), I see you've left your work.' Among us was a strong and powerful Hali named Sikh Ram. He said, 'Sudru left his work, and he's a Sippi. We will do the same.' And Tani Ram said: 'So you won't do it anymore?' And although he beat many Halis, we never did Chamar work again.

While I cannot verify this account, it was roughly corroborated by other narratives and oral histories. What is clear, however, are the myriad sociopolitical consequences of Arya conversion. There is general agreement that Arya adoption has not enhanced the social status of Halis among Gaddis or within the larger regional caste system in which Gaddis have assimilated. Their situation parallels the 1920s Arya reconversion of Gujarati Muslims to Rajputs, who failed to win acceptance from the wider Rajput community and rarely intermarried. In the case of the Halis, however, it should be noted how historical amnesia has birthed new forms of self-elevation and tribalisation. Most Hali youth are unaware of the link between the Arya Samaj and their

Arya caste name; the rituals that accompanied conversion have disappeared and the Arya Samaj has yielded most of its institutional relevance (apart from granting court marriages and offering an all-India marriage helpline).

Because their Arya caste name is so completely severed from its Arya Samaj origins, many Halis now consider it to be indicative of Central Asian ancestry. Just as the Jat community claim to be Proto-Vedic Aryans, Arya-converted Halis take pride in claiming to be scions of the 'Solar race'. In other words, the collective historical oblivion of Arya Samaj conversion has cleared conceptual space for Halis to link their caste with colonial speculation (especially by Hutchison) that Gaddis are of Central Asian origin (Shashi 1977, 13–4); the 'Aryanness' of Halis is thus 'evidence' of their inclusion in the Gaddi tribe.

At other times, however, Halis invoke their Aryanness to distinguish themselves from the decidedly less 'tribal' narrative of Gaddi Rajputs fleeing Lahore. The oft-quoted saying among high-caste Gaddis, 'After Lahore was deserted, Bharmour was inhabited' (*ujreya Lahore, te baseya Bharmour*), suggests a forced migration after the invasion of Aurangzeb in the seventeenth century (Handa, 2005, 29). In similarity with many other upper caste Hindu communities in the Western Himalayas, Gaddis attribute their migration to protecting the *dharma* from Muslim assaults. In so doing, they craft a politicized history that impacts both their relationship with Muslim Gujjars and Gaddi Dalits (Thapar, 2007, 191). With raised eyebrows and knowing smiles, Halis counter this narrative by describing their ancestral connection to Aryans; the purest nomadic pastoralists of Central Asia.

Although the designation 'Arya' was adopted between 1923 and 1950, it is popularly (mis)remembered as indexing the hoary invasion of Central Asian Aryans; the prototypical tribe of mobile pastoralists.

The context-specific instrumentalism of forgetting Samaji conversion has, ironically, furthered the egalitarian goals of the Arya Samaj, but not as Dayananda Saraswati might have intended. By associating Aryans with 'firstness' in Bharmour—the tribally protected Gaddi heartland—Halis stake a claim to autochthony that supersedes the later migrations of Gaddi Rajputs and Brahmins. Further, by emphasizing Aryan pastoralism, Halis undermine the notion that flock rearing is an exclusionary Gaddi vocation; the nexus upon which ST benefits were conferred and a primary source of historical casteism and unequal wealth accumulation.

The collective Hali 'memory' of ancient Aryan origins has obvious utility in the discursive trenches of the garnering of ST recognition; although this indexing is not *only* discursive. O.C. Handa (2005, 24) argues for an etymological link between *pashmīnā* wool production and Pushan—a Vedic Solar deity associated with the Ravi basin and pastoral ritual. He speculates that the 'primitive inhabitants of the region [such as Halis] were the cousins of the pre-Indo-Aryans, if not the Aryans themselves' (Handa, 2005, 24). The Gayatri *mantra* is virtually forgotten, the Arya Samaj temple in Chamba is a fossil relic, but the 'debatability of the past in the present'—that is, claims of Aryan heritage by lower caste communities—continues to inform social aspiration and ethnic boundary making practices (Appadurai, 1981, 218). Communal misremembrance and connotative slippage proliferate styles of self-representation and affective forms of belonging.

Whatever the symbolic benefit of these unintended meanings, they are mitigated by countervailing forms of political misrecognition that have rendered 'Arya' synonymous with social suffering and political disenfranchisement. Across Old Himachal—within the tribal belt in Bharmour, spilling over 100 kms west past Chamba and Salooni, approaching the border with Kashmir—many Halis are officially recorded as Aryas in the Revenue Record. As they migrated across the Dhauladhars into low-lying mountain villages, extending east to west from Baijnath to Nurpur, they brought their Arya caste name into the Kangra Valley.

The adoption of Arya has brought about further complications of Hali consciousness. For example, in Gaggal village in Bharmour, intermarriage between Halis, Gaddi Aryas and Aryas (variously SC, ST and general) actually highlights their social sameness. The three caste communities—all essentially Halis who self-identify as Gaddi—are saddled with mismatching official designations. Government-issued identity documents, often contradictory or illegible, have led some Halis to cleave tightly to the belief that their registered Arya caste is real and meaningful; while, for the majority, the documentary effects of the state have led to communal exhaustion and the abdication of any hope for congruence between felt identity, official classification and constitutional benefits. The erroneous but official (*aupcārik*) version of reality undergirds and, in a sense, authorizes the social identities carried by these Halis in their daily lives.

The divisive nomenclature of Hali, Arya and Gaddi Arya also shape political participation and the ability to secure reserved employment. For example, when elections are reserved for SCs, Aryas are ineligible to compete. One elder, who had corrected his caste from Arya to Hali, described to me how his daughter had to submit her newly minted family copy (*parivār nakal*) before her husband could stand for office in an SC-reserved *pancāyat* election. Further, when civil service jobs are reserved for STs, Aryas and Halis are ineligible to apply. In 2003, Dumanu Ram's son was selected for an ST-reserved constable position in the Central Industrial Security Force (CISF). For nearly a decade he provided security to government-owned industrial hydropower plants. When Dumanu corrected his caste from Gaddi Arya to Hali, his son was suspended for producing a false caste certificate and standing for ST-reserved civil service as an SC. Dumanu appealed to the state court in a case that devolved into incomprehensible minutiae about the authenticity of documents and their authorizing social identities (LAWS (HPH)—2012–3–89). This case might be lightly read as a Kafkaesque satire on bureaucracy, but for the fact that it very tangibly affected vulnerable individuals; supplanting much-needed state assistance with legal ambiguity and evincing kaleidoscopic social identities that erode Dalit solidarity, so causing considerable torment.

Chandru's Arya Problem

The thousands of Arya-converted Halis who are disenfranchised from SC benefits face the choice of either appealing on an individual basis for legal caste emendation (*duruśtī*) or continuing to swim against the tide of residual casteism. Many struggles to remain buoyant, without even the symbolic protections of positive discrimination. With life chances circumscribed by illiteracy and poverty in remote mountain villages—often kilometres away from motorable roads—the exertion required to amend one's caste cannot be overstated.

The following is an ethnographic vignette of Chandru, my Arya research assistant and longtime friend, as he quests for SC benefits via Hali recognition. Although particulars may vary in other cases, Chandru's story is broadly emblematic of the struggle for recognition faced by Halis everywhere; beginning with their almost-forgotten ancestral conversion to the Arya Samaj. While Gaddi Aryas with ancestral residence in tribal-reserved land are enumerated as ST, Aryas such as Chandru, together with many others in his village, are actually Halis thinly disguised as a *svarṇ jāt*. This dynamic first arose in Chamba, where many thousands of Halis are encumbered with Arya liminality, but often climaxes in Dharamsala where, each year, the Revenue Record Office rules on Hali caste correction appeals from across the state.

Chandru always had a way of smoothing our introduction into Hali villages and putting people at ease. It wasn't just a matter of shared caste identity; Chandru connected to villagers because of their shared experiences and rural disposition—an excitability, physical sturdiness and open-mouthed manner of chomping food that is sometimes disparaged among Dharamsala's sophistos as 'bumpkin' behaviour (*grāncar*). Affectionate informalities crept into our working relationship, and Chandru would often interlace his fingers with mine as we gambolled down the dusty backwater roads of Lower Dharamsala. He was fond of gentle teasing—known in Hindi as 'making an owl' (*ullu banānā*) of someone. 'Stephen's dream is to marry a milk-giving water buffalo and live in a mud hut with her in Ladakh', he would tell villagers to their great amusement; grinning with an unguarded authenticity I came to admire and even unconsciously emulate. I would pay him back, announcing that Chandru is an avowed vegetarian so long as you don't offer him chicken *tīkhā*.

After an exhausting day walking between villages (often spaced several kilometres apart), hours of continuous interviewing and sometimes missed meals (compensated for by a profusion of milk tea and butter biscuits), I would pay Chandru and he would try to return his hard-earned salary. 'This is too much fun hanging out with you; I don't need money. Did you see how happy those women were to speak with us?'.

We conducted fieldwork among Christian converts, those afflicted with evil spirits, and traditional healer-diviners; we canvassed entire villages of Halis who concealed their caste name because of historical stigma; we met Hali social activists; we attended marriages and got trapped in mountain temples by the monsoon rains. One day we would conduct fieldwork and the next day hang out in Chandru's rented quarters in Dharamsala's Kotwali Bazaar, translating audio recordings; a tedious enterprise about which he rarely complained and always outdid my stamina to complete.

A friendship summarily blossomed alongside our professional relationship. After a relationship break-up, Chandru consoled me with the ubiquitous Indian advice to drive away painful introspection with headlong devotion to work. When he found out, to his muted chagrin, that his parents had arranged his marriage to a 17-year-old,

I was there to lend a sympathetic ear and accompany him, bearing gifts, to a meeting with his betrothed. When I hosted a Gaddi ritual sacrifice (*nuālā*) upon the completion of my first fieldwork, Chandru laboured with me for a full 24-h, indefatigably humping mattresses and tenting between the road and the mountain temple. I also coached Chandru through each stage of a Fulbright scholarship application; editing his essays, helping him file passport paperwork, strong-arming his hesitant professors into writing recommendation letters, and accompanying him to Delhi on his first trip to a big city, for an interview and exam. However, over two successive years, our efforts fell short. While I helped two other Gaddis reach America through the Fulbright Programme, Chandru had the largest gap to close—a Hali from a mud home in a far-flung village in Chamba, speaking a dialect that has no name; his education constrained by inferior, Hindi-medium government schooling, his parents' illiteracy and the exigencies of poverty.

Work successes and setbacks naturally gave way to friendship. No doubt our brotherly affection informs my depiction of Chandru's life and the emotional immediacy of his social aspirations, but my intention is to draw objective parallels between Chandru's struggle for SC recognition and the broader issues of political misrecognition and fractured Hali ethnic consciousness.

Halis are popularly defined by their caste occupation within traditional *jajmānī* patronage roles. As ploughers, their vocation cuts across ethnic affiliations and there is tremendous regional variation among Halis: many live contiguous to Gaddi identify as tribal, while others, who live outside of Bharmour amidst non-Gaddis, have no tribal pretensions. Regardless of their tribalisation, Halis face uniform caste-based discrimination and exemplify the migratory pattern of rural villagers pulled into urban centres such as Dharamsala. Chandru's biography as an Arya illustrates the ascendency of Dharamsala as a Gaddi village turned Tibetan town turned global 'Smart City'—a place that attracts rural migrants harbouring dreams of socioeconomic uplift.

The issue of political disenfranchisement first arose when I helped Chandru and three Gaddis apply for the aforementioned Fulbright Programme. I was fortunate enough to have secured a Fulbright grant for my 2014 dissertation research, which paid me 90,000 rupees a month to live in rural villages—only a fraction of which was needed to subsist at local standards. During my fieldwork, I returned to Delhi to sit on a panel that selected Foreign Language Teaching Assistant (FLTA) candidates. Around 15 Indians, all aged below 30 and holding M.A. degrees in English, would have the opportunity to teach Hindi while taking English-language courses at American universities. Of the 35 candidates we evaluated, the overwhelming majority were from urban general castes and had been educated at some of India's elite academic institutions, such as Jawaharlal Nehru University and the University of Delhi. Recognizing that the applicant pool was weighted towards urban elites, I endeavoured to enlist Gaddis from the Dharamsala regional campus of Himachal Pradesh University for the following year's competition.

Several months later, I met Chandru and three Gaddis, who were all enrolled in the English M.A. at the regional campus. We would convene at the local computer café and, between power cuts, infected pen drives and bootlegged software prone to self-uninstallation, we completed their applications. I noticed how the Gaddi Rajput, Bhatt Brahmin, and half-Gaddi Badi/Gorkha students designated their SC/ST status on the form and proudly expanded on their marginalized identities in the required personal essays. However, Chandru was uncomfortable about divulging his Hali caste, even to us; let alone describing his caste struggle in his application (to the end of winning the sympathy of the evaluators). He left his family name blank on the application and, when one of the Gaddi applicants nudged him about this, he stared disconsolately at the screen.

For reasons explained below, Chandru did not list SC on the application. He subsequently watched on as all three Gaddi applicants were selected by Fulbright in the next two application rounds, and departed for universities including Yale. I knew from my experience sitting on the previous year's selection committees that Fulbright would identify minority students and assess their applications with more lenient criteria, with the aim of increasing diversity. I also knew that Bihari had no chance competing against JNU graduate students from elite backgrounds.

Later, in private, Chandru explained his situation to me. His official caste certificate bears only the name Chandru, without a surname; according to the revenue records, he is Arya. His 'home name' is Amrendra, and his adopted surname, Kumar, which he uses on Facebook, is simply fanciful. He sometimes uses Kashyap as a surname, which is his *gotra*. The politics behind this cacophony of names became the impetus for my fieldwork in Dharamsala in 2014 and, later, when I stayed in Chandru's village in Salooni District in 2016.

In the following passages, I link Chandru's sociopolitical liminality—being neither SC nor sharing affective attachment to Gaddi tribal culture—to the issue of caste fracturing and the problems it poses for Gaddi tribal integration. Drawing from Chandru's and cognate testimonials concerning the insurmountable difficulties of caste emendation (*duruśtī*), I highlight the social humiliations, financial encumbrances and eventual cynicism that arise from negotiating the neoliberal welfare state. The labyrinthine rules, arcane criteria and corruption at every stage of the process stymie the efforts of Aryas to unify their Hali consciousness and secure SC benefits. They also demonstrate the cultural and geographical similarities and differences between Halis and Gaddi Halis, together with the intersection of these factors in the shared quest for political recognition and cultural dignity.

Chandru, in his early 30 s, had overcome innumerable hardships to reach Dharamsala and pursue both an education and civil service employment. Such achievements would easily surpass the life of scratch farming and jungle foraging currently practised in his village. His employment history began at 14, when he spent the summer of 8th standard in Upper Mugla, levelling land for a cell phone tower. The following summer he worked in construction in an army cantonment in Dalhousie. The summer after that he remained in his village and humped (*borī utake*) potatoes from fields to trucks 1.5 kms away. 'I made the record for the most carries in a single day', he relates. '16 baskets. That fetched me 250 rupees that day'.

Each winter break and summer vacation, from 8th standard to the completion of his bachelor's degree, Chandru worked as a migrant labourer. Between sessions of his first year at Chamba College, he juggled his studies, his caste correction appeal and his migrant work. During his first year, he earned 200 rupees a day laying sewage pipes in Yol Cantonment, near Dharamsala. During his second year, he found MGNREGA work; in his home village of P, an irrigation tank had been authorized at the cost of 80,000 rupees but a team of workers had abandoned the project and 30,000 rupees remained. Chandru and two friends completed the work in two months. 'We built an underground tank from cement and gravel, and for a month there was water; then the pipes got stolen and the tank dried up'.

Chandru's household includes his mother, father and sternly affectionate grand-mother (*dādī*). He has three sisters, two of whom are functionally non-literate and were married at the age of 19. The third sister is a spritely 14-year-old who habit-ually skips school to perform housework and agricultural labour. Chandru has two brothers; one fixes mobile phones and the other is a dedicated 8th standard student who aspires to follow in Chandru's footsteps. Chandru's father ploughs around two acres (12 *bīghā*) of land—spread out over several kilometres of terraced moun-tainside—and sells his surplus yield in Salooni. He studied until 5th standard at a government school; access to which entailed fording a stream (*khad*) every day. His mother told him, 'If you go to school, one day we'll find your corpse in the *khad*'. On her advice, he dropped out. A taciturn, hardworking man, he has now taken to drink.

Chandru's village is located a strenuous 25-min hike uphill from the nearest driving road. In the regional caste hierarchy, Halis are positioned below Rajputs and above Chamars and Dhumne. The nearest contact point with Gaddi culture is a Sippi village one hour's walk away; the residents of which have either SC or ST status, depending on their ancestry in Bharmour. Chandru's family home is the middle partition of a mud longhouse in which five Hali families of the same *birādarī* live. At first, the courtyard appears to be a manicured pebble field but is, in fact, the flat rooftop of the Rajput homes beneath. Jutting out of the earth are equally spaced slate chimneys, around which children can be seen kicking around a deflated football. Chandru's partition has wooden rafters and support columns, which divide the space into three rooms, occupied by eight family members. Between each family unit, ten-inch-square holes (*tabārī*)—cut into the mud wall or shaped from slate reinforcements—allow for communication and a modicum of family surveillance. In the neighbouring partition, a 22-year-old cousin, his wife and two children live in a foetid single room, with two cows, a buffalo and several sheep tied to poles under makeshift wooden lean-tos. Each house has a tub for making *lassī*, a spinning wheel, a mud *chulhā* and cots.

Poverty manifests in the minutiae of daily life: the coarse quilts, frayed and unwashed; the parsimonious allocation of ten rupees at a time to buy *achār* and onions; the reverence given to each rupee, carefully stored in a cloth pouch; the resistance to girls' and womens' education by *dādī* and like-minded village elders (who are preoccupied with marriage alliances as a means of enhancing social secu-rity); the nonchalance with which leathery fingered villagers pluck stinging nettles (*aun*) (desensitised to the hours of discomfort caused by the myriad trichomes that line their edible leaves, injecting itch-inducing histamines); the predominance of forest-foraged herbs, vegetables (*fonfaru*), pickles and the scarcity of imported rice;

the flies that swarm like dirty clouds (one of which once settled on the sleeping Chandru's face and caused his eyelid to swell like the punched-in eye of a boxer); the billows of smoke stagnating in unventilated rooms (contributing to lung infections and exacerbating tuberculosis); the absence of flush toilets; and the farm animals defecating in the house.

I could not conceive how Chandru had ever studied in his smoky, dark, loud room, with people constantly coming in and out, his *dādī* shouting at him to go to thrash the mustard leaf. But despite these material hardships, Chandru remained, if not content, then joyful. While vigorously soaping up using the ice melt that trickles down the mountainside, he would loudly render Bollywood tunes. 'One should bathe in cold, cold water!' was his favourite refrain, from the 1978 film *Pati Patni Aur Woh.*

When I stayed in early 2016, I was the first Western visitor to P village. After respectfully touching his mother's and grandmother's feet, Chandru and I were welcomed in, fed *lassī* and given leg massages. We sat around the stove, beside which a bedraggled off-white cat luxuriated. After conversing for some time—supported by Chandru's Hindi translation of the apparently unnamed local language (neither Churahi nor Chambiyali)—*dādī* asked Chandru if I was of the Gadhvaie caste of Brahmins who live in Vishoie, northern Himachal Pradesh. The Gadhvaie sometimes visit P village as fortune-tellers; peddling divination and speaking in a bookish Hindi similar to my own. This elicited a belly laugh from Chandru, who found it impossible to explain just how far away America is. After dinner, as we sat around the stove and Chandru's sister washed our feet, a Rajput Thakur entered and announced that the next day was reserved for compulsory housework (*gharoti karne*), during which, as per tradition, every able-bodied villager must work without pay until lunchtime.

Chandru is the scholar of the village. No one comes close to his level of education: B.A. and M.A. He has become an urban sophisticate; bringing home a computer tablet, to the wonderment of his brother (who went on to disassemble it with a screwdriver in a disastrous attempt to 'fix' a software glitch), *panīr* cheese (a luxury food his mother had no idea how to cook), and even an American! Chandru's achievements should be put into context. His father and fictive kin are mostly alcohol dependent and no one places much value on education. He has had to fight for his own education, fight to leave the village, fight to delay marriage—at the age of 32, he is way beyond the socially acceptable limit. In Dharamsala, he struggles to earn 5,000 rupees a month by tutoring children. This keeps him afloat during his hibernations in the library and cramming sessions for civil service exams. In the city, Chandru is seen as an awkward yokel but back home I saw him fully embrace his village mannerisms. With a toothy grin he would twist off a walnut tree branch, mash it with his molars and brush his teeth vigorously; yellowing his mouth but apparently cleaning his teeth. 'I had never even heard of Colgate until I got to college', he would smirk; a leafy twig jutting from his mouth.

Chandru first realized he was missing out on SC benefits as a first-year student at Chamba College. At the time, he was living with a distant relative to save on rent. Whenever he filled in a government form, he paid the full fees. 'That was the first clue: last year I paid 400 rupees for the HP administration form; if I were SC, it would have only cost 200. Two months ago, I filled in a form to take the *patvāri* exam [to qualify to maintain land ownership records and collect land taxes]. That was 250 rupees for me but only 100 rupees for SCs. From my first year in college to the present, I've never received a single SC discount or reserved seat'.

Although he was only 18 years old, and living away from home for the first time, Chandru convinced his non-literate father to check with the authorities as to why his family was being deprived of SC benefits. After being rebuffed during a visit to the Revenue Record Office in Chamba, Chandru's father hired an advocate to press his case. 'That amounted to nothing. He kept saying, 'Come back tomorrow and we can talk', and every time I visited his office, he claimed not to have our file on hand'.

With lawyer's fees mounting and nothing to show for it, Chandru demanded his file and personally visited the Tonkri-language archivist (*Tonkri-vālā*) at the Revenue Record Office in Chamba. "I have no time, come tomorrow', he said, and the next day, 'I have urgent work, come tomorrow'. I realised that nothing was going to happen. So, I slipped him 500 rupees. He accepted it and told me to come back in a few days. I felt confident that he would locate our file'. Between university courses, Chandru returned to the Revenue Record Office, only to find that his file was still missing. 'Then I gave him two kilos of clarified butter (*ghī*), thinking, 'That should get me something". Although the official took both bribes, he came up with nothing and, after repeated failures, Chandru snatched back his file and screamed, 'Listen, I will handle the case myself!' Dejected, and having exhausted his options at both the village *patvār khānā* and the Revenue Record Office, he resigned himself to being indefinitely burdened with the tangible impediments bound up with his Arya caste name (despite its hypothetical social prestige).

The failed process of *durustī* demonstrated to Chandru how little his *birādarī* understood their family ancestry. Despite socially identifying as Halis, they are officially recorded as Aryas—a title which, for them, has neither any historical connection to the Arya Samaj nor any specific time frame of adoption. What Chandru does know is that his family has conventional ownership of two properties in Chamba district: the first an undocumented ancestral inheritance; the second their current residence, purportedly bought by his grandfather. Land holdings must be filed via property forms—*katuni* in Urdu, often translated to Hindi as *parcā*—at the regional Revenue Record Office. Such forms indicate the caste of a landowner at the time of purchase. Originally, Chandru's grandfather was a Hali tenant, and was only awarded the property over which he laboured because of the implementation of the Tenancy Act. For his family and countless others, the documents that might satisfy the legal requirements for caste correction are simply non-existent. For other Halis, however, there is a clearer path to caste correction: they must produce a Tonkri-language land ownership form (*nakal takra*) to prove their family was recorded as Hali at the time of the Settlement Report and the Tenancy Act, and converted to Arya at a later date.

Hali elders speak openly, albeit generally, about their landlessness, tenancy and patronage exploitation under *hāliprathā* servitude. For the younger generations, however, researching and securing admissible evidence for *durustī* is not only time consuming and financially draining; it also forces them to confront, often for the first time, the precise nature of their past exploitation. While many Halis contemporarily adopt spiritual pathways that encourage disidentification with caste, the *duruśtī* process may intensify caste identification and the logic of social hierarchy. In common with many others, Chandru was uneasy about unearthing and identifying with his ancestral link to patronage exploitation. He prefers to describe how his grandfather bought their property, as opposed to accepting that it was granted to him through legislation aimed to empower landless tenants. His eagerness to adopt cosmopolitan competencies in Dharamsala is often at loggerheads with his investigation of familial ties to patronage exploitation. Repeated and fruitless encounters with bureaucrats over his caste liminality have left him with an apparent sense of shame and bewilderment; as if social advancement were predicated on personal debasement. Chandru's engagement with the 'everyday state' during his efforts to alter his caste identity has only amplified the many humiliations of daily cultural life (Fuller & Bénéï, 2001).

In 2015, despite the frustrations described above, and having been overlooked by the Fulbright committee for a second time, Chandru renewed his quest for *duruśtī*; spurred on by the social disadvantages of Hali caste fracturing we had become aware of during our fieldwork. Together, we retraced his steps, beginning with the Revenue Record Office in Dharamsala. The first employee we met, who was processing papers amidst a mountain of scattered folders, summarily dismissed Chandru as soon as he heard that his residency was in Chamba district. 'Nothing will go here. We can't say anything about that area. Only there you can file a case'. As Chandru pressed his case, I could sense his mounting frustration and, having reached an impasse, I capitalized on my white privilege and social respectability as a foreign research scholar to arrange a meeting with the head officer.

Serendipitously, the head officer was both amicable and a trained anthropologist, with experience in tribal research. He permitted us to examine the 237 ongoing Gaddi and Hali caste correction cases being processed by his office. Around one-third concerned general caste Rajputs who were petitioning for Gaddi Kathri ST benefits; the remainder were Aryas petitioning for Hali SC benefits. The officer reviewed Chandru's documents sympathetically and found countless inconsistencies. How could Chandru's family own land without an official file existing at the Revenue Record Office? On what logical basis could Chandru be Arya when his great-uncle was recorded as a Hali in receipt of SC benefits? Why did the land number (*kasra*) on Chandru's ancestry chart not include the requisite settlement year in which the land was first given? He mocked the report: 'This is totally bogus; it neither denies nor confirms anything'. He also suggested that Chandru return to the District Commissioner's Office in Chamba and reapply using two pieces of circumstantial evidence: the *patvārī* report that testified to Chandru's Hali culture and his great-uncle's ancestry chart. 'You can arrange it through other means [other means *jo hum abhī jutā sakte hain*]'.

The officer also advised Chandru to file a Right to Information (RTI) for government information pertaining to Arya caste emendation in Himachal Pradesh. That night, Chandru struggled through the English instructions on how to open an RTI account. In his request, he asked, 'In Himachal Pradesh, the ARYA caste community is which status—SC, ST or General? I need to know in HP, is there a legal case which has determined that ARYA is in fact HALI and open for SC benefits … Before

the Settlement in Chamba, HP, ARYA were [sic] which caste—Hali or otherwise'?
The following day, he received a pro forma response: 'Since your RTI application
is meant for a public authority under the State Government, the same is returned to
you herewith. You may file the same before the concerned public authority under the
State Government'. Chandru was unsure of some of the English, I had no idea how
to proceed, and the matter died.

Months later, with diminished hope, we arrived at Chamba Revenue Record
Office to meet, once again, with the *Tonkri-vālā*. Chandru braced himself for another
contentious interaction with the official, who would likely humiliate him and stand
between him and SC benefits. In a cramped archival office, stacked from floor to
ceiling with mouldering records, Chandru once again explained his case. 'Oh, yes, I
remember you, you angrily took back your report." Placing the bogus report alongside his 2011 application, Chandru responded, 'Of course I did. I wasted six months
coming and going here and getting nothing. So now I've returned after five years to see
if we can fix this problem'. Chandru requested a copy of his ancestral chart preceding
the *bandobast*, which would presumably verify his Hali caste status. 'Give me a new
application and I'll check it within a week'. A secretary who was hovering nearby
instructed Chandru to take a serial number from the *arjanavīs* in the courthouse,
without which an archival request could not be formally lodged. Facing another
delay, Chandru pleaded with the *Tonkri-vālā*, who had turned away from our discussion. 'I did all this last time and nothing happened. I live in Dharamsala; I can't keep
coming back'. Whether due to my inquisitive presence at Chandru's side, which
often garnered the goodwill of officials, or whether because he was simply in a charitable or contrite mood—perhaps with 500 rupees and two kilos of *ghī* in mind—the
Tonkri-vālā unexpectedly announced that he would check immediately. We followed
him into the inner recesses of the archive, where he slid out a manila folder from an
unruly stack. Flipping through to the land holdings of village P, he said:

> At the time of the Raja, Halis like your family worked under a landlord … the *kastekari*
> system. The land was not registered under the famers' names. And then, after the *bandobast*,
> the farmers who seeded (*bata*) the land, they became owners (*mālkiyat*). If the land is
> registered (*agar chadi hogi*), then your record is available; if not registered, then it won't be.
> After 1978, under 104, the land was registered under the name of the farmer.

Thumbing through the P village listings, he said, 'Your family is not here. This is
not my problem. This happens all the time: people can't locate their file and become
angry'. Chandru asked, 'But with my Arya caste certificate, can't you assume that I
must be a converted SC even if you don't find my family ancestry? Isn't that obvious'?
The *Tonkri-vālā* closed the manila folder. 'Without the report, I know nothing. I
might think that, but without the file nothing happens'. 'So that means that Chandru
will never get SC benefits his whole life'? I asked. 'That's exactly (*vahī*) what I'm
saying. There are people waiting outside'. That afternoon, we conducted lacklustre
interviews; the pall of dejection and creeping cynicism overhanging Chandru's mood
(Fig. 2.1).

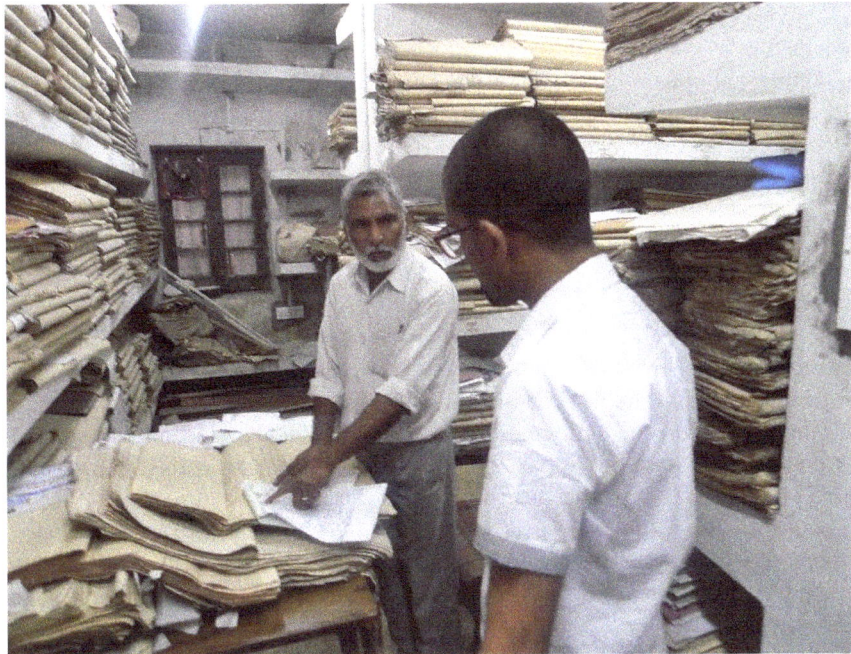

Fig. 2.1 Chandru with sloped shoulders facing more bureaucratic humiliation. *Photo* by author

Caste Correction Woes

In several villages, bookended by the Jammu border to Chamba City's northwest, and the end of the Gaddi tribal belt radiating from Bharmour to the east, we recorded dozens of similar testimonials in which caste correction lay at the centre of narratives of hardship and suffering. One morning, we met Ram Singh, a Radhasoami Hali from a nearby S village. He described his personal odyssey, which actually culminated in the acquisition of SC benefits. After tracking down his family ancestry chart (*vanśāvalī*) from a distant relative, he visited the nearest village accountant (*patvār khānā*) to obtain a copy of his family settlement records (*jamābandī*). After several subsequent abortive meetings at the Revenue Department in Chamba, he received a Tonkri-language report which showed his family was Hali before the issuance of the first *jamābandī*. Amar took the attested documents—written in Hindi, Urdu and Tonkri, none of which he could read—to the Revenue Record Office in Dharamsala. Once validated, he brought them back to the Chamba Revenue Department and finally to the Salooni Sub-Divisional Magistrate office, for the final issuance of the statutory SC certificate. It took three years and, he estimates, cost between 8,000 and 10,000 rupees. 'And I can't tell you how many days I lost (*mere bahut din ṭūṭe*) without income'. His blood brother (*sage bhāī*) was included in the *duruśtī*, although his distant and fictive Hali kin remained mired in appeals and aborted attempts at legal recognition.

Similar accounts abound in the hills. 'I used to joke, when I was a so-called *svarṇ jāt*, that we Aryas are higher than tribal Gaddis', recounted Anuj Kumar. Seven years ago, in pursuit of economic uplift, Anuj successfully amended his caste certificate to reflect his Hali ancestry, relinquishing his Arya status. Unlike Ram Singh, Anuj is educated and politically active; a longtime *pancāyat* committee member who has openly advocated for Aryas to reclaim their SC status as Halis. Yet his efforts were equally mired in corruption, misinformation and undue expenditure. Having only the vaguest idea of his family's ancestry and their migration from the Bhaderwah region of Jammu and Kashmir, Anuj's first step towards reclaiming his Hali status was to discover (from a butcher to whom he would sell sheep) the exact location of the *patvār khānā* in his supposed ancestral village of Ghata. After visiting and bribing the *patvārī* there, he returned to his village *pancāyat* committee with an attested *vanśāvalī* and drew up an official report (*prastāv*). From this starting point, Anuj gathered additional documentation from the tax officer (*tahasīldār*) and, having compiled a full portfolio, visited the *Tonkri-vālā* in the District Commissioner's Office in Saluni. After the *Tonkri-vālā* failed to locate his records (and intimated a bribe) Anuj threatened a lawsuit and invoked some of his political connections. Instantly, the *Tonkri-vālā* found Anuj's family file and forwarded his *duruśtī* appeal to Dharamsala.

A full two years passed between Anuj Kumar's discovery of his *vanśāvalī* in Bhaderwah and his being called to the SDM in Dharamsala. 'There were 150 of us bundled into one summons—Halis from Jhund and Vasua and so on'. The first summons ended unsuccessfully. Months later he was called again; this time on the day of his son's wedding procession (*bārāt*). 'I called a lawyer in Dharamsala, who said he would file on my behalf for 4,000 rupees. Who has that kind of money'? Strategically leaning on personal connections, Anuj persuaded an officer who was his 'known' to give a direct recommendation to the SDM. The SDM office requested Anuj's phone number but, at the time, he didn't own a phone. He gave the number of his Public Works Department supervisor, who received a call suggesting that Anuj's *duruśtī* petition was conditionally possible. 'The way he told me, I had the feeling I should send the SDM office a box of sweets'. After some deliberation, he decided against bribery and, on the day of his son's *bārāt*, his PWD supervisor passed his mobile phone to him. 'Are you in the wedding right now? Congratulations. I've done your work and posted your file to the Chamba DC office. You can pick it up from there after two days'.

There was one final ordeal. 'I showed up at the DC office six days later—I had to stay back in the village until then to wash the utensils—and the gatekeeper was a sister fucker (*bahancod*) who was taking bribes to get quicker access into the building. Seven people got in front of me. Instead of giving money, I grabbed his arm and shouted, 'This is not your family's DC Office. This belongs to everyone!' The commotion that ensued immediately won Anuj Kumar an audience with the District Commissioner. Using a local idiom—'bribery leads to advancement' (*banda jai, kuch pakadai*)—he demanded his file.

It was at the District Commissioner's Office, after years of anxious waiting and routine debasement, that one last administrative hiccough almost destroyed Anuj's hopes of judicial redemption—the petty officer who dispenses files from Dharamsala had taken a holiday. 'They explained that I would need to return the next day. At that point I almost went crazy. I didn't scream. I almost broke down'. In one final humiliation, Anuj Kumar announced to the District Commissioner that his son's wedding had bled him dry and that he couldn't afford food and accommodation in Chamba while waiting for his file to be returned the next day. In an act of sympathy— remembered by Anuj more as humiliation—the petty officer was dragged to the office and Anuj, having waited until the last minute before the office closed at 5 pm, received his file. Shuffling out, the DC officer apologized, slipping Anuj 100 rupees. 'I used that money to stay the night in Chamba. I remember eating alone in a *ḍhābā* that night. The next morning, I took a bus to Salooni and deposited the file in the Revenue Department. And from that day forward my family has received SC benefits'.

An Institutional Rejoinder

Accounts of villagers falling into Arya-related legal quagmires led Chandru and I to wonder if the contemporary Arya Samaj took any institutional responsibility. It is indisputable that the propagation of Arya Samaj ideology had the unintended consequence of trapping some of the most vulnerable individuals in Chamba and Kangra districts within the fluctuating ethno-logics of Indian bureaucracy. So, we visited the Arya Samaj temple in Chamba, in search of an institutional perspective. The skeleton staff of volunteers was unable to move past platitudes and generalities, so we entered instead into a wide-ranging and highly informative conversation with the headmaster of the affiliated Arya Samaj school.

Chandru introduced himself by narrating his odyssey for SC Hali recognition, while I expanded on the similar plight of Arya-converted Halis throughout Himachal Pradesh. Because Halis are virtually absent from the contemporary Arya Samaj, the headmaster was unaware of their specific dilemma. Although he was receptive to our concerns, and highly knowledgeable about regional Samaji history, as the conversation unfolded it became clear that ideological blinkers prevented him from accepting even marginal institutional responsibility. His logic hinged on three points:

First was a definitional dispute around Arya. 'The meaning of Arya is the highest person (*shresht*)', he said. 'Arya is not a caste; it is not anything. Sita called Rama [in the Ramayana] as '*Arya Putra*''. By substituting the real-world denotation of Arya as a Dalit euphemism with a range of connotative meanings—perfection, self-realization, theological abstractions and mythological references—the Arya Samaj privileges the probity of its ideology over the sociopolitical reality of its implementation. The headmaster repeatedly emphasized how government officials are to blame for not knowing the real meaning of Arya. 'Arya has been written in the Revenue Record, but the government doesn't understand its meaning. It's not a caste; it's not a religion. Ask the officials what it means—they won't be able to tell you a thing about it'.

Second, by considering Arya as a spiritual disposition and not an officially regis-tered caste, the headmaster rejected institutional responsibility by enumerating the 'natural resources' Aryans possess; foremost among them being self-respect and self-realization. He asked rhetorically, 'When you are in possession of such amazing natural resources, why would you run after reservation benefits'? I pressed him, asking whether all Arya-named Halis possess such qualities, so obviating any need for government assistance. 'In the beginning', he said, 'the Arya Samaj wanted to uplift the downtrodden who were discriminated against based on caste. In the begin-ning, it was this uplift mentality that led Dalits to adopt the name Arya. But now it depends on personal mentality—those with Arya mentalities have no need for bene-fits. Why would the best (*shreṣṭ*) need benefits'? This insistence on abstraction cuts against ethnographic reality. The Arya tag has been beneficial to Halis in only one sense; when discursively linked with Central Asian pastoral ancestry as evidence of their tribal Gaddiness. Otherwise, Arya is a mere euphemism for Dalit. Gaddis universally understand Aryas and Gaddi Aryas to be Halis by another name. Further, I have never encountered an Arya who is an active member of the Arya Samaj, or recites the Gayatri *mantra* with conviction, or wears a *janeū*. The 'natural resources' cited by the headmaster are merely an abstraction, negated by the reality of Dalit life.

Finally, the headmaster rejected the validity of caste as a system of social organiza-tion; seeing it rather as an outmoded measure for administering reservation benefits. The Arya Samaj is a liberation movement, not a religion, and certainly not a caste. Dayananda Saraswati considered the Arya Samaj to be a corrective for the post-Vedic aberration of caste, and a form of rehabilitation for Dalits oppressed by casteism. This institutional rejection of the caste system implies the definition of Arya as a caste is doubly meaningless—Arya is distinct *from* the caste system; rather, it is a personal attribute and spiritual collective identity. 'We believe all people are Aryas. Ram Sharan didn't tell people to adopt Arya as a caste name, but rather the opposite: to delete their caste names altogether! He encouraged Samajis to affix Arya to their names, such as Vikramjeet Arya, which shows allegiance to the Samaj without having any caste significance'. For the headmaster, absolute rejection of caste necessitated rejection of caste-based reservation. 'I will put it very plainly: the Arya Samaj doesn't want any reservation on the basis of caste at all. Caste shouldn't exist. The govern-ment should give reservation on the basis of IRDP [Integrated Rural Development Program] alone'.

Chandru and I were unable to penetrate the headmaster's idealist ideology. He maintained that Arya conversion entails cultivating those natural resources that lie latent in everyone; culminating in the realization of individuals of the highest moral character and the complete obviation of caste-based government reservations. Although we disagreed, I appreciated his transparency and idealistic fortitude, which seemingly derived from a genuine compassion for those oppressed by casteism. However, when the headmaster made disparaging comments such as, 'Why would Aryas run after handouts from the government'? I could sense Chandru's exas-peration. For my friend and thousands of Arya-converted Halis, Aryanness is at best an incidental resource. It primarily disenfranchises the neediest. Further, for the many Halis who strive for Gaddi inclusion, their Arya designation drives them nominally closer to discursive claims to tribal belonging, while further complicating their relationship to the state.

Conclusion

By July 2021, when this chapter was completed, Chandru had resided in Dharamsala for seven years. Before the pandemic lockdowns, his routine involved visiting the Government District Library almost daily to prepare for exams and tutoring children in the evening to pay for a cheap rental room in Kotwali Bazaar. In the past several years, he has repeatedly taken and failed exams to become a village accountant (*patvari*), Sub-Divisional Magistrate (SDM), labour inspector and Himachal Administrative Services (HAS) officer. If his caste emendation were to be approved and his SC benefits restored, he would be automatically eligible to pass state exams with reduced minimum marks. Given his scores, Chandru would have *already* passed several state exams years ago. In this alternate reality, he would also have emphasized his SC status to the Fulbright committee and been selected for their prestigious programme in the USA—as were the other SC/ST applicants I encouraged to apply. In this alternate reality, Chandru would be a respected government employee and a global cosmopolitan. His CV would boast of teaching at an American university and attending a conference for future global leaders at the U.N. headquarters. But there is a perversity in speculating how things might have gone differently with nothing more than the headwinds of a Reservation quota. In this reality, Chandru spends his days hanging around the library like so many other young men stuck in the limbo of 'timepass' (Jeffrey, 2010). When the pandemic lockdowns terminated Chandru's tutoring income, he resorted to charity and, increasingly desperate, posting amateurish videos on YouTube for students cramming for state exams.

Chandru's anguish is one stitch in the tapestry of Hali anguish, by which his fellow caste members waste inordinate amounts of time and resources bribing bureaucrats, negotiating with state administrators, excavating the archive for non-existent property documents and being hoodwinked by avaricious advocates—all in the pursuit of casting off their Arya caste name to receive SC benefits. Many are non-literate village scratch farmers, struggling against the impersonal and seemingly perpetrator-less structural violence of state misrecognition and red tape-ism (Gupta, 2012, 21). Young men and women like Chandru, compelled to prove their familial ties to patronage exploitation, are overwhelmed with feelings of worthlessness and inadequacy. Their dreams of brighter futures are predicated on cleaving closely to their exploited pasts— being paradoxically compelled to prove their Dalitness in order to try to transcend it. During my fieldwork, Halis often showed me their portfolios of disintegrating government documents with a sense of bafflement: being either unable to read the English-language forms or unsure of how some forms cancel out others; or unsure of whether their reservation status is that which is circled or that which is underlined; or which forms entail which rights. These portfolios have a range of significations for Halis, as they negotiate the material trappings of the state (Bakewell, 2007; Gordillo,

2006), and often constitute indecipherable determinants of who they are and how high they can aspire. Despite the hazy legal morass into which many Halis find themselves sunken, they are finding ways to improvise; bending the legal disadvantages of being Arya into the discursive advantages of being self-stylized Aryans—scions of Central Asian pastoral nobility with every right to Gaddi tribal inclusion—and seeking out modern social citizenship through Dalit tribal inclusion.

References

Appadurai, A. (1981). The past as a scarce resource. *Man, 16*(2), 201–219.

Asani, A. S. (2011). From satpanthi to ismaili muslim: The articulation of ismaili khoja identity in South Asia. In F. Daftary (Ed.), *A modern history of the ismailis: Continuity and change in a muslim community* (pp. 95–128). I.B. Tauris Publishers.

Bakewell, O. (2007). *The meaning and use of identity papers: Handheld and heartfelt nationality in the borderlands of north-west Zambia.* International Migration Institute.

Barnes, G. C. (1862). *Report of the settlement in the district of Kangra in the Trans-Sutlej states.* Lahore.

Bloch, N. (2018). Making a community embedded in mobility: Refugees, migrants, and tourists in Dharamshala (India). *Transfers, 8*(3), 36–54.

Bora, P. (2010). Between the human, the citizen and the tribal: Reading feminist politics in India's Northeast. *International Feminist Journal of Politics, 12*, 341–360.

Christopher, S. (2020a). Divergent refugee and tribal cosmopolitanism in Dharamshala. *Copenhagen Journal of Asian Studies, 38*(1), 31–54.

Christopher, S. (2020b). 'Scheduled tribal dalit' and the emergence of a contested intersectional identity. *Journal of Social Inclusion Studies, 6*(1), 1–17.

Fuller, C. J., & Bénéï, V. (Eds.). (2001). *The everyday state and society in modern India.* Social Science Press.

Ghai, R. K. (1990). *Shuddhi movement in India: a study of its socio-political dimensions.* Commonwealth.

Gordillo, G. (2006). The crucible of citizenship: ID-paper fetishism in the Argentinean Chaco. *American Ethnologist, 33*(2), 162–176.

Gupta, A. (2012). *Bureaucracy, structural violence, and poverty in India.* Duke University Press.

Gupta, C. (2011). Anxious hindu masculinities in Colonial North India: 'Shuddhi' and 'Sangathan' movements. *CrossCurrents, 61*(4), 441–454.

Handa, O.C. (2005). *Gaddi land in Chamba. Its history, art and culture.* Indus Publishing.

Hardiman, D. (2007). Purifying the nation: The arya samaj in Gujarat 1895–1930. *The Indian Economic and Social History Review, 44*(1), 41–65.

Jeffrey, C. (2010). *Timepass: Youth, class, and the politics of waiting in India.* Stanford University Press.

Jones, K. W. (1976). *Arya dharm: Hindu consciousness in 19th century Punjab.* University of California Press.

Newell, W. (1952). Gaddi kinship and affinal terms. *Man in India, 33*, 82–104.

Phillimore, P. (1982). *Marriage and social organisation among pastoralists of the Dhaula Dhar (Western Himalaya).* University of Durham.

Prakash, G. (2000). The Impossibility of Subaltern History. *Nepantla: Views from South, 1*(2):287–294.

Prashad, V. (2000). *Untouchable freedom: A social history of a dalit community.* Oxford University Press.

Shashi, S. S. (1977). *The gaddi tribe of Himachal Pradesh.* Sterling.

Taylor, C. (1994). The politics of recognition. In A. Gutmann (Ed.), *Multiculturalism: Examining the politics of recognition* (pp. 25–73). Princeton University Press.

Thapar, R. (2007). Secularism, history, and contemporary politics in India. In A. D. Needham & R. S. Rajan (Eds.), *The crisis of secularism in India* (pp. 191–207). Duke University Press.

Wagner, A. (2013). *The gaddi beyond pastoralism: Making place in the Indian Himalayas.* Berghahn Books.

Chapter 3
A World Inside a Pig's Stomach: Alimentary Knots of Tension Around Nutrition, Autonomy and Nationhood

Nimisha Thakur

Abstract This chapter explores how caste-based Hindu nationalist purity and pollution discourses about food align with public health variables of hygiene used to categorize nutrition for a tribal-indigenous community called the Mising in Assam, India. Several Mising communities live in inaccessible, small river island *char* regions of the Brahmaputra in the Lakhimpur District of Assam. These *chars* are visited by health practitioners from a local NGO called the Center for Northeast Studies and Policy Research (CNES) who collaborate with doctors from the National Rural Health Mission (NRHM) to provide monthly health checkups through boat clinics. While the Mising understand pigs as holding ancestral, ritual and migratory links to their religious practices, pork is categorized by state health practitioners as unhygienic and unhealthy. Increasingly, these caste-based discourses are being complicated by Hindu nationalist proselytization to incorporate northeast India into homogenous ideas of Hinduism. This chapter explores how these discourses overlook the community's assertion that traditional food sources are changing in nutritive value due to environmental change and the commercial farming of pigs. It is within this context that the Mising are attempting to acquire systemic governmental protections afforded in the Sixth Schedule. Further, it ethnographically explores how Mising community beliefs about their bio-social well-being are often at odds with public health standardizations of nutrition, which neglect their constructions of well-being and overlook the need to ensure cultural continuity affected by environmental change, riverine flows and capitalist modes of porcine farming.

Keywords Mising · Hindu nationalism · Pigs · Anthropocene · Health discourses

N. Thakur (✉)
Anthropology, Syracuse University, Syracuse, NY, USA
e-mail: nithakur@syr.edu

© The Author(s), under exclusive license to Springer Nature Singapore Pte Ltd. 2022   39
S. S. Acharya and S. Christopher (eds.), *Caste, COVID-19, and Inequalities of Care*,
People, Cultures and Societies: Exploring and Documenting Diversities,
https://doi.org/10.1007/978-981-16-6917-0_3

Introduction

A group of men gather in the backyard of the household where I am living for
ethnographic fieldwork in 2018 in a village—inhabited by Mising people, a tribal-
indigenous community—located on a river island (*char*) of the Brahmaputra river's
northern bank in Assam, India.[1] They are carrying a medium-sized, adolescent male
black pig, which they bathe using a bucket of water and then lay on a bed of straw. The
pig is to be offered for a ritual sacrifice on the occasion of an upcoming household
ceremony (*xat joniya hokam*). The ceremony is meant for the prosperity of the eldest
brother's household and his extended kin whose houses surround his *saang ghar*,
a house built on bamboo stilts. As I sift through a series of pictures on my phone
encasing this event, the first few show two cousins from adjoining households sitting
on both sides of the pig's head using a giant bamboo pincer that is meant to slowly
drain the life from the animal. Then, one of the older uncles (*Borta*), who has taken
part in this ritual slaughter several times since he was a young man, makes a small
incision at its rear end while his nephew holds up the pig's hind legs, which the
uncle explains allows faecal matter to seep out of the pig. He then makes a second
incision below the pig's stomach, removing the thick outer skin covered by hair to
meet an inch above the first incision. The large intestine which carries the pig's waste
is first removed, followed by the small intestine which contains digestive juices and
finally the heart and lungs. Emptied of its internal organs, the pig is then carried to
the kitchen fire where it is roasted to remove hair and pollutants on its external skin.
Borta explains:

> There are different ways we clean and prepare the pig for consumption, depending on
> the nature of the ritual-such as the *doha* (funerary rites), *dodgang* (funeral feast), *mitur*
> (wedding), village festivals like Ali ai Ligang or the *hokam* (household ceremony) for pros-
> perity. For instance, in the case of the funerary rites, we often insert a coin and sickle-like
> object into the pig's upper portion, near its neck. This is to ensure that the pig as offering
> appeases *opo-debotas* (evil spirits) and ancestors to keep their living kin safe. Smoking and
> burning the pig's outer skin before it is divided into pieces of meat to be cooked is always
> important to remove the toxins.

This ritual cleaning of the pig centres its importance as an alimentary conduit
between Mising community members and their ancestors where sacrifice maintains
their community's 'terrestrial wellbeing' (Pandian, 2008, 172). The alimentary care
of ensuring the pork is suitable for consumption by the Mising and their ancestors
is seen in the process that goes into this cleansing before the ritual sacrifice of
pigs to appease ancestors and evil spirits. This indicates that relationships between
Mising community members and their pigs are an 'embodied experience of being
entangled in intimate relations of care and mutual subjection' (Govindrajan, 2018,
40). The Mising also emphasize that the conversion of pigs into human food does
not take away from these ancestral relationships where pigs were seen as both their
companions and as abundant sources of food in harsher climates. These relationships

---

[1] This NGO ran a Boat Clinic program to provide immunization camps, family planning awareness,
and menstrual sanitation awareness to the river islands.

spanned travels across the mountains of Tibet to the Abor, Miri and Mishimi hills of Arunachal Pradesh and to Assam, the latter two being present-day states in the northeastern region of India.

Increasingly, the inability to maintain these same black pigs familiar to ancestors are linked by several Mising community members to contemporary gastrointestinal health problems which their ancestors did not suffer from despite eating pork. They point to changing modes of porcine production where crossbred and imported pig breeds with higher fat contents are becoming popular in Assam (Nath, 2002, 94). They also emphasize that climate change seen in increasing flood patterns and sand desertification patterns (Saikia, 2020, 509) in these river island *char* regions, impacts their crop outputs and in turn the availability of fodder crops for pigs' diets. These diminishing fodder sources are often the reason for increasing porcine malnutrition and deaths. Food security and an inability to acquire state funds meant for agricultural and husbandry schemes in remote areas such as the *chars*, is an aspect that has been emphasized by community members as one of the solutions to improve Mising nutrition.

However, medical practitioners who visit the Mising in these *chars* for health camps point out that pork is inherently unhealthy due to pigs' unclean environment and diet. This is an aspect that is seen across hegemonic global hygiene discourse which identifies pigs and communities who consume them as repositories of dirt, disease and pollution. These discourses do not take into account scientific evidence that clearly demonstrates that several common porcine diseases, such as swine flu, are not zoonotic (Davis & Sharp, 2020, 3). Mising community members emphasize that the rate of gastrointestinal problems was always low in their communities despite pork historically being an integral part of their diet. Instead, they point out that the source of these health problems could be due to the replacement of local breeds traditionally reared by the community by imported, non-local sources of pork from commercially bred pig farms.

In this chapter, I argue that the discursive framing of pork as unhygienic and unhealthy neither takes into account the complex lived experiences of the Mising nor scientifically frames disease etiologies around pork consumption. Driven by Hindu nationalist sensibilities, it incorrectly assumes that pork is the root cause of several health problems afflicting the Mising. These assumptions further overlook how actual changes in pork production impacts Mising health, specifically how imported pork has a higher fat content and is more metabolically harmful. Here, the connection made by medical practitioners I met regarding hygiene and nutrition functions according to the understanding that standardized industrial modes of production and biosecurity measures for rearing, cleaning and processing of pork for consumption are the ideal way to avoid diseases and consume pork (Thompson, 2021; Blanchette, 2020). However, communities such as the Mising who have historically reared and eaten pork often assert that these same biosecurity and industrial modes of porcine production are harmful for consumption and reduce community income and overall well-being. Changes to the composition of pork render its impact on human bodies uncertain.

For many upper caste Hindu communities who live in the region, on the other hand, pigs are inherently understood through discourses of purity and pollution, where their consumption and care has historically been seen to embody filth and a location of marginalization on the caste hierarchy (Narayanan, 2021, 1). In the case of pork consumption among the Mising, biomedical discourses on hygiene often align with nationalist framings of purity which, taken together, disregard the lived experiences of the Mising and the centrality of rearing local pig breeds as a marker of communal well-being. These claims are also not backed by any medical evidence to ascertain if pork is leading to the specific health problems pointed out for the Mising, as a result of which these biomedical claims remain discursive. The community however contends that their increasing health problems are linked to a lack of access to financial support for community pig rearing, which is possible through the systematic dispersal of government funds under the Sixth Schedule.

Sixth Schedule, Autonomy and Food Security

The Sixth Schedule was constitutionally designed for parts of the region of north-east India termed the Excluded Areas under colonial rule, an aspect that provides for autonomous districts and regions administered by elected autonomous councils. Sixth Schedule aimed for autonomy in 'the administration of customary law—justice involving tribals, and lawmaking powers on areas including land allotment, occupation or use of land, regulation of shifting cultivation, formation and administration of village and town committees, appointment of chiefs, inheritance of property, and marriage and social customs' (Baruah 2020, 39). The Mising have an Autonomous Council but the council is not under the purview of the Sixth Schedule constitutionally and was instead formed as an ad hoc addition (Pegu, 2013, 12). As a result, it has limited powers and often cannot access funds meant for Mising community area development. In a long struggle waged by the Mising for Sixth Schedule provision, the community points out that colonial classifications of tribal communities as either 'plains tribes' who lived in the Brahmaputra floodplain and 'hill tribes' (Baruah 2020, 29) that lived higher up in the mountains, resulted in several migratory communities like the Mising being forced to identify as either plains or hill tribes, as a result of which several provisions for tribal communities in the plains of Assam were not provided to them in post-colonial constitutional measures (Thakur, 2021). Across India, the monolithic classifications of SC and ST fail to address intersectional inequalities within tribal communities (Christopher, this volume).

In February 2020, Mising community organizations and leaders pushed the government to grant constitutional status to the Mising Autonomous Council (MAC), stating that this limitation causes issues of land allocation in Mising dominated areas. They asserted that with the inclusion of the MAC under the Sixth Schedule, a scientific agro-economy could be developed through the provision of skills to Mising youth and allocation of funds to sustain agricultural systems. Mising community organizations further asserted that these measures could help the community to avoid the import of resources and increase export instead (The Sentinel, 2020). The struggle for tribal autonomy has however been a long one for the community since the Mising Autonomous Movement began as early as the 1930s. The specific demand for community inclusion under the Sixth Schedule was raised by Mising Student Unions in 1982 (Pegu, 2013, 12).

A history of the Mising community reveals that autonomy in administering and cultivating land was historically important and acquired by the community in precolonial Assam. The Ahom Buranji (Barua, 1985, 23) makes allusions to uprisings of several tribes in the area against the precolonial *Ahom* state among which were the Mising. They were attempted to be contained through the *posa* system (Mipun, 2000, 18). According to this system, some marginal lands of the Ahom state were given to the Mising people on an agreement that they would help resist other tribal communities who attempted to rise against Ahom rule. Kar (2016, 47) points out that this accorded the community amongst others, a degree of autonomy over land that continued with British administrative measures. This is an aspect that the Mising point out as their history of never fully being governed by the British or converted by Christian missionaries. The term 'self-sufficient' is used in this context by community members to point out how food and everyday resources used to be adequate before riverine areas became increasingly vulnerable due to increasingly erratic floods and sand deposition. Mising people in the *chars* believe that Sixth Schedule can help combat this vulnerability through access to government resources such as seeds and capital.

During a conversation with a Mising community member regarding the current political scenario before the upcoming March 2021 elections, Hara said:

> If we had gotten autonomy according to constitutional provisions, then our access to resources would have been systematic. Now, because we do not have these guarantees in place and because state provision of funds to our Autonomous Council often do not reach us, developmental schemes and agricultural schemes for our Mising villages never happen. With Sixth Schedule, we would have been able to access these resources from Delhi (national capital) or Dispur (Assam state capital), be able to see the corruption and take action, but without it, this is how it will be, with people from our community having no access to agricultural schemes to ensure food availability.

The conversation then shifted to pig breeding for community consumption in relation to these demands for tribal autonomy measures and their possible impact on traditional food practices. Hara specified that several pig sectors have had funds under Prime Minister Rojgar Yojana, the North Eastern Regional Centre of the National Institute of Rural Development & Panchayati Raj (NIRD & PR-NERC) for villages but training and funds are not systematic or sustained by these schemes. 'Our community is not commerce oriented or trade oriented', Hara said, referring to the small-scale community rearing of local pigs for community consumption, due to which access to government schemes mentioned above remain unorganized and uncertain as long-term sustenance measures.

Across Mising migrations from Burma to the Sino-Tibetan border (Doley, 1998; Nath & Pegu, 2012) or according to another conjecture as part of Sino-Tibetan groups that formed at the confluence of China and Tibet and then moved to India

(Nath, 1998, 32), food practices often emerge as a means to ensure cultural continuity across histories of migration and retain links to places and religious traditions (Mintz & DuBois, 2002, 99). The Mising emphasize that their ideas of indigeneity and belonging continue to be linked to several present-day tribal communities under the Tani lineage groups that migrated from Tibet-India borderlands to Arunachal Pradesh in waves of migration by the fifteenth century (Blackburn 2003/2004, 46). Around the thirteenth/fourteenth centuries, Mising communities initially occupied foothill regions between present-day Arunachal and Assam (Barpujari, 1990, 41).

Pigs are often cited by community members as constant companions across these migrations with a Mising woman named Ira stating that: 'In the hills, we used to have a lot of wild pigs, they had so much forested area to graze in and were so healthy. According to our legends, pigs were our constant companions. Even in death, they appease angry ancestors or evil spirits, when they are offered as offerings'. In the harsher climate of the mountainous and hilly regions of Tibet and Arunachal Pradesh, wild boars were hunted, serving an integral part of Mising diets dependent on hunting and gathering practices. However, following the Mising community's migration to the Brahmaputra floodplain of Assam, small black pigs whose diets and lifestyle were more suited to the plains began to be reared.

In the Brahmaputra floodplain, several Mising communities began to live in small river islands, *chars* (or *sors* as they are pronounced in Assamese). They are semi-permanent sand bars that arise from the riverbeds throughout the Indus-Ganga–Brahmaputra-Meghna floodplains, as rivers move to lower elevations and deposit huge quantities of silt and sand. The *chars* become inhabitable depending upon the level of deposition (Lahiri & Samanta, 2013, 9). These smaller *chars* in the middle reaches of the Brahmaputra River in Lakhimpur District are mostly inhabited by the Mising community. The larger river island Majuli, adjacent to these smaller *chars* is currently about 350 square miles. It is much more permanent and includes Neo-Vaishnavite monasteries (Sarma & Phukan, 2004, 3) and several different local communities as compared to the smaller Lakhimpur *chars* where Mising community members are sole inhabitants. Here, community members shift frequently as homes are swept away with the floods. Many *chars* become submerged, while others emerge anew with riverine sand depositions in the monsoon months (Thakur, 2021, 3). Increasingly erratic flood cycles have created further uncertainties in food availability, particularly for staple crops such as paddy that get buried with high rates of sand desertification (Saikia, 2020, 509). In turn, this causes scarcities in food and fodder sources to rear pigs. In hegemonic caste Hindu discourses about pigs across India, however, there is a tendency to focus on the inherently dirty nature of pigs without accounting for these specific porcine life processes and the role of riverine flows.

Caste Hindu Porcine Discourses

Unlike caste Hindu communities across India, in Assam the consumption of pork is prevalent amongst diverse communities. Non-vegetarian food especially chicken, mutton and fish are consumed by all including Assamese Brahmins, many of whom have also increasingly begun to eat pork though refrain from cooking it within their homes. This is an aspect that has often been an anomaly in Hindutva attempts to incorporate Assam and Northeast India into mainland ideas of Hinduism and Savarna caste identities, across Assam (Baruah, 2019, 1). However, this region where I conduct fieldwork is home to several Neo-Vaishnavite monasteries and Assamese Brahmin families attached to these institutions cite an inherent dirtiness in the porcine alimentary tract that creates feelings of repulsion (*ghin*) due to the pig's diet and living environment. In thinking about the consumption of pork, several Assamese Brahmins I spoke to in North Lakhimpur town which is across the river at a distance of about 25 km from the *chars,* talk about a lack of hygiene in the Mising community and their food practices.

The muddiness of riverine *char* or small river island spaces of the Brahmaputra (Thakur, 2018, 2) where the Mising live conjure images of dirt and an inherent inability to practise hygiene. These discourses of hygiene though expressed at separate moments from the doctors I spoke to often echo state health practitioners' categorization of pork as an unhealthy, excessively fatty food on account of their lived environments and their cohabitation with Mising community members. Though pigs can realistically be linked to gastrointestinal diseases and parasitic diseases in humans such as ringworm infestation (*fita pelu*), many of which rise during the flood season in June and July, medical staff cited that pigs and their consumers were naturally inclined to breed these diseases due to the muddiness of their lived environment and the inherent dirtiness of their diet. Pigs and their environment were thus coded as conducive to zoonotic parasites which could be transmitted to human beings through many recent porcine diseases such as the recent African Swine Fever that occurred during the pandemic are non-communicable to human beings (The Hindu, 2020). These claims did not investigate causal factors in specific cases of Mising gastrointestinal health issues.

Instead in this biomedical rationale, mobile communities like the Mising, whose lives in the river islands are constantly shaped by the Brahmaputra's flood and soil deposition patterns, are seen to be inherently inclined towards alimentary practices that do not emphasize hygiene and nutrition. Such a rationale makes no attempt to actually find out if community-reared porcine breeds in the *chars* consume toxic material, unlike their urban and commercially farmed breeds whose diets and life cycles remain unknown. There is also no attempt to consider the fact that pork is not eaten in everyday meals and pigs are often slaughtered for community occasions and religious ceremonies. Further, this reasoning that pork is inherently harmful for consumption does not account for the contingency of riverine life and the increased risk of diseases in the monsoon that often have no relation to porcine consumption. Instead, this discourse focuses on the inherent nature of backwardness in the community vis-à-vis hygiene that is seen to make them automatically vulnerable to an inability to ensure alimentary care in cleaning and assuring that the pork they consume is suitable for consumption.

Such discourses abound across colonial and caste discourse about food seen in the case of the Musahar community in Bihar whose consumption of rats is often coded as a mark of caste inferiority, an aspect that overlooks the historical context of caste in creating the structural marginalization that the community faces in access to land and sustenance (Sahay, 2019, 30). Similarly, the consumption of small animals categorized as rodents such as guinea pigs in Peru has faced public health vitriol about indigestible and unhealthy food practices among indigenous communities (Garcia, 2013, 506). These global discourses continue to overlook the underlying systems of structural inequality as well as differing definitions of what constitutes healthy food for communities that have historically eaten these food sources. Similarly, several Mising community members point out that while pigs bred in large industrial factories in urban areas may be susceptible to consuming toxic waste, their pigs are reared in places close to their homes. The Mising also assert that imported porcine breeds that they call *saalani* or foreign had higher proportion of fat and were thus responsible for any increasing health problems. Several community members further point out that a lack of government resources to support the breeding of local pig varieties was causing their traditionally valued porcine sources to diminish. This changing nature of pork and the pig's increased indigestibility are linked by the Mising to commercial farming and environmental changes, aspects that need to be taken into consideration in government schemes to ensure food security and access to traditional sources of food that are ultimately linked to community understandings of well-being and nutrition.

Complexities of Caste and Hindu Nationalism in Assam

The state of Assam was historically located in later Vedic literature as a distant land on 'the margins of Indic culture' (Sharma, 2012, 49), in a sense locating this region as distinct from other parts of India considered 'mainland' (Baruah 2020, 26). There are records of several indigenous gatherers and Neolithic period cultivators before settlement by successive waves of caste Hindu communities around the fifth/sixth centuries according to land grants (Lahiri, 1991, 158). The thirteenth century saw the beginning of the rule of the Ahom kingdom, rulers who managed several land systems through negotiations with neighbouring hill chiefdoms of tribal communities (Sharma, 2012, 26). The Ahoms, who were initially seen as 'outsiders' due to their roots in Upper Burma were seen to commission Brahmins[2] for temple administration in Assam. In childhood stories about where and how my family came to live in Assam, my father often spoke about a similar land assignment that his father's paternal

---

[2] Brahmin communities were seen to be dated in Assam from about the sixth century CE according to the Nidhanpur inscription (Bose 1989).

ancestors had received from the Ahom King Purander Singha to travel from Kanauj in current day Uttar Pradesh, to look after rituals in a Sakti temple in present-day Sivasagar District, which was the stronghold of the Ahom kingdom (1228–1826) in Assam. However, I grew up away from these regions and others close to my field site where Neo-Vaishnavism was prevalent and where I had distant relatives whom I met for the first time during research. I grew up eating chicken, fish and pork collectively with my nuclear and extended family. While conducting fieldwork with the Mising, my comfort in eating pork during meals was often pointed out by Mising community members as a reason for speaking freely about issues of caste inequality and ostracism on account of their tribal positionality.

The sixteenth-century Neo-Vaishnavite movement in Assam is also pointed out by communities as having changed the trajectory of Hindu spirituality and understandings of Hinduism in Assam with its founder, the fifteenth-century *bhakti* preacher Sankardeb, aiming to create parity among caste Hindu and tribal populations in Assam. Many Mising practice this Sankari dharma but believe that the aspect of equality nurtured by Neo-Vaishnavite faith is threatened by increasing Hindu nationalist forces in Assam and within certain monasteries in the region. Sankardeb sought to 'improve regimes between God and man' (Sharma, 2011, 129) institutionalized in the form of the Vaishnavite monastic institution called the *satra*, prevalent in Lakhimpur and Majuli where this chapter is located. Caste and alimentary practices around it are similarly different for caste Hindu Neo-Vaishnavite societies in Assam as opposed to other followers of Vaishnavite vegetarianism across India (Sharma, 2011, 90), as Sankardeb is seen to have believed that alimentary restrictions were not required for spiritual connections with divinity. Though monastic members of *satras* eat fish, and extended families living away from the *satra* may eat mutton occasionally, chicken and pork were seen to be taboo. Further, away from the *satra* in nearby towns and cities, several Vaishnavite families do eat chicken and pork outside their homes despite thinking of these meats as taboo to cook in their homes.

This complexity of categorizing 'caste' and alimentary practices around it in Assam is specified across anthropological work in Assam (Cantille, 1984; Dowdy, 2017; Ramirez, 2014, 2013). Caste in Assam has often been explained through the lens of ethnicity and through specific eventual and occupational circumstances in which *jati* distinctly unfolds (Dowdy, 2017, 153), rather than asserting a universal caste hierarchy derived from other regions of India. Over time 'caste' structures in Assam have historically been embroiled in questions of ethno-territoriality, colonial racial categorizations of communities designated as 'tribes', post-colonial articulations of Scheduled Tribes as well as self-identifications of communities themselves as tribes (Karlsson, 2003; Xaxa, 2008; Nongbri 2003). The inability of caste in Assam to be understood through the lens of Indian heartland caste structures (Baruah, 2021, 1) has often been an aspect that thwarted the proselytization of the BJP and its Hindutva regimes among diverse communities, despite its electoral victories in 2016 and 2021.

With rising Hindu nationalist proselytization in Northeast India following the 2016 elections where BJP came to power in Assam, communities like the Mising who identify as tribal point out that proselytization against pork increased. The Mising further point out that while caste-based discrimination has historically impacted tribal communities who are located outside Hindu caste hierarchies, current Hindu nationalist discourse about caste is unfamiliar to them due to the Neo-Vaishnavite movement's role in complicating caste, Hinduism and associated alimentary practices in Assam. Several Mising community members have also increasingly stated that BJP and RSS proselytization against their food practices attempts to impose ideas of a singular Hindu nation that is heavily influenced by monolithic understandings of Hinduism that are specific to northern and western states such as Uttar Pradesh and Gujarat.

'We are unable to become Hindu': Alimentary Paths, Nutrition and Nationhood

When working on the much larger Majuli island in the summer of 2016, I increasingly saw RSS bike patrols with saffron flags flying. The Rashtriya Swayamsevak Sangh (RSS) is a pro-Hindu organization that is seen to be the ideological fountainhead of the Bharatiya Janata Party currently ruling India (Jaffrelot et al., 2019, 134). The RSS propagates a Hindutva ideology that attempts to impose monolithic ideas of Hinduism that do not account for caste and tribe positionalities, historical and spatial contexts of interpreting religious subjectivities across India. Hindutva forces have been making inroads into Assam and were strengthened following the 2016 elections when the BJP won in the state (Baruah, 2020, 16). Mising community members point out that increasingly RSS-influenced schools have appeared in different parts of northeast India to incorporate the region in more mainland ideas of Hinduism (Siddiqui, 2014, 1), targeting tribal communities whose meat-eating practices are part of their subsistence. This targeting of the Mising is enabled by various state discourses about civilizational progress through Hindu reform movements and other embodied reforms around hygiene prescribed for Dalits and STs (Christopher, this volume).

As one of these patrols whizzed past, I was interviewing a Mising farmer, Bhuben, who had begun an initiative for organic farming in the region.

Bhuben commented:

> They tell us to eat fruits, vegetables and *paneer* (cottage cheese) instead of meat for our rituals. How can we appease our gods with paneer instead of pork? The pig was seen as our companion throughout our time on earth; it is the only offering that can appease gods and evil spirits who seek to harm our kin.

Bhuben then told of the increasing advocacy of the RSS which specifically sought to prevent Mising conversion to Christianity. Further, they focused on the need to reduce the consumption of alcohol and meat prevalent in Mising rituals such as the *hokam*. The farmer expressed that though he did not agree with the RSS, he did advocate a need to stop ritual animal sacrifice performed within the community. He felt that the Mising have 'not been able to become Hindu' (*Hindu hobole para nai*) due to the practice of ritual animal sacrifice which he does not designate as religious.

He believes that these '*amangaliya*' or 'inauspicious' practices were unnecessary for spirituality and for establishing connections with divine forces such as Donyi-Polo (sun-moon worship) that is prevalent in Arunachal Pradesh among other Tani groups which the Mising fall under.

Shifting to the smaller river islands or *chars* in Lakhimpur, I heard a similar discourse of self-reform propagated mostly by Mising youth organizations such as the Takam Mising Porin Kebang (TMPK). Current TMPK members, some of whom were interviewed in 2018, spoke about the need to sanitize Mising ritual sacrifices. One member, Gana felt the need for the community to undertake self-reform through the renunciation of *apong* and the consumption of pig meat which he saw as unhealthy and cited several gastrointestinal problems prevalent among community members on the island as evidence. Another focus was that of modernity and development: 'These old rituals are socio-economically and medically obstructions to community upliftment and therefore needed to be eliminated', Gana said. More recently, they reiterated that while self-reform was important for the community to progress, they could not agree with the RSS' ideas of Hinduism that portrayed the consumption of meat and pig meat as inherently non-Hindu practices.[3]

Srirupa Prasad uses the term 'alimentary anxieties' (2015, 21) to refer to the patterns of food consumption that are associated with pollution in nationalist discourses' need to construct ideal Indian citizens. Unsanitary conditions of pig rearing are cited in medical discourse as the cause for deteriorating health and disease among the Mising as a result of which they are unable to become healthy citizens while Hindu nationalist discourse codes pigs as alimentary obstacles to becoming ideal citizens of an imagined Hindu nation. Longkumer (2018) points out how Hindutva ideas about the body around homogenized practices of food and health propagated by the introduction of a godman called Baba Ramdev's Patanjali products in the northeast Indian state Nagaland promoted a form of 'somatic nationalism' (Longkumer, 2018, 401). This is exemplified in the ways in which dominant caste rhetoric about what is idealized as nutrition gets embroiled in medical discourses. On the contrary, Mising community members assert that it is the changing life cycles and the porcine species' 'genetic manipulation that is problematic and in conflict with notions of food sovereignty' (Garcia, 2013, 519), and in their case inter-generational well-being. Here, the pig "becomes a site of a medium and a message of conflict" (Appadurai, 1981, 501). It is on account of the everyday materiality of eating and rearing local pigs that medical discourses, fixated on hygiene in prescribing nutritional sources of food, need to account for community-specific understandings of well-being while also establishing more scientific causal links for their claims.

---

[3] Non-Hindu practices emphasized by the RSS usually target Mising and other tribal communities who had recently converted to Christianity.

Medical Discourses About Hygiene and Nutrition

Unlike the traditional Mising methods of cleaning the pig which are deemed inadequate, hygiene is described by medical practitioners and pig breeders as a process that needs to follow a 'prescribed standard or purity' (Prasad, 2015, 29) to enhance nutritive value. Doctors I met during my first visit to the region often pointed out that a lack of systematic cleaning measures amongst the Mising led to several health problems such as bacterial infections in human beings. While bacterial infections such as tapeworm infestations are a reality, I am pointing out that references to systematic cleaning measures do not address specific health issues or cleaning measures used by the Mising but instead assume that the community does not have the required knowledge to ensure sufficient cleaning of pork before consumption. This is the knowledge that is automatically assumed for the middle class, upper caste communities who live away from the *chars* and buy meat from commercial farms.

Here, standards of purity in understanding the nutritive value of food impose elite health discourses without scientifically interrogating how biological health is impacted by pork consumption. Hygiene emerges as a means to dictate the terms of pork rearing, cleaning, and consumption without scientifically demonstrating how the assumed dirtiness of pigs affects its nutritive value. Instead, porcine diets, upbringing and muddy domiciles are seen as clear evidence of their harmfulness (Cortesi, 2018, 617) for Mising consumption. Despite pork consumption by communities other than the Mising, their spatial location in the remote river island region and their positionality as a tribe is ultimately linked to civilizational backwardness and an inability to ensure the cleanliness of rearing environments for pigs as well as the safe preparation of pork.

In commercial porcine farming, technological interventions are seen to increase purity compared to traditional Mising methods of drying and smoking pork to ensure healthy consumption. This is outlined in a recent conversation with Maitreya Goswami who is involved in a pig farming livelihood initiative organized by the National Hydroelectric Power Corporation (NHPC)[4] for farmer producer organizations in the Subansiri river region where my field site is located. Goswami describes that the pig manufacturing and slaughtering process has to be strictly hygienic to add value to the meat, which is why the pig is killed instantly using an electric shock treatment, blood is seeped out of the pig by hanging it upside down to reduce contamination and the insides of the pig are cleaned using machines that can ensure maximum hygiene. Several Mising community members however argued that they always took utmost care to ensure the cleaning of pork including the removal of internal organs that might be toxic for consumption. They pointed out the use of intergenerationally passed-on methods such as smoking and drying of pork in the sun to ensure the removal of bacteria that can cause gastrointestinal issues. They also point out that tapeworm infestations were historically low in community-reared

---

[4] The NHPC was also embroiled in Mising community protests when it proposed the Lower Subansiri hydel project in the early 2000s, a project that was passed for resumption in December 2019.

pigs. Instead, they assert that imported, industrial varieties and the uncertainties of knowing the environments and diets that these non-local, commercially farmed pigs are reared in bring in new health repercussions for the community.

According to the Livestock Census 2012, Assam's total pig population is 1,636,022 which is approximately 15.89% of the country's total pig population. The Animal Husbandry and Veterinary Department runs about 19 Pig Breeding Farms across the state with several other independent pig farms (Animal Husbandry and Veterinary Department Strategy Report 2019–24, 7). This is on account of the fact that a majority of the state's population eats pork accounting for a total annual require-ment of pork of about 3,63,000 tones (Integrated Sample Survey Report 2016–17). The government aims to develop commercial pig farms to increase farmers' income due to which chosen pigs bred at these industrial farms are mostly crossbred varieties of Hampshire, Large White Yorkshire and Large Black and Duroc pigs which are popular in the UK and the US. These breeds are focused on commercial farming programs as they achieve optimum meat outputs while they are increasingly pointed out by the Mising as the cause of diseases in their community.

Hygiene and nutrition emerge as keywords in several sets of ethnographic conver-sations around 'porcine worlds' (Blanchette, 2020, 4), described here as the different ways in which pigs are semiotically discussed and the material ways in which they become different forms in Mising community diets. In contrast to medical, caste and nationalist discourse that highlights the pig's low hygiene and nutritive value, Mising community members I spoke to emphasize that it is the industrial production of the pig in its imported, *saalani* (non-local) form that lowers its nutritive value. This is seen to be further exacerbated by an accompanying inability to sustain small-scale pig rearing due to a lack of systematic funds for tribal community development from the federal government. The 'indigenous' varieties which provide lesser amounts of meat per pig are generally seen to be the Ghungroo and Smaller Black pigs which in themselves are increasingly becoming crosses between Large Black Pigs and Hamp-shires. The community's experience of nutritional deficiencies emphasizes required systems for Mising tribal autonomy among which several community members point out the Sixth Schedule. They believe access to funds for the rearing of local pigs at home will increase through this tribal autonomy measure. These lived relationships with pigs in the Anthropocene and the increasing problems pointed out about the inability to rear local porcine breeds is at odds with the medical discourse that echoes caste and Hindu nationalist tropes of pigs as sites of embodied pollution.

Muddiness, Dirt and Disease: Medical Discourse About Porcine Lives

A popular story narrated by Borma's sister-in-law was recently reiterated by Juwel Pegu.

In a popular story often told to children, pigs and dogs were told to cultivate the fields. The pig actually did the work but fell asleep behind the fields. As a result, the dog took credit by leaving its footprints. When the master came, he believed that the dog had done the work because the pig's footprints were nowhere. So, pigs are kept under the *saang ghar* in a dustbin type area, but dogs are allowed to come up to the house. The lack of intelligence in the pig made it lesser in value but it is still important because it appeases evil spirits (*opo debota*) and gives peace to dead ancestors.

This story of porcine appeasement is often repeated by Mising community members when they are asked about their cohabitation with pigs. This cohabitation becomes a point of focus in relationships between monsoons, human illnesses and pigs that medical professionals whom I met pointed out. These doctors and nurses were clear that pigs are inherently dirty, living in muddy environments and believed to eat unsanitary muddy matter that consisted of discarded human food and excretal waste. They would point out that Mising community members suffered from diarrhoea and tapeworm infestation due to this cohabitation, without any medical evidence linking all these cases to pigs.

Assamese Brahmins associated with local Neo-Vaishnavite monastic institutions in Lakhimpur and Majuli reiterated this belief. Many said: 'The Mising live in unsanitary, small spaces shared with their livestock'. They pointed out that Mising *saang ghars* housed pigs, hens and ducks underneath them. The bamboo and cane floors of the *saang ghars* with their gaps made it easy to see and hear the animals living underneath creating a feeling of cohabitation and proximity that was imagined as unnatural and unhygienic. Food remains after family meals were thrown through the cracks, a system of sharing that the Mising saw as easy waste disposal and a lack of wastefulness.

The reality of hygiene as a measure of civilizational differences between Mising and upper caste communities is seen in rural health initiatives that target Mising populations for population and disease control primarily based on the rationale that the community has no knowledge or desire for hygiene and hence needs to be sanitized. Further, the dichotomy created between the upper caste mainland vis-à-vis Mising inhabited river islands, is impacted by the rhetoric of hygiene which assumes that the river island is the contact zone 'teeming with hundreds of potential microbes' (Prasad, 2015, 1), from where infection can spread to other areas. In public health and caste Hindu reiterations of livestock as creating zones of contagion, the emphasis is similarly on pigs and their lived environments where purity and pollution and hygiene discourses often become parallels due to the lack of concrete evidence linking pigs as causal factors for all Mising diseases. Pigs are considered dirty creatures who live in mud and eat polluting substances such as faeces, both of which reiterate the inherently embodied dirtiness of muddy environments (Cortesi, 2018, 617) and the Mising bodies who care for and inhabit them. Mising community members contradictorily point out that pigs residing in the same dwelling places make it easy to supervise their diets and living environments. As a result, the same toxicity that medical discourse imagines of pigs and human beings cohabiting is seen by the community as a marker of control over what the pigs ate and how they dwelt.

The inherently dirty nature of pigs as linked to their muddy environments in hygiene and nutrition discourse among doctors, nurses and many Assamese Brahmins underlies the notions of dirt that are attached to bodies inhabiting these riverine spaces, an aspect that Narayanan explains is the process through which casteism is sustained through the dehumanization (Narayanan, 2021, 14) of intertwined human and non-human lives. Muddy soil which makes up Mising *char* lives is seen by the community as having the power to make (*bonai*) and break (*bhange*) land and life. This making refers to the formation of the *chars* by these soils, the life that grows in the form of crops in the fields, and the human and animal lives it sustains. But in upper caste discourse and medical discourse, mud takes on connotations of 'dirt and pollution, particularly when present on the bodies of people associated with lower castes' (Cortesi, 2018, 619), and in this case through the interconnected bodies of pigs and human beings. In the case of the Mising community where I lived pigs mostly stayed in the vicinity of the household. The area under the *saang ghor* was generally swept dry and during the rainy summer seasons, the pigs dwelt there. They occasionally ventured into muddy puddles towards the rear of the *saang* but were frequently chased towards the drier areas.

I argue that medical discourse brings up caste tropes of the muddiness and dirtiness of pigs but fails to account for the ways in which the changing riverine ontologies due to increasingly erratic floods shape animal and human health. In addition, their claims that pork is unhealthy based on the environments in which they dwell fails to account for the actual lifeworld of the pig—both local and imported, the composition of their diets and changes due to ongoing environmental and technological changes in porcine farming. In this chapter, ontology refers to the philosophy of being that is used in anthropology and other social sciences to refer to the multiple ways in which objects—human and non-human—become what they are through their participation in socio-material practices. Here, this conception is indebted to Annemarie Mol (2002, 6), who states that 'ontology is not given in the order of things, but that, instead, ontologies are brought into being, sustained, or allowed to wither away in common, day-to-day, socio-material practices'. Ontologies of riverine environments and pigs are constantly shaped and modified through environmental change and commercial farming, respectively, both of which interact to change the composition of the pig as the Mising have historically known it.

Mising demands for systematic fund dispersal for small pig farmers through proper tribal autonomy measures to remote areas such as the *chars* also remain unheard as the state instead focuses on standardizing large-scale pig breeding, focusing on breeds that the Mising believed to have caused disruptions in their alimentary and ritual systems. Further, as the African Swine Fever hit during the pandemic and decimated the pig population in Mising villages, community members were more attuned to how food inaccessibility due to lack of tribal autonomy was more a cause of social harm than the impacts of COVID-19 itself. Their critique of government inadequacies was similarly prevalent in other tribal communities across India (Sharma, this volume). I further argue that a focus on these lived gaps in chains of food production, quality and distribution of culturally imbued food sources, governmental ambivalence and the materiality of riverine lives in the Anthropocene do not get accounted for in medical variables of nutrition for marginalized tribal communities in India.

Climate Change and Nutrition in Riverine Mising Lives

When asked about these medical discourses about pigs as sites of contagion, the Mising often asked me the question: 'If pigs cause so many diseases, why have they not caused them before for all our ancestors who ate them from the time they were in the hills?'. Across these Mising conversations about pork, three reasons are cited for why this meat is becoming unhealthy even though historically it was a source of community sustenance. First, the community points out rising flood patterns amidst climate change that threaten to bury crops in *char* regions, making food and fodder sources scarce which makes it difficult to continue breeding smaller, local and less fat producing pig breeds without state funds. Second, community members mention that it is the lack of traditionally used herbs with medicinal properties (Sharma & Pegu, 2011, 1) that once grew along riverbanks and were used to absorb fat in pork to make it more suitable for digestion. Third, the increasingly non-native breeds of pigs such as imported cross-breeds which are termed *saalani* have a higher fat content.

In the discourses criticizing the consumption of pork that I heard from the NGO doctors, nurses and Assamese Brahmin community members I met, the muddiness of pigs and Mising lives were seen as a marker of shared unhealthy diets. This meant that muddiness was coded as breeding an environment conducive to unhygienic diets for pigs and in turn Mising communities who consumed them. Here, absorption which refers to the porosity between bodies and their environments (Solomon, 2016, 6) is seen as the process through which the inherently embodied dirtiness of muddy environments that pigs imbue transfers to Mising community members. Caste hierarchies and their associated bodily pollution are then seen to be extended through the alimentary tract through Mising consumption of pork. The Mising point out that any changes in the pig's diet are on account of the scarcity of traditional fodder sources due to increased flooding, the burial of crops, and the uncertainty of knowing what diets are being fed to pigs under industrial farming. Discourses about hygiene that resonate in both caste Hindu communities and among medical practitioners overlook these changing ontologies of the industrial pig as compared to the local pig. These discourses further fail to account for any material connections between pigs' diets and their ramifications for human consumption, as industrial pigs are never interrogated with regard to their lifecycle, lived environments, and diets due to the assumption that commercial porcine farming maintains standards of purity, where purity is conflated with nutritional value.

Solomon (2016) asks some key questions about how ideas about nutrition are never static and instead impacted by interactions with the lived environment- 'Who and what become the eater and the eaten? What is nutrition and what is poison? Who and what set the boundaries of inside and outside, delineating organism and environment?' (Solomon, 2016, 5). In making these value judgements about what constitutes suitable kinds of food, nutrition in medical discourse asserts the unsuitability of pork as a form of sustenance contrary to Mising assertions that it is healthy and will continue to be if state systems provide stability to small-scale pig breeding. While excessive consumption of red meat such as pork may affect gastrointestinal health, medical discourse about Mising consumption of pork does not outline specific health issues and their causes but instead focuses on perceptions of inherent dirtiness in the pig and its lived environment, thus concluding that it cannot be a suitable source of nutrition. Further, caste and hygiene discourse gets extended through increasing Hindu nationalist discourses that assert that porcine consumption in northeast India keeps it from integrating into mainland ideas of Hinduism. It is at this juncture that further tensions emerge between alimentary worlds and the need to forge national health, without accounting for the fact that intimate human–animal relationships impact Mising health. Pork is essential for Mising community well-being which they express is part of their definitions of health, as food and as a link to places of migration and ancestors who protect the community from ill-health from their afterlives.

"We do not eat the Mother": Intimate Human–Animal Relationships

In February 2021, I called Borma to ask about their celebration of *Ali ai Ligang*, which is the festival associated with the beginning of the *Ahu* variety of rice cultivation, celebrated in the Assamese calendar month of Phagun, in February.

Me: *Did you eat smoked pork with mati dayl (a black gram lentil curry accompaniment to rice) for Ali ai Ligang?*

Borma: *'Where would we get pork? All the pigs died and there was none to feed the village for Ligang'.*

Me: *'What happened to the big female pig and her piglets that you were rearing for the festival? Remember, I had met her last year before the pandemic'.*

Borma: *'Oh! That mother pig that we used to chase, she died, and all her children also died, so long back. They all died from the disease'.*

When I asked her husband about this pig, he said: *'But we wouldn't have eaten her anyway, we don't eat the mother'.*

During my stay in the *char*, I was often given the responsibility of feeding the pigs, ducks and hens in the evening before the younger women returned from the fields. *Borma* (Assamese word for eldest aunt) spoke of this pig mentioned above fondly, talking about how she slept too much and often tried to eat the other animals' feed. She also pointed out that since the pig fed so many piglets, she needed the extra food. In talking about this particular sow who recently died due to the African Swine Fever epidemic in 2020, *Borma* often remembered many others who came before her and whose piglets had been offered at *hokams* and cooked for funerary feasts, these relationships at once intimate and valued for consumption.

Govindrajan (2018) talks about the intimate and 'affectively proximate lives' (2018, 80) of humans and animals, that make their connections deeper, the smells and sounds of each other's lives intermingling as it did in the case of the Mising. Pigs here are sacrificial and often take on the sins of the immediate family and extended kin. However, the 'sacrificial victim needs to be understood as more than just symbol' (Govindrajan, 2018, 39). Mising understandings of pigs as sustenance emphasizes that their death and sacrificial connection is not fixated on an embodied kinship (Govindrajan, 2018, 37) with the animal itself. Instead, relationships between pigs and humans are based on the knowledge that the pig has the power to provide nutrition and maintain cultural ties to lineage groups and ancestors even in the afterlife. In contrast, however, the pig in its industrial *saalani* form has minimal nutrition value or socio-cultural familiarity as it is imported from and processed in places where there is no 'sensory or sacrificial relatedness' (Govindrajan, 2018, 38). Instead, the industrial pig is embroiled in 'consumptive desires to meet the offerings of industrial alimentary capitalism' (Benson and Fischer 2007, 808).

Porcine Industrialization as Disrupting Ancestral Connections

During a conversation with Juwel Pegu, a Mising community member and former secretary of a Mising literary association called the Mising Agom Kebang, he commented that:

> Whenever we visited our relatives in Arunachal, they would feed us smoked pork from local pigs bred in their village. We used to carry parcels of smoked pork when we left for the city. But lately, everyone eats and feeds guests *saalani* pork. That is the reason we are getting so many diseases. We also used to smoke our pork after burning the outer skin to remove hair and dirt and then boil it. Smoking pork on our porches traditionally for 3–4 days dries it and kills germs. But now we have to buy pork from the market and all these imported pigs have high fat content, often there is no time to smoke it as less pigs are bred locally. In tribal societies, we always lived with animals in shared spaces, but the environment our ancestors lived in was not conducive to creating diseases. There were so many forests to graze and now there are so many floods. So, diseases are more and there is more scope for exposure and transmission from animals to human beings.

Pegu's wife, Pratibha Kuli, who remembered rearing pigs as a young woman with her sisters and mother pointed out that increasingly pigs were fed 'veterinary college-approved feeds and vitamins to make them bigger that were nothing like their traditional fermented feeds', as taught to them by mothers and grandmothers. They used to give rice and *tuguri* (ground rice husk), boiled *bon kosu* (taro or *Colocasia esculenta*), plants that cannot be easily found now in the forests where women used to gather them. Pratibha also pointed out that increasingly these substitutes have to be used due to the scarcity of food and fodder sources.

What is described here is a change in the nature of the pig in its imported, crossbred, differently fed, climatically vulnerable and 'industrialized' porcine form (Blanchette,

2020, 4). This is seen in questions about biosecurity emphasized by pig breeders and veterinary doctors in the region. A local pig breeder, Manoj points out that diseases are more prevalent amongst pigs in Mising villages as compared to other tribal communities. This is seen to be mainly due to open range grazing systems and feeding systems that involved unhygienic feed or water systems, though most of these common diseases were not transmitted from pigs to human beings. With the more recent African Swine Fever, several veterinarians and pig breeders pointed out that it was predicted to have spread via the Brahmaputra river's flows from the Tibetan region due to the disposal of diseased pig corpses in the river and riverine transmission (Ahmed, 2020, 1). As most Mising villages had very few pigs and most of them were housed without built enclosures with most housed under their *saang ghar*, the risks of diseases spreading through contact between pigs, especially in the monsoon, was high as a result of which epidemics such as the African Swine Flu wiped out several Mising pigs.

Here again, the non-Mising 'experts' emphasized that humans and pigs dwelling in proximity was a reason for the transmission of zoonotic diseases. The superior nature of the industrial pig was emphasized while citing that confinement was key to managing diseases in pigs, seen in industrial pig rearing systems (Blanchette, 2020, 27), and as a result central to assuring food security for the Mising. In contrast to these claims, Ghanakanta Doley, a veterinarian in nearby Dhemaji district who has done extensive work on the recent African Swine Fever and is from the Mising community, noted that while the newly introduced breeds were economically viable, they were not biomedically resistant. 'Due to the global food market and privatization, all these imported pigs have really changed people's diets', he said. Doley went on to talk about the indigenous pigs that his community had been eating for generations, an aspect that is repeated by several community members in the *char*, demonstrating that a push for the industrial pig is not desired by Mising communities. Rather they seek to retain the ties that their migratory ancestors had developed with pigs in their corporeal forms as meat and in incorporeal ties enabled with ancestors in their afterlives, a connection that is often overlooked in medical discourse.

'We ate pork with herbs that cut its fat': Co-Produced Lifecycles of Pigs and Herbs

'In our grandparents' and great grandparents' time, we always ate pork with *bon xak* (herbs) that could cut its fat. There was the *dermi gos*, the *ombe pat*, spices were less as we only used ginger and garlic. Everything was balanced, but where will we find these herbs anymore? There are no forests left and plants that grew by the riverbank all get uprooted in the floods. The balance is lost in our food preparations', said Lalit as we talked about the food he ate growing up in the *char*.

This description reflects on the myriad ways in which food systems amongst the Mising challenge medical claims that pinpoint pork as unhealthy, fatty meat while asserting that the imbalances brought about by the industrial nature of the *saalani* pig is further offset by the imbalances in plant systems as a result of changing riverine flows. The co-produced lived in worlds that Mising community ancestors are seen to have built with pigs and herbs in their food preparations (Sharma & Pegu, 2011, 1) are breaking down due to changes in the industrial nature of food production but also in conjunction with increasingly erratic fluvial geomorphology and biogeography. Community members talk about their inability to rear pigs due to reduced crop and fodder outputs impacted by floods submerging them. Further, they pointed out the difficulties of finding medicinal herbs that grew by the riverbank but were no longer possible to find, thus pointing out the interlinked impacts of changing life cycles of pigs and herbs.

This reflects some of the concepts of the dwelling perspective (Ingold, 2011, 9), where human and non-human beings constantly co-produce their shared environments. This is seen in Mising struggles with climate change's impact. In this context porcine and herb life-worlds are both being impacted by industrial food export systems and riverine flows that transform traditional Mising foodways into indigestible, toxin-inducing environments in the body. All these reveal the 'dire social inequities of environmental, human, and animal degradation at the hands of industrialization' (Weiss, 2011, 440). Alimentary anxieties over national belonging, cultural continuity and autonomy revealed in the knots of a pig's stomach asserts that porcine paths (Weiss, 2011, 440) can trace a whole set of interrelated blocks in Anthropocene food systems.

Juwel Pegu reflected on a recent conversation he had with his relatives in his childhood village who talked about moving back to the hills of Arunachal Pradesh citing the repercussions of environmental change for riverine life in the Brahmaputra's floodplain:

> We always lived by the river and felt the floods. But it also gave us food and a life that could sustain the crops our ancestors grew. Now, the river gives less and less, floods more, and has more sand deposits that bury crops. Plants have disappeared. Pigs, hens and ducks have become difficult to rear [...]. Moreover, with rising government initiatives that tell us to follow North Indian ideas of Hinduism that we cannot relate to, our culture is at a risk.

This idea of imbalance is central in the narratives I hear from doctors and nurses, pig breeders, veterinary doctors, Mising community members and nationalist proselytizers regarding pigs. For medical professionals, this imbalance is in the pathways of consumption: in both porcine and human stomachs causing a block in Mising communities being able to avail of nutrition. For pig breeders, this imbalance is in the need for biosecurity to ensure optimum pork output to reach optimum economic viability. For veterinary doctors, this imbalance lies in the lack of bio-resistance of crossbred pig breeds. The Mising emphasize that the imbalance lies in the fact that they cannot recognize the pork they put into their bodies. They emphasize that their intergenerational ancestral links, migratory connections and cultural cosmologies of well-being are impacted by a lack of sufficient autonomy to govern their own livelihoods and funds to properly raise 'indigenous' pig varieties. Hindu nationalists emphasize that the imbalance is due to the inability of tribal communities like the Mising and other communities who ate pork to 'clean up' their food systems to become more truly Hindu.

Conclusion

Across these discourses, the pig becomes an alimentary, 'cultural site' (Sutton, 2000, 121) where different discourses about nutrition by non-Mising 'experts' overlook the community's assertion that their health and well-being can only be realized through systematic government measures that recognize their knowledge practices and retain them in ideas of nutrition. Pigs emerge as' localized cultural wholes that become points of identification for people displaced by migrations caused by larger global processes' (Fog & Hastrup, 1996, 11). This is the setting in which the Mising retain connections to places of migration, cultural knowledge and struggles for autonomy. Here, rearing the 'indigenous' black pig and cooking it in the ways in which the ancestors prepared it, using herbs and spices that were grown and available in places of migration, becomes a part of what is counted as healthy and nutritious food for the community. The community's struggles to retain these practices amidst the industrial production of the pig (Blanchette, 2020, 4) and erratic fluvial flows, reveals how nutrition is embroiled in processes of commodification. As pig breeders and state pig breeding programs aim to make the sector more economically viable, pigs become further cultural sites of capitalist production where crossbred, non-local pig breeds become dominant. These are the commercial varieties pointed to by the Mising community as increasingly available in the market and leading to the gastrointestinal problems that doctors blame on pork consumption. This dual interpretation of the current world in Assam shows how food reveals connected knots of tension around health, environment and nationhood.

Public health discourse often corroborates dominant upper caste tropes of hygiene regarding nutritious food but fails to make connections with the ways in which disease is linked to the increasingly changing riverine landscape inhabited by human and non-human communities. The multi-species world of water that makes up its materiality influences public health experiences in the Brahmaputra River Valley but is not taken into account by public health discourse and policies. As the River Brahmaputra floods annually during the monsoon months of June–August, the composition of water also changes. An NRHM doctor who lived for 5 years with these Mising communities in the *char* I visited, stated that the stagnation of water as a result of flooding often changed the nature of the water itself which in turn caused several skin-related diseases. However, several other doctors who occasionally visited were quick to point out pork consumption and tapeworm infestation as related to these same skin diseases, thus revealing the gaps in lived realities of disease causality amidst riverine flows.

During the time I spent on the river island, I remember the young women, mostly daughters and daughters-in-law of the household who would return every evening, their clothes drenched from the rain-soaked rice fields. I would often hear older women approaching the young women returning to advise them to wash their clothes and selves by the pump well before coming into the kitchen for dinner as this would ensure the removal of *letera* (dirt) and *juk* (leeches) that were prevalent in the stagnant water. At this juncture, I find that 'fluid subjectivities' (Sultana, 2009), defined as the ways in which changing water ontologies make and unmake inhabitant human bodies, need to be taken into account in-state public health programs for riverine regions such as the Brahmaputra River Valley. There needs to be a shift in current rural health programs from discourse on the inherent nature of contagion among riverine communities like the Mising to a focus on the ontologies of water, the built ontologies of the industrial pig and the lack of systems of accountability for agricultural and porcine rearing in riverine spaces such as *chars,* that make and unmake bodies that live enveloped in waterscapes (Anand, 2017, 48).

Across these divergent discourses about pigs vis-a-vis Mising health and this example above, what emerges is the prioritization of upper caste, middle class and caste Hindu nationalist ideas of what constitutes national health and ideal, healthy citizens of a nation. Here, industrial pig farms and medical teams seek to transform traditional Mising religious and alimentary practices by framing them as caste and 'tribal' backwardness. In contrast to discourses of blame, which result in further situations of food deprivation and poor health among riverine Mising communities in increasingly climate change impacted *char* lives, attention needs to be directed towards lived experiences and resulting demands for tribal autonomy that Mising communities insist will be a move towards accessing land, food and capital for their long-term biocultural well-being.

References

Ahmed, F. (2020). In Northeast India, African swine flu causes an epidemic among pigs. *The Wire.* Retrieved January 12, 2021, from https://science.thewire.in/environment/northeast-india-african-swine-flu-pigs/. Accessed 12 January 2021.

Anand, N. (2017). *Hydraulic city: Water and the infrastructures of citizenship in Mumbai.* Duke University Press.

Animal Husbandry and Veterinary Department. (2019). Strategy report 2019–24. *Government of Assam.* Retrieved January 12, 2021, from https://animalhusbandry.assam.gov.in/sites/default/files/swf_utility_folder/departments/ahvetdept_webcomindia_org_oid_3/portlet/level_1/files/piggery.pdf.

Appadurai, A. (1981). Gastro-politics in hindu South Asia. *American Ethnologist, 8*(3), 494–511. https://doi.org/10.1525/ae.1981.8.3.02a00050

Barpujari, H. K. (1990). *The comprehensive history of Assam* (Vol. III). Nabajiban Press.

Barua, B. K. (1985). *A cultural history of Assam, early period.* K. K Barooah.

Baruah, S. (2020). *In the name of the nation: India and its Northeast.* Stanford, CA: Stanford University Press.

Baruah, S. (2019). The fire in Assam. *The Indian Express.* Retrieved January 3, 2020, from https://indianexpress.com/article/opinion/columns/assam-protests-citizenship-amendment-bill-nrc-5538446/lite/.

Baruah, S. (2021). BJP's Assam triumph has one caveat: Akhil Gogoi. *The Indian Express.* Retrieved May 20, 2021, from https://indianexpress.com/article/opinion/columns/akhil-gogoi-assam-bjp-win-caa-hindutva-7306342/.

Benson, P., & Fischer, E. F. (2007). Broccoli and desire. *Antipode, 39*(5), 800–820.

Blackburn, S. (2003/2004). Memories of migration: Notes on legends and beads in Arunachal Pradesh, India. *European Bulletin of Himalayan Research,*15–60.

Blanchette, A. (2020). *Porkopolis: American animality, standardized life, and the factory farm.* Duke University Press.

Bodhisattva, K. (2016). Nomadic capital and speculative tribes: A culture of contracts in the Northeastern Frontier of British India. *The Indian Economic and Social History Review, 53*(1), 41–67.

Bose, M. (1989). *Social history of Assam: Being a study of the origins of ethnic identity and social tension during the British period, 1905–1947.* Concept Publishing Company.

Cantille, A. (1984). *The Assamese: Religion, caste, and sect in an Indian village.* Curzon.

Cortesi, L. (2018). The muddy semiotics of mud. *Journal of Political Ecology, 25*(1), 617–637.

Davis, A., & Sharp, J. (2020). Rethinking one health: emergent human, animal and environmental assemblages. *Social Science & Medicine, 258.*

Doley, D. (1998). *History of the Tanis or Amis.* Ayir Publications.

Dowdy, S. M. (2017). Ichthyonomics, or fish and humans in the time of floods: Rethinking speciation in Assam. In Y. Saikia & A. Baishya (Eds.), *Northeast India: A place of relations* (pp. 135–158). Cambridge University Press.

Fog, K. O., & Hastrup, K. (Eds.). (1996). *Siting culture: the shifting anthropological object.* Routledge.

Garcia, M. E. (2013). The taste of conquest: Colonialism, cosmopolitics, and the dark side of Peru's gastronomic boom. *Journal of Latin American and Caribbean Anthropology, 18*(3), 505–524.

Govindrajan, R. (2018). *Animal intimacies relatedness in India's central Himalayas.* The University of Chicago Press.

The Hindu. (2020). Amid pandemic, 1,300 pigs die of swine fever in Assam. Retrieved December 12, 2020, from https://www.thehindu.com/news/national/other-states/amid-pandemic-1300-pigs-die-of-swine-fever-in-assam/article31403558.ece.

Ingold, T. (2011). *Being Alive: Essays on movement, knowledge and description.* Routledge.

Jaffrelot, C., Chatterji, A. P., & Hansen, T. B. (2019). *Majoritarian state: How hindu nationalism is changing India.* Hurst and Company.

Karlsson, B. G. (2003). Anthropology and the 'indigenous slot': Claims to and debates about indigenous peoples' status in India. *Critique of Anthropology, 23*(4), 403–423. https://doi.org/10.1177/0308275X03234003

Lahiri, N. (1991). *Pre-ahom Assam: studies in the inscriptions of Assam between the fifth and the thirteenth centuries AD.* Munshiram Manoharlal.

Lahiri-Dutt, K., & Samanta, G. (2013). *Dancing with the river: People and life on the chars of South Asia.* Yale University Press.

Longkumer, A. (2018). 'Nagas can't sit lotus style': Baba Ramdev, Patanjali, and Neo-Hindutva. *Contemporary South Asia, 26*(4), 400–420.

Mintz, S. W., & Bois, C. D. (2002). The anthropology of food and eating. *Annual Review of Anthropology, 31,* 99–119.

Mipun, J. (2000). *The Mishings (Miris) of Assam: development of a new lifestyle.* Gian Pub. House.

Mol, A. (2002). *The body multiple: Ontology in medical practice.* Duke University Press.

Narayanan, Y. (2021). Animating caste: Visceral geographies of pigs, caste, and violent nationalisms in Chennai city. *Urban Geography.* https://doi.org/10.1080/02723638.2021.1890954

Nath, D. (1998). *The Misings, their history and culture.* Ayir Publications.

Nath, J., & Pegu, N. K. (2012). *A cultural history of the Misings of Assam.* Prithibi Prakashan House.

Nath, D. R. (2002). Piggery development in Assam. In *Proceedings of the Seminar on Agriculture in 21st Century.* Assam Science Society.

Nongbri, T. (2003). *Development, ethnicity and gender: Select essays on tribes in India.* Rawat Publications.

Pandian, A. (2008). Devoted to development: Moral progress, ethical work, and divine favor in South India. *Anthropological Theory, 8*(2), 159–179.

Pegu, M. (2013). On questions of identity and the Mising autonomous movement. *Daltri Journals, 1*(2), 15–26.

Prasad, S. (2015). *Cultural politics of hygiene in India, 1890–1940: Contagions of Feeling.* Springer.

Ramirez, P. (2013). *People of the margins: Across ethnic boundaries in North East India.* Spectrum.

Sahay, G. R. (2019). Substantially present but invisible, excluded and marginalised: A study of Musahars in Bihar. *Sociological Bulletin, 68*(1), 25–43.

Saikia, A. (2020). *The unquiet river: A biography of the Brahmaputra.* Oxford University Press.

Sarma, J. N., & Phukan, M. K. (2004). Origin and some geomorphological changes of Majuli Island of the Brahmaputra River in Assam, India. *Geomorphology, 60*(1–2), 1–19.

The Sentinel. (2020). NEPPFA opposes transportation of pigs from Punjab & Haryana. Retrieved December 12, 2020, from https://www.sentinelassam.com/topheadlines/neppfa-opposes-transportation-of-pigs-from-punjab-haryana-491504.

Sharma, U. K., & Pegu, S. (2011). Ethnobotany of religious and supernatural beliefs of the Mising tribes of Assam with special reference to the 'Dobur Uie'. *Journal of Ethnobiology and Ethnomedicine, 7*, 16. http://www.ethnobiomed.com/content/7/1/16

Sharma, J. (2011). *Empire's garden: Assam and the making of India.* Duke University Press.

Solomon, H. (2016). Metabolic living: Food, fat, and the absorption of illness in India. Durham: Duke University Press.

Siddiqui, F. A. (2014). Target northeast: How RSS plans to make region saffron. *Hindustan Times.* Retrieved December 15, from https://www.hindustantimes.com/india/target-northeast-how-rss-plans-to-make-region-saffron/story-YZGPkOBXb6tS301BvpunpJ.html.

Thakur, N. (2021). The struggles of a "river people" in Assam. *SAPIENS*, April 14.

Sultana, F. (2009). Fluid lives: Subjectivities, gender and water in rural Bangladesh. *Gender, Place and Culture, 16*(4), 427–444.

Sutton, D. E. (2000). Whole foods: Revitalization through everyday synesthetic experience. *Anthropology and Humanism Quarterly, 25*(2), 120–130.

Thakur, N. (2018). River song: Caste and cultural assimilation in the Brahmaputra river Valley, Assam. *Ancient Asia, 9*, 1–7. https://doi.org/10.5334/aa.159

Thompson, R. (2021). Penning pigs: Pig rearing practices, biosecurity measures, and outbreaks of African swine fever in Central Uganda. *Human Organization, 80*(1), 017–026.

Weiss, B. (2011). Making pigs local: Discerning the sensory character of place. *Cultural Anthropology, 26*(3), 438–461.

Xaxa, V. (2008). *State, society and tribes: issues in post-colonial India.* Pearson Education.

Chapter 4
The Role of Caste Prejudice in Hampering Infection Control Efforts in Government Hospitals

Payal Hathi and Nikhil Srivastav

Abstract While poor hygiene in a hospital setting can always have serious consequences, the risks are even higher during the COVID-19 pandemic. In this chapter, we describe a problem that goes deeper than the unique concerns of the current moment: among both medical and paramedical staff, many do not adhere to practices in line with the germ theory of disease. We use observations and in-depth interviews with cleaners and health staff in 22 government hospitals and health centres in Uttar Pradesh, Bihar and Madhya Pradesh to detail practices of poor hygiene that prevent the successful implementation of infection control standards, and the reasons these practices persist. With the hospital as the central institution of focus, we highlight the treatment of Dalit cleaners, and the practices and behaviours that demean them and expose cleaners, staff and patients to risk of infection. Further, misperceptions of the probability of contracting an infection, a lack of resources and systemic corruption and negligence all continue to make hospitals and health care facilities less safe from infection than they can and should be. In addition to addressing deeper issues of caste prejudice, it is critical that we professionalize the work of infection control and hygiene in hospitals, and make sure that staff understand the importance of abiding by the germ theory of disease. During this pandemic and afterwards, this is a lesson that can help address the ways that social inequality manifests in our institutions of health care, and that can serve to protect the health of everyone.

Keywords Hygiene · Caste inequality · Medical institutions · Dalit cleaners

P. Hathi (✉)
Departments of Demography and Sociology, University of California, Berkeley, US
e-mail: phathi@berkeley.edu

N. Srivastav
Research Institute for Compassionate Economics (R.I.C.E.), Lucknow, India
e-mail: nikhil@riceinstitute.org

Introduction

COVID-19 has highlighted important concerns about infection control within hospitals across the world. Hundreds of thousands of healthcare workers worldwide have contracted the COVID-19 infection and have even lost their lives while providing care to their patients (Erdem & Lucey, 2021). In light of the pandemic, it is encouraging that governments and the healthcare industry have responded with urgency to the threat of Hospital Acquired Infection (HAI, also called nosocomial infections). But even beyond COVID, health workers and patients continue to face many other infections while giving and receiving care in hospitals.

Unhygienic conditions are known to be hotbeds of infection, and Indian officials are beginning to recognize extremely high rates of hospital-acquired infection as a serious health system problem. Although we are unaware of population-level, representative estimates of the burden of HAIs in India, multiple small-scale studies have documented the phenomenon in India (Choudhuri et al., 2017; Kamath et al., 2010; Kumar et al., 2018; Pai et al., 2006; Rosenthal et al., 2020; Thamby, 2013). Given these conditions, it is possible that some patients suffer more by choosing to visit a hospital to seek care, than if they had avoided such a visit. This is unfortunate, as healthcare facilities are intended to be places of wellness and healing.

In this chapter, we present findings linking the lack of infection control to the way that public health facilities and hospitals serve as sites of institutionalized marginalization. During COVID, many have called for increased safety measures and protection for healthcare staff. But these calls leave out an important group of people who are responsible for the functioning of hospitals (Srivastav et al., 2020). These are the cleaners, who are almost always Dalits, whose work is largely invisible, and yet so essential. The lack of respect and protection they have always faced, and continue to face, puts them at risk of infection, which puts everyone else at risk too.

Through qualitative interviews with cleaners and staff at 22 government health facilities across Bihar, Uttar Pradesh and Madhya Pradesh, we show that the combination of caste prejudice and a lack of infection control endangers the health of all Indians. We highlight the treatment of cleaners within the hospital system, and the practices and behaviours that both demean cleaners while also exposing cleaners, staff and patients to the risk of infection.

With or without an ongoing pandemic, our public health facilities are neither taking seriously the imperative of infection control, nor are they equipped to implement the necessary precautions to prevent HAIs. We find that among both medical and paramedical staff, many do not adhere to practices in line with the germ theory of disease. At times this is because of the influence of casteist notions of purity and pollution. At others, it is because of a lack of resources or because of a misunderstanding of the probability of infection based on past experience. And at other times, negligence and corruption make it easy to cut corners on the crucial work of infection. Beyond infection control, casteism in public healthcare facilities reinforces structures of institutional exclusion for patients who do not have the means to access health care outside of the government system.

Background

This project began with an interest in why hygiene in government hospitals remains so poor in India, despite greater government investment and attention to the health system. In 2013, in the form of the National Health Mission, the government launched several initiatives aimed at improving health in underserved areas. One focus was improving maternal and child health, and so Indian health policy increasingly emphasized hospital births as a means to reducing maternal and neonatal mortality. Based on the assumption that hospital births are cleaner and safer than home births, India's Janani Suraksha Yojana (JSY) cash transfer programme provides a cash incentive to encourage women to deliver their babies in public hospitals. As a result, between 2005 and 2015, hospital births increased dramatically from 40 to 80% (IIPS and Macro International, 2007; IIPS and ICF, 2017). Still, rates of maternal mortality (SRS, 2018) and infection rates among mothers and babies remain high (Chaurasia et al., 2019; Malhotra et al., 2014; Manjula et al., 2011; Qadri et al., 2015).

One reason that implementation of the JSY has not clearly translated into improved health outcomes may be that as the JSY brings in so many additional women into the hospital system, great pressure is placed on public facilities that they are not equipped to handle. Many studies have documented the deficiency of sanitation infrastructure and maintenance in government hospitals in India (WaterAid, 2016). These problems are no doubt exacerbated as more women turn to health facilities to give birth, and under-resourced facilities become more crowded, resulting in falling standards of care, and increased risk of infection (Hussein et al., 2011).

In 2015, the Indian government launched another health initiative called Kayakalp, which awards cash to the cleanest public health centres in each state in an effort 'to promote cleanliness, hygiene and infection control practices in public health care facilities'. The creation of this programme demonstrated an understanding that cleanliness in hospitals is important.

However, the Kayakalp initiative falls short in addressing infection prevention, which is one of the most critical purposes of hospital cleanliness. Kayakalp guidelines (NHP, 2015) state that verification of wards and procedure areas are to be done by direct observation, and include checks for visible dirt or dust, cobwebs, grease, stains, dried human tissue, body fluid, etc., as well as asking cleaning staff about the frequency of cleaning. The government checklist tends to prioritize what can be plainly seen, relying largely on documents and staff reporting to make assessments. Only a handful of items ask reviewers to watch what health workers do as they work. This means that as long as documents are in order, and staff knows the right answers to give, actual behaviours can be largely neglected, while cosmetic cleanliness can earn a facility a glowing review. All this while hospital-acquired infections continue to affect patients and health workers.   .

In previous work, we have shown that discrimination against cleaning staff, who are most directly in charge of keeping facilities clean, prevents the professionalization of those services, leaving hospitals and patients gravely at risk from deficient infection control practices and standards of care (Hathi & Srivastav, 2020). We found that because of the associations between low-caste workers and traditionally assigned cleaning work, cleaners are not given training for the important job of keeping hospitals clean. They are also rarely given protective equipment to protect themselves from infection, though they are legally mandated to have these protections. Additionally, workers higher in the hierarchy often delegate their own tasks to cleaners, which they feel they have to do, even though they are not trained for those tasks. At the same time, casteist rules of purity and pollution make other staff feel that they cannot do the work of a cleaner, leaving cleaners overburdened and making it difficult to maintain high standards of hygiene for the purpose of infection control.

Here we expand this research on the caste dynamics of work in government hospitals to focus on how hospitals are important but overlooked sites of institutionalized marginalization rather than sites of care. We turn our focus to details about the behavioural practices and beliefs that are shaped in part by traditional caste prejudice, and corruption in the health system that takes advantage of the low status of cleaners, both of which make progress in infection control difficult. In light of COVID-19, these findings are ever more urgent.

Methods

Our original study began with a focus on maternal and child health; thus, we used the 2011–12 Annual Health Survey reports to select the divisions in Madhya Pradesh, Bihar and Uttar Pradesh with the highest maternal mortality rates. Within each division, we selected the most populated district within the division. We first visited the main district hospital in that district, and then additionally visited at least one Primary Health Center (PHC) or Community Health Center (CHC) in that district. We purposely selected health centres that were easily connected by road in order to the main district hospital to see the places where medical supplies and staff are most likely to reach. In each division, we also visited at least one other district hospital in the division, and in some cases, nearby PHCs/CHCs also.

We spent approximately four to six days in each division, and between three and six hours per hospital, interviewing staff and walking through hospital wards and grounds. Each interview lasted for approximately one hour. Out of a total of 55 interviews, 26 were conducted with cleaners, using a question guide to direct the conversation. Topics of inquiry included challenges to doing their jobs well, job responsibilities, what cleaning procedures exist and which are enforced including glove use, cleaning floors and latrines, changing sheets, and needle and biowaste disposal, knowledge and understanding of infection and infection control policies, nature of interactions with other hospital staff, job-related health concerns and family work history and aspirations. The remaining interviews were conducted with *dais* (midwives), ward attendants, *ayahs* (female staff) nurses, doctors and hospital administrators.

A breakdown of interviews by state is given in Table .4.1

Table 1 Count of interviews by state, facility type and hospital staff position

	Cleaner	Cleaning staff supervisor	Ward boy	Dai	Ayah	Dhobi	Lab technician	Nurse	Doctor	Hospital manager/health manager	Total
Madhyapradesh (August, 2016)											
District	3	1			1			1			6
phc/chc	4						2		1		7
Medical college											0
Bihar (March, 2017)											
District	6	1	2			1		1		2	13
phc/chc	2							3	1	2	8
Medical college	2						1		1		4
Uttarpradesh (April, 2017)											
District	7	1			2			1			11
phc/chc	2			1				3			6
Medical college											0
Total	26	3	2	1	3	1	3	9	3	4	55

Findings

We arrived on a weekday in the late afternoon at the very first facility we visited. As we walked through the dimly lit halls of the hospital, we were pleasantly surprised at how tidy the place seemed: it was not overly crowded, there was no garbage on the floors and there were cleaners mopping. Towards the back of the hospital, we ventured outside, where we came upon the first of many trash pits that we would encounter. A large mound of used gloves, pieces of old sari fabric covered in dried blood, empty IV bottles, empty blood bags, red biohazard bags, broken glass medication vials, gauze packaging and discarded syringes were heaped upon the muddy floor near the hospital's perimeter wall and in the drains that lined the building.

A few minutes later, as we approached the general, paediatric and maternity wards, a middle-aged woman walked out of the room with a steel bowl in her hands. She walked straight past us, and into a large courtyard, dumping the watery contents of the bowl onto the cement floor. Some of it splashed up and onto her bare feet and her sari, but she didn't seem to notice, and she walked back into the hospital. Upon further inspection, we saw that it was watery diarrhea—human faeces—that she had left on the floor. It could have been the case that this woman didn't know how dangerous those faecal germs could be to the babies, children and new mothers nearby, or to anyone in that hospital. But we were surprised to find that many hospital staff that we would speak with in the coming months would hold beliefs, either misinformed or deeply prejudiced, that would affect their ability and willingness to maintain standards of hygiene that should be commonplace.

The behaviours and practices that we saw in maternity wards and delivery rooms make it clear that knowledge and training are often clouded by prejudiced beliefs about cleanliness, or trumped by the practicalities of an under-resourced health system.

Unhygienic Practices and Lacking Infection Control

In 1846, a Hungarian doctor named Ignaz Semmelweis discovered that the reason that so many women in his maternity clinic were dying of puerperal fever was that germs on the doctors' hands were being transferred to women during delivery, causing disease and ultimately death. Although he did not know of the germ theory of disease, he addressed the problem by requiring hand washing and instrument cleaning with chlorine, which dramatically reduced mortality. Today, we understand that germs can spread anywhere, not simply on patients or hospital staff, and medical guidelines for maternity patients ubiquitously include glove use, handwashing and instrument cleaning as standard protocol.

And yet, across multiple delivery rooms, across multiple states, stories abound of behaviours that were serious cause for alarm. In a delivery room of a district hospital in Bihar, two women lay on bare metal delivery tables. As a third woman came into the delivery room, the senior nurse had her climb onto the only remaining delivery table. She did a quick internal exam on the woman with a gloved hand and asked her to come back later. As the woman walked out, another woman walked in. This time, without explanation, the nurse asked her to lie on the floor. As the woman clumsily got into position, the nurse turned the faucet on, held the used glove under the water for a few seconds, knelt down, and performed an internal exam on the woman on the floor using the same glove. In addition to not changing gloves between patients, she also did not wash her own hands before, during, or after these examinations.

At a delivery room at a district hospital in Uttar Pradesh, after performing an episiotomy to deliver a woman's baby, a nurse took a piece of gauze in a set of forceps and inserted it into the woman's vagina as part of the cleaning procedure. Subsequently, she took a piece of sari cloth from near the mother and pushed that inside as well. In a larger district hospital in Uttar Pradesh, where many women were delivering simultaneously, an *ayah* assisting the nurses removed metal instruments for use on one of the mothers from water in a rusty metal container with her bare hands. And at a smaller CHC in Uttar Pradesh, a nurse mentor explained that before she came to the facility in 2016, instruments were simply cleaned with water, and that she is now encouraging staff to use bleaching solutions. In reality, the standard recommendation is to wash, boil and autoclave instruments in order to sterilize them (ICMR, 2016).

Stories like this abound: examining women on the floor, hanging used gloves on sinks, leaving delivery tables bare with no sheets or mattresses, sheets not getting washed regularly, rodents and animals running around near patients, cleaners using just water and cloth to wipe down delivery tables, keeping soap inside cabinets or none visible, not having sinks or soap in the delivery room, sterilization only by boiling instruments, placing instruments on unclean surfaces after cleaning, pulling instruments out of sterilizers with bare hands and putting cloth and instruments in women's vaginas to clean them after birth. Each of these behaviours is cause for serious concern, and we saw them many times, across facilities and across states.

Dangerous conditions and practices in hospital wards more generally were also numerous. Across health facilities in various wards, toilets were often left uncleaned for several days. This could have been the result of cleaners who are unwilling to deal with faeces, or of a lack of time as cleaners are often called upon to do tasks for *ayahs* or nurses. For patients, including newly delivered mothers in maternity wards, it meant that they either had to expose themselves to faecal germs in a latrine, or by going out in the open.

Several cleaners who worked in delivery rooms and maternity wards mentioned that they are responsible for changing soiled clothes for women post-delivery, and for inserting and removing catheters, both of which take them very close to the sites of open wounds. In the maternity ward at a district hospital in Bihar, a cleaner had been working for a full shift, sweeping and mopping the ground, and going in and out of the delivery room, talking with patients and their families. She didn't wear gloves throughout her entire shift, including when she went into the latrine. At the very end of the shift, right before leaving, she put on gloves and removed a patient's catheter, discarding it out the window along with the gloves. It is not her job to be handling catheters for newly delivered women, and although it is good that she wore gloves, gloves can have holes or break, and she should have washed her hands prior to any kind of patient contact.

At a CHC in Madhya Pradesh, a government employee who started out as a cleaner was now also in charge of doing post-mortem examinations. As he was getting ready for his main responsibility of dressing wounds for patients, he used his bare hands to take the gauze out of the packaging, cleaned three people's blood and pus-filled wounds without washing hands or tools in between and threw trash and needles out of the window. Over the course of the observation, it became clear that he also does many other tasks, such as putting in IV bottles for patients and changing them if needed.

Such unsafe behaviour clearly puts patients, particularly newly delivered mothers, and also hospital staff and cleaners, at risk of infection. And so, we must ask—why do such behaviours persist?

Persistence of Unhygienic Conditions

The Role of Caste Prejudice

India's rigid system of caste hierarchy continues to play an important role in society today. Caste is a hereditary system that is defined by ritual purity and maintained by endogamy (Vaid, 2014; Allendorf & Panadian, 2016). Although its ties with occupational status and class are complex in the present day, caste-based inequalities remain deeply ingrained (Desai & Dubey, 2012; Thorat & Neuman, 2012). Dalits, or the lowest caste in the Indian caste system, have traditionally been expected to perform tasks considered dirty and impure, such as cleaning faeces and garbage, handling animal carcasses, preparing dead bodies for cremation and cleaning after childbirth. Contact with them was considered to be polluting, and even today, this work is used to justify the widespread oppression of Dalit communities (Shah et al., 2006).

In the hospital setting, cleaning work continues to be done by the same marginalized Dalit communities across generations. In all of the facilities that we visited, we never found any non-Dalit person in the role of a cleaner, and a majority of the cleaners that we interviewed mentioned that others in their families, both younger and older, did or do similar cleaning work in hospitals, in the railways or in other government and non-government offices.[1]

---

[1] This reality is reflected in government documents (GOI 2010): given that Dalits are the ones taking cleaner positions, they separate out the caste-wise counting of sweepers from other group D employees because including sweepers 'results in inflating the figures of representation of SCs in group D posts'. However, the reasons for Dalits taking these jobs are complicated. Many of the cleaners we met lamented that they were not educated enough to do other work. Indeed, socioeconomic disadvantages and social discrimination in the labor market (Thorat & Attewell, 2007) do

The stigma around cleaning work is still strong: cleaners explained that while people of non-Dalit castes are in cleaning work, they often refuse to do the dirtiest work of cleaning blood and latrines, and only actually do sweeping and mopping. These tasks are not just considered physically dirty, but also ritually polluting in society more broadly (Khare, 1962; Srinivas, 1978). Such beliefs continue to drive this hierarchical separation of tasks in hospitals today. At a CHC in Bihar, a health manager explained that the tradition of certain types of workers, like *Dais* from the *Chamar* caste and barbers from the *Nai* caste, has been going on since the Vedic period. A district hospital manager in Bihar explained that many cleaning jobs stay vacant because 'normal' people 'naturally' would not want to do this work, and only those of a certain caste are willing to take the jobs. Their explanations demonstrate the complete internalization of the hierarchical social order.

When asked directly about the discrimination they face in their work, cleaners mostly denied that it happens. However, caste discrimination is disguised in the form of an internalized hierarchy in the hospital institution, and both upper and lower caste people act according to tacitly understood rules of power. For example, our attempts to speak to cleaners were sometimes met with outright hostility because many staff and administrators seemed to believe that cleaners were not worth talking to and were offended by how much attention and importance, we were giving them.

Another manifestation of the hierarchy can be found in day-to-day interactions, in which cleaners know that they are never supposed to sit in front of their high-ranking, upper-caste superiors. A cleaner at a CHC in Uttar Pradesh explained that they cannot sit at the same level as other staff, even if there is a chair available. A cleaner at another CHC in Uttar Pradesh described how decades earlier, when he came for his job interview, he sat on the floor and touched the feet of his interviewers to show that he was as small as they believed him to be. He explained that only by giving sufficient respect to the privileged people in charge are marginalized individuals able to get anywhere. He described that older cleaners pass down the rules to newcomers as they join the staff, making sure that norms stay intact and that hierarchy is maintained:

> We follow the path that our elders lay out, because we are not going to go in a separate direction from them. If they showed us the wrong way, then we will go that wrong way.

These sentiments were echoed by many of the cleaners that we spoke with. Based on their life experiences, they understand the negative consequences of a Dalit individual breaking social norms. While they may not face physical violence in the hospital setting, there is always the threat of losing their job.

This internalization of prejudice is similarly seen among those perpetrating the discrimination. Non-cleaning staff, of higher caste, openly admit to the discrimination and justify it. Using circular logic, a nurse at a CHC in Bihar explains that there is a distance because this distance has existed for so long:

---

prevent upward mobility. Many spoke of bigger aspirations for their children, but also seemed to be aware of the barriers that their children would face, conceding that if the opportunity arose to secure a cleaning job, they would absolutely take it. Thus, these cleaning jobs are also valued by Dalit communities. What is required is dignity in their work.

> This is Bihar, and there is a greater adherence to tradition here, as this has been going on for a long time, people have been divided. For example, they shouldn't come [and sit in this room] here. We should not eat with them. Since this has been going on for so long, one doesn't get satisfaction unless we follow the rules. They are also not clean, and so the distance remains.

In several instances, we found that the rules of caste hierarchy override what makes sense for hospital hygiene, infection control and patient well-being. For example, most cleaners we met had received no training at all for their work. Whatever they knew how to do, they learned by watching others already in the same job. This is in part because cleaning jobs are not considered important enough to warrant special training, and in part, because it is assumed that since they are all from the sweeper castes, those who take the jobs already know what to do. As a cleaner in Bihar explains:

> What training? I'm being open here. We are of a low caste, and from childhood we have been doing this work. You can see this as training. We have been doing this work since we were young, and what better training than this could there be.

When training happens, it is not always given to the right people. At a CHC in Madhya Pradesh, a lab technician explained that the technicians are the ones who are sent for any government training (in fact, under the Kayakalp initiative, it is the lab technicians who are responsible for infection control in hospitals). They are taught about proper cleaning practices and procedures and are supposed to train others. But the lab technician admitted that it is difficult to communicate everything accurately and in detail to the cleaners. He justified this by implying that low-caste cleaners are not intelligent enough to understand the details of technical training, suggesting that it was not worth the effort to make sure cleaners had sufficient information. In practice, this means that cleaners, even though they are the ones most actively doing the work of infection control, sometimes do not even know what the protocols are for hygiene maintenance.

Even without training, the list of tasks that cleaners are responsible for is long and ever-growing. It is commonly understood that officially, they are responsible for what is 'below the windowsill'. For cleaners in the wards, this includes taking out the trash, sweeping and mopping the floors and cleaning latrines. For those in the delivery room, tasks additionally include cleaning blood off sheets, mattresses, and beds and removal of the placenta to an outside location. Unofficially, however, workers at all levels aspire to do the work of their bosses, and so task shifting, in which cleaners help those above them in the hierarchy with many of their assigned tasks, is common. Thus, cleaners often change sheets for ward boys or *ayahs*, clean and dress infected wounds for dressers, insert IV lines and put in and remove catheters for nurses and clean newborns fresh out of the womb for nurses or doctors. In some cases, they even deliver babies. While this gives their bosses some free time, this leaves less time for cleaners to do cleaning work, and sometimes puts patients at further risk because cleaners are untrained in performing the medical tasks that they are sometimes asked to take on.

Conversely, even when there is too much cleaning work to be done, task shifting in the opposite direction is never done. This is problematic because, in reality, cleaning in hospitals should be done frequently, consistently and in a timely manner (GOI, 2015). Instead, a doctor in Madhya Pradesh explained that if he could not find a cleaner, 'the dirtiness will stay'. A cleaner at a CHC in Uttar Pradesh described how the delivery room sometimes stays dirty all evening and night because he is the only cleaner and he comes in the mornings to clean once per day. An *ayah* at a district hospital in Madhya Pradesh pointed out that if there is no sweeper available right away, they will put gloves on both hands, wrap everything in a rubber sheet and put it on the side. She said that if there is anything dirty on the ground, someone will use their feet to wipe it up. Then eventually they'll find a sweeper to do the cleaning.

Hospital staff and administration were not worried about the implications of waiting for cleaners, and how delays are problematic for hygiene. Rather, we were assured that eventually, cleaning would get done because cleaners could ultimately be found if needed. The cleaning staff is given vacation only if other cleaning staff will be available to do the work. But more importantly, families and entire communities of cleaners commonly live together, so if one person is not available it is easy to find another. Repeatedly, we heard, 'Only the sweeper will do the sweeper's work'. A nurse in a Bihar CHC explains how there is no need for her to worry about doing cleaning work because cleaners manage within their own communities:

> Here, whoever is the sweeper has her whole family with her, and they all live here. So, if one needs help, another will come. Like those three… mother-in-law and her daughter-in-law take shifts, like that. They all live nearby. If there is an emergency, then all of them come. Among themselves, they manage.

Some nurses at a PHC in Bihar similarly explain that cleaners depute other cleaners (including their children) to finish their work if they can't do it themselves, but that the nurses themselves will not do the cleaning work under any circumstances:

> They will delegate to someone. We can move the placenta, but we won't do any of the other cleaning work. We won't do it. At any cost. I'm telling you clearly.

One might argue that a separation of tasks is efficient. However, when cleaners are doing the work of others while no one is willing to do the critical cleaning work that keeps a hospital clean, the result is a lot of pressure on underpaid cleaning staff, with subpar results for hygiene.

Casteism plays a more direct role also, as everyone from patients to caregivers to hospital staff treats cleaners poorly because of their low status. This lack of respect is problematic from a human interaction perspective, and also because it prevents cleaners from doing the work of keeping hospitals hygienic.

One way in which this lack of respect manifests itself in the hospital setting is the general lack of concern from the public about keeping public spaces clean because of the assumption that cleaners will ultimately clean everything up. This is true in hospitals, and other public spaces as well. For example, Anand (2007) describes that Indian city planners have never needed to design more humane systems of managing garbage and sewage because 'they rely on an unending source of disposable, cheap, Dalit labour'. Gatade (2015) says that the only explanation for the long-standing indifference to the deaths of sewer workers is that 'caste and related discriminations have become so common and ingrained in our psyche that nobody finds anything abominable. Perhaps this unique system of hierarchy—legitimized by the wider society and sanctified by religion—which has condemned a section of its own people to the 'profession' of cleaning, sweeping, and scavenging, has become a part of our thinking'.

Overcrowding in public health facilities puts great pressure on cleaners. One of the most consistent sights in large district hospitals is the crowd. While hospitals were created with, for example, 50 patients in mind, they must cope with 200 people on the premises because it is customary for patients to bring several attendants with them, particularly those coming from further away. This makes sense because the system requires that patients purchase their own medications, so while a patient rests or keeps a bed so it is not taken by anyone else, the attendant is needed to procure supplies and do paperwork.

There is a stark contrast between the overcrowding seen in larger facilities and the relative emptiness of PHCs and CHCs. Efforts to get PHC/CHC level facilities functional have been unsuccessful, as seen by how empty they are. People are aware that the larger hospitals have better facilities and more staff, and will be open at night, and so rather than protesting or complaining about non-functional PHCs/CHCs, people opt to go to district-level hospitals, further adding to the overcrowding problem. Many cleaners complain about the lack of courtesy that families show. A cleaner at a CHC in Madhya Pradesh explained:

> If this was their home, they would throw the garbage outside. This is a hospital, and they should also understand it to be their home. Those who come for delivery stay for three days, and they themselves have to live in this.

We met one cleaner who felt empowered to ask families not to make the spaces in the hospital dirty. She explained the disrespect she faces:

> Lots of people throw [their garbage] on the floor. [If I ask them not to] they get angry and tell us to do our job [of picking up the trash]. They just throw it.

Similarly, a cleaner at a Bihar district hospital explained that he and other cleaners try to fight with patients to keep things clean, like asking them not to go into a room with shoes while it is still wet from being cleaned. But he said that they do not understand or cooperate, they just get angry and tell the cleaners to do their work. He explains that every patient brings ten people with him/her, and they do not keep things clean:

> There could be lots of problems. The dirtiness can spread. When patients come, they can also get an infection.

There is a general lack of concern about keeping public areas neat, and a lack of awareness of how hygiene is connected to infection, and this lack of cleanliness is seen in every facility that we visited. Such dynamics of disrespect between the public and cleaners exist even outside the hospital setting (Gatade, 2015). However, this prejudice in the healthcare setting is particularly dangerous to health and well-being for those working in and seeking care at these facilities.

In addition to the lack of public concern and consideration, hospital staff's behaviour demonstrates an underlying assumption that cleaners will pick up after them. Even though waste disposal systems have been put into place, these are also undermined by the same carelessness and lack of respect for cleaners. Different coloured bins are seen in various places in wards and delivery rooms. In some cases, healthcare staff use them diligently, while in others, they do not. When they do not, it is another responsibility left to the cleaner to sort through that trash and separate it into the bins. Cleaners do not feel they can push nurses to follow the rules, as it is not their place. A cleaner at a Bihar CHC explains:

> What can we say, what can we say to the nurses? They are above and we are below. If someone is higher up in the hierarchy, they can throw things anywhere, and they do. We just clean as we were told.

Misperception of the Probability of Infection

In many cases, we saw that health workers' decisions were often based on misperceptions of the probability of infection. Hospital staff and cleaners often exhibited a version of the 'gambler's fallacy', which comes from a belief that small samples are representative of a larger population: in this case, many believed that their own experiences of the past were indicative of what was likely to happen in the future. For example, we met two doctors who said that they do not worry so much about infections because they can tell before examining the patient what they have. They only take precautions, such as wearing gloves and washing their hands afterwards, if the patient is contagious. It is possible that their decisions are being impacted by their short-term experiences of not having yet caught an infection. But it is unclear what rules they use to determine which individuals can be safely examined without gloves and which cannot, given that it is impossible to know who is contagious just by looking at them. Again, these are practices that do not adhere to rules of infection control and patient safety, that leave healthcare workers, hospital staff and patients all at risk of infection.

Similarly, and perhaps because hospital staff face such real danger or risk, many hospital staff turn to their faith to feel like they are protected from infection, even if, in reality, they are not. It is documented that hospital staff and patients are at risk of exposure to diseases like HIV, Hepatitis A, B, C and E, varicella, influenza, pertussis, diphtheria and rabies (WHO 2002). However, many had the attitude that as long as one stays *bindaas* (carefree) then no sickness will come. This is precisely the opposite of the meticulous care and attention to detail that infection control requires (Gawande, 2007). While handling tuberculosis slides without gloves on his hands, a lab technician at a CHC in Madhya Pradesh explains:

> If you remain carefree, nothing will happen. If you worry a lot, then something will happen. I stay carefree, and nothing will happen, and in 36 years nothing has happened.

Cleaners also use their faith to elevate their work to a type of *seva*, or public service, in spite of the exploitation that they face. Unfortunately, this distorted image of cleaning work as noble and sacred has been used by government leaders for decades (Gatade, 2015). It is a cruel system indeed that not only exploits Dalits but then also makes them believe that they should keep doing the work they're doing because it is their *dharma* (duty). As one cleaner at a district hospital in Bihar put it:

> Why be scared, we'll die today or tomorrow. It's best that we at least die serving the public.

At a district hospital in Uttar Pradesh, we met a retired cleaner who was working in the burn unit. Without gloves, he was dressing wounds, with a tin of brackish water by his feet, which he later poured on the floor to clean everything away. We soon learned that he also takes care of patients who were homeless and had no one to care for them. He had retired several years earlier, but the hospital administrator had called him and asked him to come back and continue working. He took us to the room where the homeless patients stayed: there was urine and faeces on the floor, one man had almost no clothes on and one bed had no mattress. He was asked to work with these particular patients because it required dealing in human fluids, a job which is generally passed on to cleaners because casteist beliefs prevent those of higher castes from being willing to take on the work. He described his motivation:

> When the government called upon me, I came. Without them asking, I would not be doing this work. But from me, I want to be able to be of service to the poor, the homeless. This is my religion.

Lack of Resources

Large district hospitals face severe overcrowding, as mentioned above. From the perspective of health workers, this translates into a lack of time, which often means that infection control is deprioritized. A health manager at a district hospital in Bihar explained that if someone comes from a faraway rural area for an emergency, it is difficult to tell the patient and her attendants to wait in order for instruments to be cleaned, and so rules sometimes have to be bent. Many cleaners admitted that when the delivery room becomes busy, rules for infection control are not always followed. A cleaner at a district hospital in Madhya Pradesh explained the impracticality of using gloves all the time:

> When there is a lot of work, what can we do? Should we look after the baby, or pay attention to gloves, or to infection? So first, we hold the baby, and it sometimes happens that we're not able to wear gloves.

Additionally, public health facilities face serious supply constraints that both health workers and cleaners must contend with. Nurses at a district hospital in Bihar explained that the problem with wearing gloves is having to change them so many times. They sometimes have a shortage of gloves, and so they only wear them for the most critical situations, like when a patient has AIDS or hepatitis. Of course, it is not always possible to know right when a patient walks in what they are infected with. Like the doctors above, this practice puts everyone at risk of infection. Decisions around glove use also tend to follow casteist notions of purity and pollution rather than germ theory. For example, gloves are required for traditionally 'dirty' work, such as cleaning blood in the delivery room, or cleaning latrines that involves faeces, but not required for tasks such as inserting IVs, doing jhadu/pocha, or handling trash, which is not considered polluting, though they can certainly expose a person to infection. Such rules leave gaping holes in efforts to strengthen infection control measures. For example, a cleaner from a CHC in MP told us:

> Let's say that there is some dirty work, like dressing a wound or if there is a sudden accident and there is a lot of blood, then we wear gloves. But for other normal work, we don't wear them.

Another reason for the rationing of glove use is that hierarchy in the context of supply shortages prevents cleaners from asking for what they need to do their jobs well and safely. One cleaner in Bihar explained that she wears a glove only on one hand for each delivery, and then as per the rules, throws it away. She uses the gloves that are for the nurses because the contract owner does not supply gloves sufficiently. Many cleaners mentioned that it is often difficult to ask nurses for supplies and that nurses give gloves only for the tasks they do not want to do themselves, not for the cleaner's protection. A cleaner in Bihar also described how cleaners like him are too afraid to ask for protective gear that they are legally entitled to because they might be seen as insolent, and fired:

> There is no one who is willing to speak. You must understand, if I speak up then they would think I am being an activist, and I would be the first to go, to be fired. Out of fear, no one speaks. If we do say something, they will say—punk, are you trying to be a leader? Let's get rid of him. Knowing this, no one says anything. Whatever they give us is fine.

Ultimately, it is clear that infection control is simply not a priority in these states' health policies, which leads to fundamentally flawed ways of framing the issue for staff. The focus of infection control measures also often centres on health staff's self-protection, rather than also incorporating the protection of patients. When asked about the purpose of gloves in a clinical setting, almost every single cleaner or healthcare worker we spoke with said that the primary purpose was for their own protection. Very few mentioned the fact that gloves also protect the patients. This was clear in practice as well, as evidenced by a nurse in a district hospital in Madhya Pradesh who put in an IV without washing her hands and with no gloves, but then washed her hands immediately afterwards. A health manager that we spoke with in Bihar admitted that in talking with staff about the importance of glove use, they do emphasize the idea of self-protection because it is a more powerful motivator than patient safety, thus perhaps this is a reflection of those messages. Cleanliness of the hospital, loosely defined, is understood to be good for patient health, but across states and facilities, infection control is largely about protecting oneself.

The lack of prioritization of infection control can also be seen in systems of waste disposal. While waste disposal systems also appear to be in place on paper (GOI, 2016) they are often not working in reality (Datta et al., 2018). Across facilities, we found varying systems for placenta disposal, and at one CHC, we learned of a placenta that had been left out and eaten by dogs. We saw many hospital staff dispose of garbage and medical waste outside of windows onto the floor. In almost every facility, we heard about a car that comes daily to pick up waste, but every facility we visited also had a trash pit, oftentimes located near the delivery room. Cleaners sometimes told us that the system that is practised is to burn trash outdoors. However, according to the WHO, improper handling of hospital waste and burning waste is hazardous for health: 'Health-care waste contains potentially harmful microorganisms, which can infect hospital patients, health workers and the general public' and 'Health-care waste in some circumstances is incinerated, and dioxins, furans and other toxic air pollutants may be produced as emissions' (WHO, 2018).

There is no question that many health facilities are overburdened and undersupplied, putting intense pressure on health workers and cleaners, often leaving them little option but to cut corners when it comes to infection control. However, it is also the case that infection control does not seem to be a priority in practice. These problems alone, and as they intersect with caste prejudice, make health facilities unnecessarily prone to infections that can spread to workers as well as to patients and their families.

Systemic Negligence and Corruption

From our very first visit, it became clear that hospital administrators are very aware of the need for cleanliness, hygiene and infection control. Unfortunately, we also saw that these things became much more a priority when administrators felt that someone was actually watching.

In one district hospital in Madhya Pradesh, we walked through the general ward as we were finding our way to the maternity ward. 114 patients were crowded into a space that allowed for 62 beds, not counting the multiple attendants that accompanied each patient. There were needles, bandage wrappers and plastic bottles on the floor in the spaces that patients hadn't yet laid their mattresses. Right outside the ward, in front of the toilets, was an enormous heap of trash, next to an empty trash can, as well as faeces on the floor. An old man was crouched on the ground, eating from a paper plate right next to the garbage. After conducting interviews at the facility, we left. When we visited the hospital the next afternoon, we saw that the place was spotless. This was not the only facility that this happened in. These overnight transformations—likely not unrelated to our presence and questions—demonstrated an awareness of what a clean facility is supposed to look like, and what is possible if implementation and enforcement are prioritized.

At a separate district hospital in Uttar Pradesh, we were not allowed into the female ward when we arrived, which was out of the ordinary. We were told that a government official was there, 'from outside', although we were unable to learn who it was. We then went to the maternity and c-section wards, and saw the same thing, with many families sitting outside on the ground. We learned that these were all attendants of patients, who had been kicked out because cleaning was happening.

Among the attendants were seven newborn babies, who had already been separated from their mothers for close to five hours. When we finally were let in, the ward was incredibly clean and smelling fresh, but some of the mothers were complaining about how hungry they were. In this instance, for the sake of the visiting government official, cleanliness seemed to be such a priority that it came even at the expense of mothers and babies who had come to the hospital for care.

There is also corruption in how cleaners are treated. From the administrators that we spoke with, there does not seem to be much serious concern about the public health implications of the lack of hygiene. Given that cleaners by and large come from the same marginalized communities that are easy to exploit, corruption appears to be particularly easy with respect to cleaning jobs. For example, a cleaner in a district hospital in Uttar Pradesh described how the Chief Medical Superintendent (CMS) at the facility had told the cleaning staff that they would have to work for a month without pay because she did not have the funds to pay them. The CMS said that it was their choice if they wanted to stay or go, but as the cleaner explained, she had a family to feed, and leaving was not a real option for her. At a CHC in Uttar Pradesh, a *dai* does the work of the cleaner, even though there is a cleaner post that is vacant. She is not paid, but is given a room, and so she feels she cannot leave. Cleaners are compelled to continue working, in the hope that there will be payment or some kind of remuneration in the future, however, these are exploitative practices. Such practices do not inspire workers to do high-quality work, but in the hospital setting, cleaning standards must be high to prevent infection. Thus, while such labour exploitation may occur in other sectors, it is particularly dangerous in hospitals where people are coming for health care.

Cleaning work is also simply not seen as requiring professional level status. Those in charge of cleaning, or those given contracts to manage facility cleaning are not hired based on knowledge, skill or experience. For example, in a district hospital in Madhya Pradesh, the supervisor of the cleaners clearly had no experience or background in what is uniquely required for maintaining cleanliness and infection control in a hospital setting. He used to work as a guard in Delhi, and he was hired because the contractor is his relative.

Across all three states, there is a move from permanent staff in cleaning jobs to contract positions. This process is also rife with problems. Cleaning jobs in Madhya Pradesh have been cut, and remaining cleaners often face payment delays for months. In Bihar, there seem to be sufficient cleaners through the contractors, but there are inconsistent wages paid to different cleaners, even within the same hospital. And in Uttar Pradesh, we even found a facility with no cleaners at all, and *dais* doing the cleaning work with zero pay. These practices continue since cleaners are not in a position to protest much, thus siphoning off funds from their jobs or their supplies is unlikely to raise any alarms.

The differences between contract and permanent workers are also telling. Most of the cleaners we met were on contract agreements. Wages for contract workers range from 1500 Rs. per month to 7000 Rs. per month, paid daily, with no job security and no clear linkages to seniority or responsibility in determining the amount paid. In comparison, government staff cleaners receive 20,000 Rs. to 25,000 Rs. per month, with additional job security. There is clear animosity between permanent and contract cleaning staff in many facilities, which may have a negative impact on the cleaning work that gets done.

Many people say that cleanliness has improved with the contract system since it is easier to get cleaners to show up and do the work. It is not clear if this is true, or if this is also a belief borne of prejudice against cleaners. But the shift to contracts comes at a cost. From the cleaners' perspective, those in contract positions expressed staying for the promise of a permanent job, feeling that if they just do a little more, maybe they will get lucky. But that seems unlikely given the general trend of the government system moving to contracts for many types of non-healthcare positions. While someone higher up may benefit monetarily from this trend of cutting corners in the hiring and payment of cleaners, the silent but deadly consequence is that hygiene and public health are also hurt as a result.

Conclusion

In this chapter, we use observations in government hospitals, and qualitative field-work with government hospital cleaners and health workers to detail practices of poor hygiene that prevent the successful implementation of proper standards of infection control, and the reasons that these practices persist. Casteist beliefs and caste prejudice against Dalit cleaners, misperceptions of the probability of contracting an infection, a lack of resources and systemic corruption and negligence all continue to make hospitals and healthcare facilities less safe from infection than they can and should be.

While poor hygiene in a hospital setting can always have serious consequences, the risks are even higher during the COVID-19 pandemic, when a lack of adherence to the germ theory of disease could turn medical practitioners into super spreaders. In India, many Covid patients first encounter practitioners in non-Covid OPDs and small clinics, before knowing whether or not they are contagious, and before knowing whether they will ultimately need to go to a hospital. Thus, poor hygiene practices in smaller health facilities potentially put an even larger number of people at risk than just those at hospitals, including staff, patients and their family members. COVID-19 has led to the writing of new and updated guidelines on clinical management of infection (DGHS, 2020a, 2020b), the use of personal protective equipment (DGHS, 2020a) and handling waste disposal (CPCB, 2020). Hopefully, these new guidelines will raise awareness about the importance of these practices.

These issues are relevant even beyond Covid. In addition to addressing deeper issues of caste prejudice and systemic corruption, it is critical that we professionalize the work of infection control and hygiene in hospitals, and make sure that staff understand the importance of abiding by the germ theory of disease. More emphasis must be put on the use of protective equipment, the practice of hand hygiene, proper training and accurate knowledge about the fact that these measures of infection control serve a dual purpose in protecting both staff and patients. These are lessons that can help address the ways that social inequality manifests in our institutions of health care, and that can serve to protect the health of everyone.

References

Allendorf, K., & Pandian, R. K. (2016). The decline of arranged marriage? Marital change and continuity in India. *Population and Development Review, 42*(3), 435.

Anand, S. (2007). Life inside a black hole. *Tehelka, 4*(44). https://assam.assamnet.narkive.com/wn9 fVQst/from-tehelka-life-inside-a-black-hole.

Central Pollution Control Board (CPCB). (2020). Ministry of environment, forest, and climate change. *Guidelines for handling, treatment, and disposal of waste generated during treatment/diagnosis/quarantine of COVID-19 patients.* https://www.mohfw.gov.in/pdf/639486095015 85568987wastesguidelines.pdf.

Chaurasia, S., Sivanandan, S., Agarwal, R., Ellis, S., Sharland, M., & Sankar, M. J. (2019). Neonatal sepsis in South Asia: Huge burden and spiralling antimicrobial resistance. *BMJ, 364.*

Choudhuri, A. H., Chakravarty, M., & Uppal, R. (2017). Epidemiology and characteristics of nosocomial infections in critically ill patients in a tertiary care intensive care unit of Northern India. *Saudi Journal of Anaesthesia, 11*(4), 402.

Datta, P., Mohi, G. K., & Chander, J. (2018). Biomedical waste management in India: Critical appraisal. *Journal of Laboratory Physicians, 10*(1), 6.

Desai, S., & Dubey, A. (2012). Caste in 21st century India: Competing narratives. *Economic and Political Weekly, 46*(11), 40.

Directorate General of Health Services (DGHS). (2020a). Ministry of health and family welfare. *Revised guidelines on clinical management of COVID-19.* https://www.mohfw.gov.in/pdf/Revise dNationalClinicalManagementGuidelineforCOVID1931032020.pdf.

Directorate General of Health Services (DGHS). (2020b). Ministry of health and family welfare. novel coronavirus disease 2019: Guidelines on rational use of personal protective equipment. https://www.mohfw.gov.in/pdf/GuidelinesonrationaluseofPersonalProtectiveEquipment.pdf.

Erdem, H., & Lucey, D. R. (2021). Healthcare worker infections and deaths due to COVID-19: A survey from 37 nations and a call for WHO to post national data on their website. *International Journal of Infectious Diseases, 102*, 239.

Gatade, S. (2015). Silencing caste, sanitizing oppression. *Economic & Political Weekly, 50*(44), 29–35.

Gawande, A. (2007). *Better: A surgeon's notes on performance.* Metropolitan Books, Henry Holt & Company.

Government of India (GOI). (2010). *Office memorandum: Issue of instructions on reservation for the schedule caste, scheduled tribes, and other backward classes in services under the Government of India.* https://documents.doptcirculars.nic.in/D2/D02adm/36011_6_2010-Estt.(Res).pdf.

Government of India (GOI). (2015). *National guidelines for clean hospitals.* https://main.mohfw. gov.in/sites/default/files/7660257301436254417_0.pdf.

Government of India (GOI). (2016). Ministry of environment, forest, and climate change. *Biomedical waste (Management and handling) rules.* https://dhr.gov.in/sites/default/files/Bio-med ical_Waste_Management_Rules_2016.pdf.

Hathi, P., & Srivastav, N. (2020). Caste prejudice and infection: Why a dangerous lack of hygiene persists in government hospitals. *Economic & Political Weekly, 55*(16), 38–44.

Hussein, J., Mavalankar, D. V., Sharma, S., & D'Ambruoso, L. (2011). A review of health system infection control measures in developing countries: What can be learned to reduce maternal mortality. *Globalization and Health, 7*(1), 14.

ICMR (2016). Hospital infection control guidelines. *Indian Council of Medical Research.*

IIPS and ICF. (2017). National family health survey (NFHS-4), 2015–16: India. *International Institute for Population Sciences.*

IIPS and Macro International. (2007). National family health survey (NFHS-3), 2005–06: India: Volume II. *International Institute for Population Sciences.*

Kamath, S., Mallaya, S., & Shenoy, S. (2010). Nosocomial infections in neonatal intensive care units: Profile, risk factor assessment and antibiogram. *The Indian Journal of Pediatrics, 77*(1), 37–39.

Khare, R. S. (1962). Ritual purity and pollution in relation to domestic sanitation. *The Eastern Anthropologist, 15*(2), 125–139.

Kumar, S., Sen, P., Gaind, R., Verma, P. K., Gupta, P., Suri, P. R., ... & Rai, A. K. (2018). Prospective surveillance of device-associated health care–associated infection in an intensive care unit of a tertiary care hospital in New Delhi, India. *American journal of infection control, 46*(2), 202–206.

Malhotra, S., Sharma, S., & Hans, C. (2014). Prevalence of hospital acquired infections in a tertiary care hospital in India. *International Journal of Medicine and Medical Sciences, 1*(7), 91–94.

Manjula, N., Shivannavar, C. T., Patil, S. A., & Gaddad, S. M. (2011). Incidence and antibiogram patterns among nosocomial pseudomonas aeruginosa isolates from maternity wards and labor rooms in Gulbarga Region, South India. *Journal of Recent Advances in Applied Sciences (JRAAS), 26*, 47–52.

National Health Portal (NHP). (2015). Kayakalp—Swacchta guidelines for public health facilities. *National health portal, Government of India.* https://www.nhp.gov.in/kayakalp-swacchta-guidelines-for-public-health-facilities_pg.

Pai, M., Kalantri, S., Aggarwal, A. N., Menzies, D., & Blumberg, H. M. (2006). Nosocomial tuberculosis in India. *Emerging Infectious Diseases, 12*(9), 1311.

Qadri, S., Sharma, K., Siddiqui, B., Ehsan, A., Sherwani, R. K., Sultan, A., & Khan, F. (2015). Microbial profile in females with puerperal sepsis: A major threat to women's health: Study at a tertiary health care centre. *International Journal of Current Microbiology and Applied Sciences, 1*, 248–255.

Rosenthal, V. D., Gupta, D., Rajhans, P., Myatra, S. N., Muralidharan, S., Mehta, Y., ... & Patel, M. (2020). Six-year multicenter study on short-term peripheral venous catheters-related bloodstream infection rates in 204 intensive care units of 57 hospitals in 19 cities of India: International nosocomial infection control consortium (INICC) findings. *American journal of infection control, 48*(9), 1001–1008.

Sample Registration System (SRS) (2018): Special Bulletin on Maternal Mortality in India, 2014–16, Sample Registration System, Government of India.

Shah, G., Mander, H., Baviskar, A., Thorat, S., & Deshpande, S. (2006). *Untouchability in rural India.* Sage.

Srinivas, M. N. (1978). *The remembered village.* Oxford University Press.

Srivastav, N., Priya, A., & Hathi, P. (2020). Our essential workers need essential care. *Economic and Political Weekly, 55*(31), 13–16.

Thamby, S. A. (2013). A prospective survey and analysis of nosocomial infections in a tertiary care teaching hospital in South India. *Journal of Pharmaceutical Sciences and Research, 5*(11), 231.

Thorat, S., & Attewell, P. (2007). The legacy of social exclusion: A correspondence study of job discrimination in India. *Economic and Political Weekly*, 4141–4145.

Thorat, S., & Neuman, K. S. (2012). *Blocked by caste: Economic discrimination in modern India.* Oxford University Press.

Vaid, D. (2014). Caste in contemporary India: Flexibility and persistence. *Annual Review of Sociology, 40*, 391–410.

WaterAid. (2016). India needs a healthy start as healthcare facilities across the country have poor water. *Sanitation and Hygiene.* https://www.wateraidindia.in/media_release/india-needs-healthy-start-healthcare-facilities-across-country-poor-water-sanitation-hygiene-finds-wateraid/.

World Health Organization. (2002). *Prevention of hospital-acquired infections. A PRACTICAL GUIDE*, 2nd edn. Availalbe at: https://www.who.int/csr/resources/publications/drugresist/en/whocdscsreph200212.pdf

World Health Organization (WHO). (2018). *Fact sheet: Health care waste.* https://www.who.int/news-room/fact-sheets/detail/health-care-waste.

Chapter 5
Public and Corporate Health Sector Disparities: Reflections on COVID-19 Experiences in India

Sunita Reddy

Abstract Health care inequities in India are well documented. Being the second most populous country in the world with 1.3 billion population, the health care resources in India are limited and need to be distributed equitably. Being a mixed economy, health care services, in India, are provided by both public and private health sectors. The poor seek medical care from the government-run resource-crunched public sector and the economically well off sections of the population go to the private and corporate sector. Health care policy and planning in India, historically, led to inequitable health care services and the dichotomous health care service provisioning in India. This paper is based on the author's empirical research in the past decade on the corporatization of health care services and medical tourism in India. Further, it is also based on a review of literature, analysis of health policies, five-year plans and media reports on COVID-19.

Keywords Health care inequalities · Medical tourism · Structural inequalities · Institutional reform · Pandemic response

Introduction

Private health sector has always existed. However, post health sector reforms, there was a budgetary cut into public health systems and there was a rise in super specialty corporate hospitals. Various public subsidies went into setting up, supporting and promoting the corporate health sector, without any mechanism to plough back profits into the general healthcare for the larger masses. The dichotomous and polarized healthcare evolved, where the private and corporate healthcare goes into serving those who can pay and the public health care services cater to those who cannot pay. The corporate sector, which works on business models, opened its doors for economically well off sections of the society, foreigners. These hospitals were build with the state support and subsidies given but NRIs and did not fulfil the lease

S. Reddy (✉)
Centre of Social Medicine and Community Health (CSM&CH), Jawaharlal Nehru University, New Delhi, India

© The Author(s), under exclusive license to Springer Nature Singapore Pte Ltd. 2022
S. S. Acharya and S. Christopher (eds.), *Caste, COVID-19, and Inequalities of Care*,
People, Cultures and Societies: Exploring and Documenting Diversities,
https://doi.org/10.1007/978-981-16-6917-0_5

conditions put forth for taking the subsidies. The already polarized health sector, with low budget and resource-crunched public health services which were overstretched in normal times, in the Pandemic COVID-19, exposed the health care fault lines even more starkly. The poor and the excluded social groups, who are also the front-line workers, struggled to get basic health facilities such as beds and oxygen and the corporate health sector overcharged its patients. Disasters like COVID-19 become an opportunity for some of the private and corporate hospitals as institutions to earn money, forgetting the ethos of humanitarian service during the disasters, as it is not mandated in the Disaster Management Act 2005. Increasing the public health care expenditure and mandatory role by the private sector in times of emergencies is the only way out to make healthcare more equitable.

India is a welfare state and health is a state subject. Being a mixed economy, there is a presence of both State-run public health care sector and profit oriented private health care sector. Post health sector reforms in the 90s, with the paradigm shift in cutting down on the budget for public health care expenditure, healthcare became even more dichotomous. The public sector is overburdened and dependent on limited and poor resources with huge vacancies at all levels of human resource. The profit-oriented corporate hospitals, built on the public subsidies with no mechanism to plough back profits into general healthcare, led to inequitable distribution of health care services. This paper traces the historical development of inequitable and dichotomous health care services, which further led to the exclusion of the poor in the pandemics. Based on the author's empirical research in the past decade on corporatization of healthcare, medical tourism in India and review of secondary literature, the paper critically looks at the policy shifts in the government's financial plans and health care policies. The paper, in the later section, looks at how the marginalized social groups experienced corona in the limited health care resource set up. Due to the lack of desegregated data on the COVID-19 on the basis of caste and class, the second part of the paper depends on the media reports of the last one year related to the response from the hospitals. The social categories of SC and ST, based on the socio-economic status and caste hierarchy, are clubbed together as 'proxy' for the 'poor'. The paper ends with a number of recommendations such as the need for investment in public health care services, healthcare mainstreaming into the Disaster law and making it mandatory for the private and corporate hospitals to provide healthcare during disasters and pandemics.

Hospitals are the most complex organizations in modern societies with a multi-faceted structure and perform various important functions. Hospitals are institutions of learning, practising medicine, cure and care of the patients and also have dynamic hierarchical relationships between the doctors, paramedic staff and patients, based on the knowledge, status, power and authority. Hospitals are characterized by division of labour, skill sets, state of art technology and infrastructure to cater to the health care needs of the population.

Hospitals are social institutions. Replicating the social structures of society, the hierarchies of caste, class and gender are well laid out. The doctors mostly come from upper caste and classes (Baru, 2003) and the nursing and paramedic staff come from lower class (Madan et al., 1980; Oommen, 1978). The sanitation and cleaning staff in the hospital comes from the Dalit social groups. The gender dimension is also reflected quite clearly where mostly the nurses are women and there are few women doctors in any hospital. Hospitals, as social institutions, also replicate the social structures. In the public hospitals with fewer resources, the vulnerability is much more for the paramedic staff who have to deal with patient care and the sanitation workers, who largely come from the lower castes, are at risk for handling the infectious hospital waste. The study titled 'Risk stratification as a tool to rationalize quarantine among health care workers exposed to COVID-19 cases' showed a total of 321 positive cases reported to the Central Contact Tracing Team from April 11 to June 8. Among the Covid positive health care workers, there were 35.3% hospital attendants followed by 17.2% nurses and 13.3% (n = 32) security personnel. On the other hand, 12% of doctors and laboratory staff were Covid positive and the administrative staff was the least affected with 5.5%. These lowest rung workers, who come from lower classes and castes, are denied basic protection and also provided low-quality PPE. A staff member said, 'It's a fact that they are the most exposed workers in hospitals who are also the most neglected lot'.[1]

The COVID-19 experience also shows that not all workers are equally susceptible to the infection. There are a number of other factors such as exposure, lack of PPE, caste-based hierarchies within medical institutions and among government hospital staff (Hathi and Srivastav, this volume). The topmost public tertiary hospital, All India Institute of Medical Sciences (AIIMS), Delhi, showed that mostly sanitation workers and attendants bear the brunt of infection and many doctors died due to infection from the public hospitals.

India has been an independent country for the past 75 years. There are a few important achievements, like the increase in life expectancy from 41 years in 1960 to 65 years in 2015.[2] The IMR has gone down from 165 deaths per 1000 in 1960 to 38 deaths in 2015. However, the decline in the case of IMR has been slow. India's overall health security index score is 46.5 as compared to 83.5 in the US.[3] This low health security index can be attributed to many factors like inequitable distribution of resources, hierarchical social structure, public policies and misplaced priorities.

India is divided on the axis of caste, class, ethnicity and gender lines. The disparities are so wide and historically deprived that the social groups are taking a very long time to come out of poverty and penury. The wide disparities will continue if we do not address intersectionalities and the multiple deprivations in education, healthcare, livelihoods, safety and security. Largely, if there are sincere efforts to bridge the wide gap of resources between the rich and the poor, one can think of achieving a decent and dignified life for everyone, as envisaged in sustainable development goals.

---

[1] https://www.newindianexpress.com/nation/2020/aug/10/sanitation-workers-attendants-most-vul nerable-to-covid-19-among-hospital-staff-aiims-study-2181595.html.

[2] https://www.firstpost.com/india/70-years-of-independence-indias-life-expectancy-literacy-ind icators-look-up-while-imr-income-inequality-are-worries3928501.html#:~:text=In%2055%20y ears%2C%20India's%20infant,available%2C%20according%20to%20the%20World.

[3] https://sites.uci.edu/energyobserver/2020/02/07/the-global-health-security-index-of-2019-for-the-us-and-key-countries/.

The themes of this edited volume, *Caste, COVID-19, and Inequalities of Care,* focus on caste-based disparities, in both daily life and in the context of the current pandemic. The poor largely come from Scheduled Castes (SC), Scheduled Tribes (ST) and other backward caste groups. Among these, SCs and STs are historically marginalized, discriminated against, exploited and humiliated. Addressing caste inequality and development in India, Borooah (2005) concludes that one-third average income generation difference is because of unequal treatment by the upper castes. Further, among the poor, SCs comprise the largest section of the deprived people (Sundaram & Tendulkar, 2003).

Despite various poverty alleviation and social welfare schemes, the low socio-economic position continues for the SC population. As per 2011 Census Report, 16.6% SCs of the total population of India have very few assets. They are largely engaged in manual, unskilled work and form a workforce in the unorganized sector. 71% of them work as agricultural labourers, leatherwork and migrant labourers (Hindustan Times, 2018). Their literacy level is only 66.1% as compared to the all-India literacy level of 73%. Most of the other SC population are engaged in sanitation work as sweepers, scavengers, tanners, fishermen, toddy tappers, washermen, artisans, vendors, drummers, carpenters and other petty occupations (National Commission for Scheduled Castes Chap-3) (end note: http://ncsc.nic.in/files/Chapter%203_2.pdf). In addition, the status of the 8% ST population is in a worse situation.

Economic developments in India have so far failed to address these social groups, who form the majority of the poor, for the purpose of development not only in terms of income but also in terms of human development index. Behind the glaring statistics of economic growth in India in recent years such as increased FDI, foreign exchange and profitability of companies or for that matter soaring BSE index upon economic liberalization, Indian development scenario hides the suppressed voices and deplorable poverty of one-third of its Dalit and ST population who remain bypassed in asserting their rights for a normal life of human being (NCSC, n.d.).

In the words of Nancy Scheper Hughes (1993), 'poor facing the structural violence', most of the SC and ST in India also face violence in their everyday life due to their position in the social structure and poverty. Apart from facing the deprivation in income, education, healthcare and lack of opportunities for decent work and wages, they also experience violence and heinous crimes in their everyday life. The health indicators are very poor and discouraging among the Dalit rural women. Around 46.5% of Dalit women never got antenatal and post-natal care. 54.8% of Valmiki sub-caste, who are the manual scavengers, never received antenatal and post-natal care, as reported by Navsarjan Trust (2013).

Poverty is both the driver and consequence of disasters. Past three decades research shows that though most disasters do not discriminate and take a toll on people irrespective of being rich and poor, it is the poor who tend to suffer the most due to the post-disaster response which, in inequitable structural hierarchies inbuilt in the societies, further pushes them down, especially those with no insurance and other means of social protection. While all those who are living in hazardous areas are vulnerable, the social impact and social vulnerability is much more for the poor (Wisner et al., 2004, 2012). Due to lack of data, it is difficult to say how many poor suffered Covid infection and how many succumbed. However, the observations and media highlighted that it is the rich and the middle-income groups who are succumbing to the pandemic, much more than the poor. However, the poor and the labour class, who are working in the unorganized sector, are facing loss of work, wages and livelihoods, leading to mass exodus from the cities, as seen in 2020. Poverty and pandemic, thus, combined together are increasing the risk of starvation and food insecurity among the poor.

Development of Health Care Services in India

In the colonial period, bio-medicine was confined to the British population and Indians serving in British until 1868, till a separate civil medical department was formed in Bengal.[4] The general population was dependent on traditional and folk healing practices. Before India got independence, Bhore Committee was set up in 1946 which proposed comprehensive primary healthcare, which includes preventive, promotive, curative and rehabilitative care, irrespective of the ability to pay (GOI, 1946). However, before it could be launched, the Selective Primary Health Care approach was proposed by Walsh and Warren (1980), which was more targeted and outcome-based. Four vertical programmes targeting children and women were added. UNICEF GOBI i.e. Growth monitoring, Oral rehydration, Breastfeeding, Immunizations were proposed. Later, FFF—Female education, Family spacing and planning, Food supplementation were added, targeting countries like India with a 'huge' population. The targeted approach continued post-Independence and continues till today at the cost of comprehensive health care services. Most resources go in family planning, Reproductive Child Health and disease-specific programmes.

The joint WHO UNICEF (1978) international conference at Alma Ata (USSR) declared, 'the existing gross inequalities in the status of health of people particularly between the developed and the developing countries as well as within the countries is politically, socially and economically unacceptable'.[5] Alma Ata declaration called on all the governments to formulate National Health policies according to their own circumstances to launch and sustain primary healthcare as a national priority. Primary healthcare is essential healthcare based on practical, scientifically sound and socially acceptable methods and technology, universally acceptable to individuals and families, in the community through their full participation and at a cost that the community and the country can afford.

However, after 36 years post-independence, the first National Health Policy (NHP, 1983) in India came into existence. The NHP 1983 was in a spirit of optimistic empathy for the needs of the people, particularly the poor and the under-privileged, and had hoped to provide 'Health for all by 2000' through comprehensive Primary Health Care services. However, the subsequent national health policies of 2002 and

---

[4] https://www.ncbi.nlm.nih.gov/pmc/articles/PMC2763662/.

[5] https://www.who.int/publications/almaata_declaration_en.pdf.

2017 clearly mandated the increasing role of the private sector towards healthcare and also promotion of 'health tourism' attracting foreign patients, despite the already overburdened and limited health care resources. The health policies (2002) promoted medical tourism and during VIIIth Five Years Plan announcing new economic policies, further IXth Plan, XI Plan, onwards clearly indicated the growth of the private and corporate health sector and promotion of 'medical tourism'. The following section looks at the organization of public health care services and health care spending.

Three Tier Public Health Care Services

Within the biomedical systems, India has a robust three-tier public health care service sector and an equally robust heterogeneous private sector. The public health care services, were well conceived to reach out to rural India. At the village level, there are Sub-Centres (SCs) where there is no doctor but two paramedical staff to cater to the primary level care, who provide basic drugs for taking care of essential health needs of men, women and children. As of 2019, there are 153,655 SCs. Above this level, there are Primary Health Centres (PHCs), which is the first referral where a medical doctor is present. Under each PHC, there are around 6 SCs. Presently, there are 28,863 PHCs in India (2019). For four PHCs, there is one Community Health Centre (CHCs), with 30 indoor beds, Operation Theatre, X-ray, Labour Room and Laboratory facilities. As of 2017, there are 5,624 CHCs in India. However, despite such a robust three-tier system of public health care services, it has many gaps, lacunae and challenges to provide healthcare to people.

Health Care Spending

India spends less than 1.5% of GDP (2018–19) on healthcare and ranks at third-bottom in the list of countries in terms of spending on health. India spends lower than the other South-East Asian countries like Nepal, Srilanka, Bhutan, Indonesia, Thailand. Though by mid-1990s, our health care spending was 6% of GDP, it reduced to 0.9% in 2005. In 2015, it was increased to 3.89% and again reduced to 1.15% of GDP in recent years. This Out-Of-Pocket Expenditure on health, especially among the poorer households, exacerbates poverty. Without financial protection, a large section of Dalits, who fall into an unorganized sector, do not have any health insurance and thus, it worsened the poverty levels in many households and they are pushed down into indebtedness (Yip & Mahal, 2008). Half of the households fall into poverty due to health expenditure (Balarajan et al., 2011; Krishna, 2004). Selvvaraj and Karan (2009) reported that in 2004–05, about 30.6 million rural and 8.4 million urban people fell into poverty as a result of Out-Of-Pocket Expenditure (OOPE). They also reported that both absolute and relative poverty has been increasing due to OOPE.

Rural population in poorer states suffers much more than the urban and the heavy burden of health expenditure is on SC and ST population. One of the main reasons for poor health performance in India is the dismal financial health budget.

The financial allocation in healthcare shows that the State Governments contribute 15.2%, the Central Government 5.2%, third-party insurance and employers 3.3%, and municipal government and foreign donors about 1.3%. For the year 2015–16, Total Health Expenditure (THE) for India was Rs. 5,28,484 crores (3.84% of GDP and Rs. 4116 per capita). Government Health Expenditure (GHE), including capital expenditure, was Rs. 1,61,863 crores (30.6% of THE, 1.18% GDP and Rs. 1261 per capita).[6] Of these proportions, 58.7% goes towards primary healthcare (curative, preventive and promotive) and 38.8% is spent on secondary and tertiary inpatient care. The rest goes for non-service costs (WB report 1995). While a huge burden of health care spending remains on the individuals, the Out-Of-Pocket Expenditure (OOPE) on health accounts for about 78% of the total expenditure on health in the country (World Bank, 1997).

Paying for health services out of pocket is a major hindrance to access health service and it pushes them further into poverty (Balarajan et al., 2011). 55 million people were pushed into poverty in a single year in 2017 due to out-of-pocket expenditure on healthcare and 38 million people fell below poverty line.[7]

Human Resource Vacancies in Public Health Sector

The public sector is left with minimum financial resources and huge vacancies at every level for human resources. As of February 2021, India's doctor population ratio is 1:1,404, whereas WHO recommends, 1:1000. In rural India, this ratio is abysmally low with 1:10,926 doctors as per the National Health Profile 2019. The staff nurse position in PHC and CHC shows the highest vacancies across states— 75% vacancy in Jharkhand, 62% in Sikkim, 50% in Bihar, 57% in Rajasthan, 43% in Haryana and 41% in NCT Delhi. The vacancy of medical officers at PHCs is 64% in Bihar, 58% in Madhya Pradesh, 49% in Jharkhand, 45% in Chhattisgarh and 43% in Manipur. The similar status of vacancies in the public sector for specialists and lab assistants at various levels is a grave concern. With so many vacancies of human resources and absence of doctors and nurses, the poor and the marginalized take the maximum brunt, who cannot afford private care. This vacuum is seen in the COVID-19 situation where there are not enough staff to serve the people.

Further, with these limited resources in public health care services, putting the onus of healthcare only on public systems is not appropriate. Rather, realizing the need and importance of a very robust heterogeneous private and corporate health care

---

[6] National Health Accounts Estimates for India, 2018.

[7] https://economictimes.indiatimes.com/news/politics-and-nation/health-spending-pushed-55-million-into-poverty-in-a-year-study/articleshow/64568199.cms?from=mdr.

sector and the important role it can play, in general and during disasters in specific, is not just desirable, but also obligatory and prerequisite.

Private and Corporate Health Care Services

India always had a mixed health care system with both public and private sectors. However, the private sector emerged as strong and further grew leaps and bounds after health sector reforms (Baru, 2003; Qadeer et al., 2001). In the private sector, the diversity is quite varied ranging from one-man clinics to 10 bedded hospitals and further to 650 bedded super and multi-specialty hospitals. The share of the private sector in health infrastructure is also quite significant with 57% hospitals and 32% of hospital beds are in the private sector. Moreover, most qualified doctors are also in the private sector. The data shows the presence of 80% of 3,90,000 qualified allopathic doctors registered in Medical Council of India and 6,50,000 providers from other systems work in the private sector (Bhat, 2000; Duggal & Amin, 1989). Many doctors moved from public to corporate hospitals, one of the doctor in public hospital mentioned, "The public hospitals work like a 'nursery' for getting good training and experienced doctors are handpicked and offered positions in the corporate hospitals, leading to internal brain drain" (Reddy & Qadeer, 2010). The cost of providing training to the doctors in government medical colleges is very subsidized, and after a few years of experience, they leave the public hospitals and join the corporate health sector.

Delhi has more than 50 super specialty private hospitals, and one can call them corporate hospitals. The corporate hospitals work on the corporate principles of management with set targets and profit-making is the basic agenda. Doctors set the financial goals for specialties like cardiology, orthopaedics and transplant centres. Thus, the doctors are given salaries and incentives based on the revenue they generate for the department. The doctors have to share the conversion rate as to how many patients they visited and how many patients were advised to undergo surgeries. Profit-driven hospitals compel the doctors to meet the targets or leave the job. As the doctors are asked to meet these targets, they over-prescribe unnecessary diagnostic tests, hold on to the patients for longer and performing avoidable procedures and surgeries.[8]

The doctors are at the mercy of the hospital management to be hired and fired at will and wish, especially those doctors who do not get the 'business' with low conversion rates. The subsidies from public to private sector go in many ways, and one such example is the, so-called, 'internal brain drain' where doctors leave government hospitals after getting the required medical training and join corporate hospitals for better salaries. This salary has to come from the income they generate for the hospitals, and that is by 'over' charging the patients (Qadeer & Reddy, 2010). This situation became much more pronounced in the pandemic situation.

---

[8] https://www.physiciansweekly.com/doctors-losing-publics-trust/.

In urban areas, especially the metropolitan cities, where there are multiple health care provisions available, the big corporate hospitals compete with each other and look for patients not just from within the city, but from other states and also target international patients. There are efforts to promote their services for international patients through social media, websites, word of mouth, international tie-ups and collaborations.

There is also a shift in the nature of the hospital ownership, where it's not just the professionals and doctors who are owning the hospitals like Dr. C Pratap Reddy of Apollo or Dr. Naresh Trehan of Medanta, or Dr. Devi Shetty of Narayana Health, but a host of business houses are also owning hospitals like Max, Fortis, Artimis and other such hospitals (Qadeer & Reddy, 2006). In such a business venture, the dynamics of health care changes from 'service' to 'trade'. They work on the corporate model, that is maximizing profits, where hire and fire at will policy is adopted for most of the staff and they expect doctors to bring 'business', leading to overdiagnosis, overtreatment and in a few cases, unethical practices of holding patients for longer to generate income. The doctors are handpicked and paid handsomely for the business they bring in. COVID-19 further brought out an opportunity for expensive corporate healthcare, and in pandemics, many patients not only lost lives but also all the wealth they had saved.

Public Subsidies to Corporate Hospitals

The health policies of 2002 and 2017 promoted the corporate health care sector, and from the eighth five-year plan onward, there has been a shift in promoting the private sector. The following section looks at the growth of corporate healthcare, the functioning of these services, the misplaced priorities to serve the international patients at the cost of local patients and the ways through which public subsidies go to the private sector. State promoted Medical Tourism in many ways and therefore, public subsidies are going to the corporate sector. There is a direct and indirect shift of subsidies for the corporate sector. The former itself is calculated to be Rs.57,000 crores (Chanda, 2002). The following changes suggest the promotion of the corporate sector,

(a)   To ease the movement of patients from other countries, 'Medical' Visas are facilitated.
(b)   State further gave a boost to promote the private sector by giving land on subsidies,
(c)   Duties were exempted on the import of medical equipment,
(d)   The tax exemptions are given for registering the medical and research institutes. However, most of the hospitals are more into clinical care than any research.
(e)   Buying health care services from the private sector for the government employees in the form of Central Government Health Scheme (CGHS) as insurance.

(f)   Other states supported schemes like Arogyasree and Yeshasvi, and national insurance schemes like Pradhan Mantri Swathya Suraksha Yojana (PMSSY) are also ploughing public money into the private sector.

It is suggested that the model of public–private partnership in healthcare will work better, but it is always public investment and private provision where the public sector invests and the private sector reaps the benefit. It is important to examine the public policy goals of the PPPs with an objective to protect the poor. Experiences in programme implementation suggest that it has always been a problem to target the poor. Research has shown that it is difficult to address equity issues and protect the poor through PPP initiatives (Bhat, 2000). There is an absence of effective monitoring systems and regulation for checking the private and corporate health sectors as seen in the case of land subsidies (Qadeer & Reddy, 2010).

The land-owning agencies like Delhi Development Authority (DDA) have put forth certain conditions on the hospitals which got land on lease at throw-away prices. The lease conditions were to treat the poor free of cost (25% indoor and 40% outdoor patients). However, all the corporate hospitals violated the clause (Qureshi report, 2001). None of the hospitals were fulfilling the lease conditions. In some cases, the nature of 'trust', for charity hospitals, changed to commercial nature and in one case, the Ayurvedic hospital changed to an allopathic hospital (Qadeer & Reddy, 2013). There is no official mechanism to see the trickledown effect where the profits earned by the corporate hospitals benefit the general healthcare in any way (Qadeer & Reddy, 2006, 2013).

Medical Tourism and Misplaced Priorities

India is hailed as a 'Medical Tourism' (MT) destination for foreigners, NRIs and also patients coming from neighbouring countries. The corporatization of the Medicare sector has brought with it five-star facilities and world-class treatments. The country can now boast of a number of corporate hospitals. India has become a medical tourist destination, largely because of the cost differences, which is around one-tenth of the developing nations as compared to the exorbitant prices in developed nations, offering a business and a value proposition, caption saying *'First World Treatment at Third World Rates'*. All the metropolitan cities can now boast of having a chain of super and multi-speciality hospitals. India offers world-class medical facilities, comparable with any of the Western countries, with state-of-the-art hospitals, highly qualified doctors, best infrastructure and facilities, accompanied with the most competitive prices.

Medical tourism is seen as a forex generator after the IT sector has gone down. India was projected to be worth $9 billion by 2020 and became 20% of the global market share in 2020 (Reddy & Qadeer, 2010). Globalization led to MT, which is a cross-border trade in medical care, transfer of technology, manpower, and knowledge that favours the elite and not necessarily the ordinary users of public sector tertiary hospitals (Qadeer & Reddy, 2013). MT is overshadowing the poor state of Indian public hospitals as the 11th Plan focused on the former and glamorized the institutions catering to foreign patients (GOI, 2008). Given a huge number of hospitals and doctors largely congregated in cities, these corporate hospitals attract patients from other countries to sustain and thrive as there is huge competition in corporate sectors. Under medical diplomacy, the country opens its already scarce resources to treat overseas patients at the cost of its own poor patients.

Those who are proponents of medical tourism envisage that trade in health services can have positive impacts on the national health system as foreign investors can bring in additional resources and new technologies, and new management techniques can be adopted to improve the provision of services and financing of the system. The corporate sector can improve the working conditions and therefore, encourage the health professional not to leave the country. The private hospital doctors feel that the health of the masses and the poor is the state responsibility and the corporate sector has nothing to do. However, not realizing the huge subsidies going from public to private sector in a welfare state, they consider health being the state subject (Qadeer and Reddy, 2013).

At a time when India is being hailed as a medical destination, it is ironic that patients in government hospitals are suffering due to the non-availability of emergency drugs/ lifesaving drugs costing less than a dollar even in normal times. Pandemics have exacerbated this situation much more. The government has decided to treat medical tourism as 'deemed export category and all incentives shall be given'. However, financing private corporations with public money is unjustifiable when GDP spending is so low. The trade in the health care sector can be harnessed to benefit the whole health system only by strengthening the stewardship and regulatory functions of national governments (Adlung & Carzaniga, 2001), which is not happening in the case of India.

As the corporate sector is built on government subsidies, it should be bound to benefit general healthcare. However, considering that there is no mechanism built to harness these profits, the corporate sector should be either purely private in nature or built on purely business models with no public subsidies, and the government resources should be limited to strengthening the public health sector only.

There is also a belief that competition is beneficial for any business. However, contrary to the general perception that competition is beneficial to consumers and society at large, there seems to be only partial truth (Godwin, 2004). The competition in the health sector can prove detrimental, especially for the poor and the marginalized, where profit is the underlying principle of any trade. Considering the fact that there are a number of corporate hospitals, there is also huge competition among them to attract patients not only local and regional but also overseas in the form of medical tourists.

However, not realizing the link that the policy shifts are favouring the expansion of the corporate sector and cutting the resources for public hospitals, there is no mechanism to ensure the trickledown effect. Moreover, the government has subsidized their input prices. With less resources in public health care services, the subsidies going to the corporate sector is unethical until a mechanism is built to make sure that the profits earned by the corporate sector go into treating poor sections of the society, at least during emergencies, disasters and pandemics.

With public subsidies going into building the corporate health sector, it is the poor who are subsidizing the rich in terms of the uses of public health resources in the country. (Godwin, 2004, p. 3983). Ethical issues have become significant (Borman, 2004), both in terms of equity and in the more competitive involvement of the market in medical care. There are examples from other countries which are doing well in medical tourism like Malaysia that show that their health care delivery is also increasingly inequitable (Connell, 2006), and in Thailand, 'there is a huge drain on the public health sector'.

Disaster Capitalism: Private Hospitals and Unethical Behaviour

A quote by Groucho Marx 'hospital bed is a parked taxi with the meter running' shows the ground realities of the private health sector. Though there is a huge presence of the private sector in the country, there are no guidelines or mention of the role of the private sector at the time of disasters in the Disaster Management Act 2005 or any other policy document. It is imperative that under corporate social responsibility, the corporate hospitals should pitch in at the time of disasters and there should be some policies, guidelines and Standard Operating Procedures (SOPs) for all the private sectors. For the first time, 'The Epidemic Diseases Act' of 1897 was invoked for the whole of India to combat COVID-19 and many restrictions were laid out on the movement of people. Despite the overwhelming dedication and heroic courage of health care workers in treating COVID-19 patients, people faced violence and were stigmatized. This led to the introduction of a new ordinance 'The Epidemic Diseases (Amendment) Ordinance 2020', in which violence against health care workers is considered as a punishable offence with 7 years' imprisonment.[9]

As P. Sainath (1996) in his book 'Everybody loves a good drought' shows how certain sections benefit due to the disasters. Similarly, the private sector took the pandemic as an opportunity to do brisk business. Naomi Klien's (2007) book, 'Disaster Capitalism' (2007), also analysed the unethical practices during disasters and the capitalist class making brisk business. Many corporate hospitals, which boost themselves as a 'Medical Tourism' destination, turned away their own patients who were not in a position to pay and those who could pay got the beds and other facilities. Many unethical practices, by some of the private hospitals, came out in the media as there were no standard costs of consultancy, beds, PPEs and ICU care. Many hospitals were overcharging their patients whereas many patients were turned

---

[9] https://blogs.bmj.com/bmj/2020/06/19/covid-19-indian-healthcare-workers-need-adequate-ppe/.

down as the beds were less and those who could pay got on priority. Some hospitals were holding patients for payment.[10]

Out of anger for not saving lives and lack of oxygen and beds, the patient's kin started abusing the doctors. This led to the amendment in the Epidemic Diseases Act 1897 which, to protect the medical staff, introduced punishment to those who abuse doctors and medical staff. Similar amendments in the DM Act 2005 should immediately be made for patients to save them from overcharging, and some reservations should be introduced such as beds for the poor in the corporate sector.

The contradiction between the public and private health care sector continued. While the private hospitals were charging patients for PPE and the health care staff as high as Rs. 10,000 per day, and the public sector, which was not charging from patients, was falling short and struggling to meet the requirements—both quantity and quality. 'A 60 years old man was admitted to one of the private hospitals in Delhi, in April 2020, after 30 days, the family was given a bill of 122 pages and charged Rs. 16,14, 596. The bill had charged 18% (2.9 lakhs) on PPE of the total bill. They charged Rs. 10,000 per day for PPE worn by medical staff treating the patient'.[11] This shows that there was no capping on the prices, and with no standard price for procedures and equipment, the hospitals were free to charge any amount, without considering the pandemic and crisis on household income at this juncture.

While the private sector could charge more for PPE and procure, the government hospitals' central procurement agency—HLL Life care told the hospitals that they are short of the supply of raw materials required for making PPE and thus orders have been delayed. The only place where the poor and the marginalized can go is the public hospitals, which are perpetually lacking essential equipment and even basic drugs. An acute shortage of beds in hospitals and a long wait for ambulances followed in the public sector. Media also reported the shortage of essential medicines from pharmacies, and the black marketing of the same was happening (TOI, 19th April 2021). Reports of hoardings, black marketing of medicines and oxygen were reported.

Role of Private and Corporate Sector in Disasters

When the private sector started fleecing the pockets of the patients, public interest litigations demanding 'cost-related regulation' started pouring in and the courts had to take cognizance of the situation. The centre, however, replied in June 2020 that they do not have legal powers to ask the private sector to give free treatment and it is in the domain of the States. The Supreme Court also asked the private sector to provide treatment at the government insurance rates, such as the 'Ayushman Bharat'

---

[10] https://health.economictimes.indiatimes.com/news/hospitals/government-asks-private-hospitals-to-stop-unfair-practices/46893730.

[11] https://www.indiaspend.com/ppe-priced-high-in-private-hospitals-while-public-hospitals-face-shortage/.

scheme. Chief justice also asked the hospitals to treat the poor, if they have taken land on subsidy.[12]

Despite the plea of the Supreme Court, the corporate sector continued to make brisk business in the pandemic. Even though the DM Act suggests that the District Commissioner (DC) can involve the private sector in disasters, it is not mandated. Very few DC in Andhra, Mumbai and Orissa took over the private sector and passed orders to convert into COVID-19 beds or treat the Covid patients free of cost. However, it is not done across the States. Thus, it is imperative to make it manda-tory for the private/ corporate sector to treat patients in emergencies, pandemics and disasters with an approved cost to be paid by the government. The DM Act should be amended by adding the role of the private sector in the disasters, without waiting for the disasters to happen in order to avoid any knee-jerk reactions, exploitation and overcharging of the patients. This has to be amended in the current DM Act to be followed though it will be opposed by the private/corporate sector. However, the terms and conditions can be worked out with the government, to pay off- no-profit no loss cost to these hospitals in emergencies.

Good Practices by Some States

In some states like Andhra Pradesh, the current Chief Minister, Jagan Reddy, announced not to take money from patients in Covid hospitals and also to cancel the registration of the hospitals if they charge. Government bearing the entire cost for Covid patients is an excellent example of a welfare state standing up to emergen-cies. This will definitely have public popularity as it was in the case of earlier Chief Minister, Y S Rajsekar Reddy, for bringing in Arogyasree State health insurance scheme. Other states also tried to regulate their own capacities. Kerala and Andhra Pradesh reached the doorsteps of people to provide services during the lockdown. The Delhi government, in June 2020, also ordered capping of cost to treat the COVID-19 patients. The National Accreditation Board for Hospitals and Health Care provider (NABH) accredited hospitals charged 10,000 for isolation bed, 18,000 for ICU with ventilator. Seeing the overcharging of COVID-19 patients and complaints pouring in, the Delhi government wrote to all the private hospitals to refrain from unethical prac-tices. The notice went to the hospitals, but there was no way to monitor and regulate them, as there is no law to bind them to follow such instructions. The Health Minister of Delhi, however, said that they are working on the grievance redressal mechanism, where the patient can approach the government or Delhi Medical Council with their complaints.

In the second phase, on 18 April 2021, courtesy Indian Army, DRDO and Tata Group, the Indian Armed Forces, in collaboration with DRDO, set up a state-of-the-art, 1000-bedded Covid Care Hospital right in the heart of Delhi without any

---

[12] https://health.economictimes.indiatimes.com/news/hospitals/supreme-court-asks-private-hospit als-if-they-are-ready-to-charge-covid-19-patients-at-ayushman-bharat-rate/76215864.

fanfare. Meant to extend a helping hand to civilian brethren and ex-servicemen, the Vallabhbhai COVID Hospital admits any person who is symptomatic and who is Covid positive. This has been done by the defence services for the service of the people of the nation.

Discussion and Recommendations

COVID-19 pandemic has led to huge losses, not just in terms of lives but also economy. The pandemic has challenged the public health systems, economic resources, food systems, work and livelihoods. The disruptions in economic and social life are devastating. The estimation is that the current undernourished world-wide population of 690 million can go up by 132 million by the end of the year.

Oxfam reports that as a result of the pandemic, the number of people living in poverty has doubled to more than 500 million. Thomson Reuters Foundation estimated that the collective wealth of the world's billionaire, however, rose to $3.9 trillion between March and December 2020 to reach $11.95 trillion. India with 1.3 billion population has a good number of poor populations with 21.9% who are under the National Poverty line. COVID-19 has further aggravated the situation where the households living on subsistence are facing acute crises. A report by Pew Research Center, using the World Bank projections of economic growth, estimated that India's middle class shrunk by one-third due to the pandemic but the poor who are earning less than two dollars have doubled, i.e. 7.5 crore population.[13] The inequality virus, as published in World Economic Forum's Davos Agenda, reports that the world's 1000 richest people recouped their COVID-19 losses within just nine months, but the world's poorest will take one decade to recover from the pandemic, as reported by Oxfam. The disparity is so stark to share that only ten richest men can provide free vaccines to the entire world. However, still many people in developing nations are not getting the vaccine shot either due to non-availability or non-affordability. India however, could reach 1 billion mark of vaccine dosses against COVID 19, on Oct 21, 2021, achieving an important milestone (Gupta and Mangal 2021). In the past 90 years, so many people were never observed as either unemployed or underemployed.[14]

The worst sufferers are the poor and the migrant workers, who live on subsistence and have lost their jobs and work. In addition, self-employed or wage labourers in the unorganized sector, with no social benefits, who live on daily wages are also at the brink of impoverishment and starvation. Loss of work has further pushed them to work in extreme and unsafe conditions and take further risk.

---

[13] https://www.thehindu.com/news/national/coronavirus-pandemic-may-have-doubled-poverty-in-india-says-pew-study/article34110732.ece.

[14] https://www.thehindu.com/news/national/coronavirus-pandemic-may-have-doubled-poverty-in-india-says-pew-study/article34110732.ece.

Given such a huge population who are poor in India can only resort to public health care services, given the poor conditions of public hospitals, with staff shortage and lack of essential drugs, oxygen and beds, the poor suffer the worst. Considering the huge population of India who is poor and can only report to public health care services and the poor conditions of public hospitals with staff shortage and lack of essential drugs, oxygen and beds, it can be said that the poor face the worst consequences.

Though, India was hailed for its well-managed strategies in the first wave in 2020, the second wave in April 2021 was not well managed. It is ironic that despite the experience of the first phase, after a year in the Second Phase of COVID 2021, still the services in the public sector have not been improved. The situation is the same and people suffer a shortage of beds, oxygen and PPEs, leading to many casualties, especially of youth. However, the death toll is more in the second wave than in the first wave. There is no data to see who are the people who are dying, young or old, rich or poor, men, women or children.

The discussion in the first part of the paper shows how the policy shifts and promotion of corporate health sectors, over the past three decades, led to dichotomous and inequitable healthcare. Further, the public subsidies going into the corporate sector, with no monitoring and regulation, led to misplaced priorities to treat international patients and the poor Indian people were left with poor public health care services. Further, low spending in the public sector left the public health sector resourceless, with significant human resource vacancies and lack of protective equipment for the nurses and sanitation staff (Hathi and Srivastav, this volume). Further lack of essential drugs, beds and basic technology for treating the patients. Consequently, the poor public health sector, which was already crippling in normal times, was overwhelmed during the pandemics.

Considering the limited economic and human resources in healthcare, the policy should be made to keep the equitable distribution of healthcare.

1. There is no other alternative to strengthen public healthcare in India when 27.9% of the population is under multidimensional poverty and many more in the middle-income group who cannot afford private medical care, especially in crisis situations.
2. It is imperative that the State government invests in public healthcare.
3. The private sector should be monitored and regulated in general and in crisis situations in particular.
4. If the corporate sector is not treating the poor according to the lease conditions, there should not be any public subsidies and it should be purely private with no public investments.
5. Or the treatment of the poor should be part of the CSR, especially where the public subsidies are going into the private sector. It should be mandated in the DM Act.
6. The DM Act should be amended to add the roles and responsibilities of private healthcare in times of disasters and pandemics.
7. The pandemic experiences and the lessons learnt thereby should be documented and prepared for future pandemics.

8. The States and the Centre should have an emergency plan to provide social security for the lower classes and the scheduled caste social groups. Social security schemes should be ensured and assured during such crisis situations.
9. The poor, migrants, unemployed, Dalits and tribal population should be given social security during the pandemics to recover from the crisis period.
10. Given the well accepted and recognized plural healing systems in the country, the government should recognize, support and mainstream folk and traditional healing practices as they play an important role in building immunity and also provide cure at the primary level care in the communities.
11. There is also a need to invest in primary and secondary level care, increase more tertiary care in all the districts and fill all the vacant positions of doctors and paramedical staff in public sector.
12. Emphasis should also be given on overall social security, employment guarantee, minimum and equal wages to the poor and the marginalized.

Pandemics and disasters are opportunities to learn lessons and make some structural changes in the society. COVID-19 has taught us that no power and/or money can save lives, then why do we have this rat race, hoarding and greed. All are mortal beings and all of us have to go, then why can't we see an equitable society and live in harmony, peace and empathy for the poor and the marginalized.

References

Adlung, R., & Carzaniga, A. (2001). Health services under the general agreement on trade in services. *Bulletin of the World Health Organization.*

Balarajan, Y., Selvaraj, S., & Subramanian, S. V. (2011). Health care and equity in India. *Lancet, 377*(9764), 505–15. Epub 2011 Jan 10.

Baru, R. V. (2003). Privatisation of health services: A South Asian perspective. *Economic and Political Weekly*, 4433–4437.

Bhat, R. (2000). Issues in health: Public-private partnership. *Economic and Political*

Borman, E. (2004). Health tourism. *BMJ, 328,* 60.

Borooah, V. K. (2005). Caste, inequality, and poverty in India. *Review of Development Economics, 9*(3), 399–414.

Chanabasappa, B. S. (2000). Caste system. Retrieved April 4, 2018.

Chanda, R. (2002). Trade in health services. *Bull World Health Organisation, 80*(2), 158–163.

Connell, J. (2006). Medical tourism: Sea, sun, sand and… surgery. *Tourism Management, 27*(6), 1093–1100.

Duggal, R., & Amin, S. (1989). *Cost of health care: a household survey in an Indian district. Bombay: Foundation for Research in Community Health.*

Qureshi, A. S. (2001). *High level committee for hospitals in Delhi: Enquiry report.* Maulana Azad Medical College and Government of India.

Godwin, S. K. (2004). Medical tourism: Subsidizing the rich. *Economic and Political Weekly*, 3981–3983.

GOI. (1946). *Report of the health survey and development committee,* Vol. II, (Chairman: Bhore). Manager of Publications. http://shodhganga.inflibnet.ac.in/bitstream/10603/94652/11/11_chapter%205.pdf.

GOI. (2008). Eleventh five year plan, 2007–2012. 2008, *New Delhi: Chapter on health*, Vol. 2. Government of India.

Klein, N. (2007). *The shock doctrine: The rise of disaster capitalism. Macmillan.*

Krishna, A. (2004). Escaping poverty and becoming poor: Who gains, who loses, and why? *World Development, 32*, 121–136.

Madan, T. N., Wiebe, P. D., Said, R., & Dias, M. (1980). *Doctors & society.* Vikas Publishing House.

MoHFW. (2002). National health policy. *Ministry of health and family welfare.* Government of India.

NCSC. (n.d.). Economic development of scheduled caste. *National commission for scheduled caste.* Retrieved April 05, 2018, from http://ncsc.nic.in/files/ncsc/new3/202.pdf.

Oommen, T. K. (1978). Doctors and nurses, Macmillan Co. of India, Delhi. Pp Xi+ 256.

Qadeer, I., & Reddy, S. (2006). Medical care in the shadow of public private partnership. *Social Scientist*, 4–20.

Qadeer, I., & Reddy, S. (2013). Medical tourism in India: Perceptions of physicians in tertiary care hospitals. *Philosophy, Ethics, and Humanities in Medicine, 8*(1), 1–10.

Qadeer, I., Sen, K., & Nayar, K. R. (Eds.). (2001). *Public health and the poverty of reforms: The South Asian predicament* (pp. 548). Sage Publications.

Reddy, S., & Qadeer, I. (2010). Medical tourism in India: progress or predicament? *Economic and political weekly*, 69–75.

Scheper-Hughes, N. (1993). Death without weeping: The violence of everyday life in Brazil. Univ of California Press.

Selvaraj, S., & Karan, A. (2009). Deepening health insecurity in India: Evidence from national sample surveys since the 1980s. *EPW, 44*, 55–60.

Sundaram, K., & Tendulkar, S. D. (2003). Poverty among social and economic groups in India in the 1990s. *Economic and Political Weekly*, 5263–5276.

Navsarjan Trust (2013). *The situation of dalit rural women.* Retrieved April 12, 2017, from https://www.ohchr.org/Documents/HRBodies/CEDAW/RuralWomen/FEDONavsarjanTrustIDS.pdf. https://doi.org/10.1177/2455328X19898449.

Walsh, J. A., & Warren, K. S. (1980). Selective primary health care: an interim strategy for disease control in developing countries. *Social Science & Medicine. Part C: Medical Economics, 14*(2), 145–163.

WHO and UNICEF. (1978). Primary health care: report of the International Conference on Primary Health Care, Alma-Ata, USSR, Sept 6–12.

Wisner, B., Blaikie, P., Cannon, T., & Davis, I. (2004). *At risk: Natural hazards, people's vulnerability and disasters.* Routledge.

Wisner, B., Gaillard, J., & Kelman, I. (2012). Framing disaster: Theories and stories seeking to understand hazards, vulnerability and risk. In: B. Wisner, J . Gaillard & I. Kelman (Eds.), *Handbook of hazards and disaster risk reduction* (pp. 18–33). Routledge.

World Bank. (1997). India new directions in health care development at the state level: An operational perspective. *Population and human resource division.* South Asia Country Department II.

Chapter 6
Knowledge Accumulation During COVID-19: Increasing Digital Divide and Vulnerability Among Indian Students

G. Dilip Diwakar and Visakh Viswambaran

Abstract Quality education is a significant aspect of human development, but all the people in a country do not uniformly access it because of the existing structural inequality in society. The exclusion and marginalization in education are exacerbated in a country like India by geographical location, class, caste, gender, religion and ethnicity. In such a scenario, the COVID-19 pandemic further exacerbated marginalized children's condition, as digital online education replaced direct school education. The government of India has issued an order to start online classes, suddenly all the schools both government and private started the online education. Though it is good that schools continued to work on the one end, but on the other end, we need to examine how many people could make use of this online education facility. While we see access to online education, we need to remember about 22% of India's population are living below the poverty line, as per the Tendulkar Committee during 2011–12. Because of their poor living condition, many of them lack access to basic facilities to acquire education through the digital platform. The majority of the poor and marginalized students, because of the lack of smartphones, laptops and television, could not attend online classes. This has not only affected their studies but also affected their psychological well-being. According to the National Sample Survey (2017–18) report, only 23.8% of Indian households have internet access, especially it is very less in the rural areas. The objective of the paper is to examine the existing digital divide in the education sector, problems encountered by the students and factors which increased the vulnerability and forced the students to commit suicide. The paper assessed 11 case studies of the student who committed suicide due to online education. Content analysis using the Atlas Ti was used for analysis purposes. The study finds students have committed suicide because they did not have smartphones, laptops and other gadgets; also some committed because they could not cope with the online education. Studying the pandemic's impact in the domain of education in a developing country like India can be effective for public policy learnings to face contingent situations. This research will help in furthering our understanding of providing better public policy solutions.

G. D. Diwakar (✉) · V. Viswambaran
Department of Social Work, Central University of Kerala, Kasaragod, India

Keywords Digital Divide · Education · Suicide · Pandemic response · Inequalities

Introduction

The twenty-first century is undoubtedly the age of information networks. Humans now live in a world connected by invisible threads that facilitate the transfer of information. These information networks are now becoming the nervous system of our society and greatly influence the kind of lives people live (Van Dijk, 2005). The term 'digital divide' was coined by Lloyd Morrisett and first appeared in the US newspapers in 1996, when Steve Lohr wrote an article for the New York Times (Compaine, 2001; Lohr, 1996). A series of reports, titled 'Falling Through the Net', by the National Telecommunications and Information Administration (NTIA) of the United States, provided conclusive evidence to validate the claim that a particular set of haves and have nots exists in the digital sphere (NTIA, 1995; NTIA, 1998; NTIA, 1999). Soon after releasing these reports, the US undertook public policy initiatives to bridge the gap between digital haves and have nots. Following the lead, other developed and developing countries also recognized the need to eliminate the digital divide (Srinuan & Bohlin, 2011).

Digital divide refers to a division between people who have access to and use digital media and those who don't. However, it is essential to understand that this division is not a simple division between two separate social categories. Instead, it should be seen as a range of positions that extends across the whole population—from people having no access and use to those having complete access and multiple benefits (Van Dijk, 2020). The digital divide is linked to existing social, economic and cultural divisions of society. The differential access to the digital services overlaps with various intersecting factors such as geographical locality, income status, gender, educational status, skill set, ethnicity, etc. (Van Dijk & Hacker, 2003; Enoch & Soker, 2006; Hanimann & Ruedin, 2007; Borgonovi et. al., 2018; UNCTAD, 2019).

The digital divide is primarily an issue of access. The concept of access needs to be taken broadly as it encapsulates physical access, skills and usage (Van Dijk, 2017). Physical access refers to the availability of the hardware required to access the internet. Physical access should not be understood as a one-time decision to adopt and purchase a particular technology but instead as a continuing process of getting access to updated versions of hardware and software, peripheral equipment and subscriptions. Besides physical access, people also need specific skills and competencies to command and use digital media, which are referred to as digital skills. The third aspect of access is 'usage', which refers to how individuals use the available hardware, resources and skills to accomplish their tasks (Van Dijk, 2017). The physical access can be measured by inspecting the hardware, and its relevance and usage can be tracked by measuring the time spent online and the time allotted for each function. In comparison, digital skill is a complex concept to measure because most digital skills are not the result of educational courses but are gained by learning through practice in a particular social user environment (Van Dijk & Van Deursen, 2014).

The digital divide is not a bipolar social split between the haves and have nots. Instead, it should be understood as gradation based on different degrees of access to information technology (Warschauer, 2003). Van Dijk's Resources and Appropriation theory argues that the pre-existing categorical inequalities in society produce an unequal distribution of resources. This unequal distribution of resources causes unequal access to digital resources (Van Dijk, 2005). The existing social hierarchies of oppression contrived out categories of class, gender, caste, ability and geographical location which are reflected in this gradation of access to Information and Communications Technologies (ICTs). Therefore, the notion of the digital divide should be stretched to encompass a broad array of factors and resources, and society must realize that the context and purpose are critical to providing meaningful solutions to the digital divide problem (Warschauer, 2003).

During the COVID-19 pandemic, the noxious effects of the digital divide were exacerbated. The crisis robbed the world of its momentum, and people started looking up to Information and Communication Technologies (ICTs) as an authentic solution to the challenges mounted by the COVID-19. Business enterprises were forced to embrace work from home protocols. Government institutions had to take up remote working arrangements to discharge their functions and similarly, educational institutions also started imparting education via digital platforms as a substitute to the existing classroom teaching–learning process. These transitions have been far from being smooth.

Digital transfer of information is not available and accessible to all people, thus creating a digital divide. According to the UN's International Telecommunication Union, the global internet user penetration stands at 53.6%. This figure is 87% in the developed world, but it drops to 47% in developing countries (ITU, 2019). The digital divide issue is a persistent issue that affects developing countries in a more exasperating manner as compared to developed countries.

Apart from this divide between the developed and developing nations, even within the country itself, there is an apparent regional and rural–urban divide, where certain regions or urban areas have more digital access to information as compared to other regions or their rural counterparts. Even in the developed nations, the digital divide exists and it has been reported that rural Americans are 12 percentage points less likely than Americans overall to have broadband connections at home (Perrin, 2019). Similarly, in the case of the European Union, there is a regional divide in digital access because of ICT policy, cultural practice and available infrastructure facilities in certain regions (Vicente & López, 2011; Kos-Łabędowicz, 2017). Along with the rural–urban availability and regional divide, the income differential among people also plays an important role in creating the digital divide among the people (Vicente & López, 2011; Fong, 2009). The digital divide was reported in the UK (Philip et al., 2017), Japan (Nishida et al., 2014), China (Fong, 2009) and other developed countries.

Though the digital divide has its influence in various sectors, this paper will examine its effects only in the education sector. In the education sector, about 94% of ministries of education across the globe have tried to solve the COVID-19 related educational challenges by adopting digital and/or broadcast instruction. However, the irony is that 31% (463 million) of school children worldwide are excluded from these remote learning programmes due to the lack of necessary household assets and/or the absence of policies geared towards their needs (UNICEF, 2020). Quite predictably, the wealthier countries have made more use of the potential of remote learning possibilities. As per UNICEF (2020), only 60% of ministries have devised remote learning policies for pre-primary education, which means that an estimated 40% of the students at the pre-primary education level do not have any digital or broadcast access to remote learning opportunities.

However, in the case of India, there exists a greater digital divide, and the factors contributing to this divide need to be understood. Furthermore, the COVID-19 pandemic exacerbated the digital divide issue by forcing people to go online to adjust to the new reality. Not all people have the means to adapt to this new reality. This paper focuses on how the digital divide in India affects knowledge accumulation during the COVID-19 pandemic. As a result of being deprived of educational resources and unable to cope with this new reality, 11 students have died by committing suicide in different parts of India. This paper attempts to make sense of the digital divide and its patterns by analysing these suicide cases. The first section of the paper looks at the existing digital divide in India and the second section examines the government initiatives to address the digital divide. The third section explores gender and e-learning accessibility. The fourth section proposes a framework to study the cases of students who committed suicide. Based on the analysis of data, the discussion is carried out in the following sections.

Digital Divide and Indian Social Inequalities

Information communication technology (ICT) is considered as one of the key factors and driving forces in the modern era. It supports rapid development and accelerates economic growth and social change. ICT reduces the hindrance of distance, saves time and resources, and helps to communicate faster (Fletcher et al, 2000). Moreover, studies have pointed out that ICT helps in good governance. E-governance has been promoted by the governments and administrators to provide services at the doop steps of the citizens as it provides convenience and increases efficiency. It is believed that E-governance brings effectiveness, efficiency and transparency in the system (World Bank, 2016).

Even though ICT and e-governance have been promoted among both the developed and developing nations to bring rapid development and better governance, there is a need for infrastructure facilities to use and implement ICT and e-governance effectively. The developed nations have the required infrastructure and resources to invest in that. However, the developing nations do not have either the resources or the required infrastructure. This has led the developing nations way behind in governance and development. In the case of India also, even till the beginning of the millennium, the infrastructure to facilitate online digital technology was poor. Singh

(2010) has pointed out that we can understand the digital divide in India through teledensity, mobile usage and internet availability.

Telephone Regulatory Authority of India (2009) gives data on teledensity, which helps to understand the penetration rate. The data shows that the majority of the states have teledensity less than 15%, and only very few states like Gujarat, Himachal, Karnataka, Tamil Nadu, Punjab and Maharashtra have teledensity more than 30% (Singh, 2010). There is a huge teledensity divide between the urban and rural areas. The data shows that during 1999, the national average was 2.52 per 100 inhabitants and in the case of urban areas, it was 6.94 whereas in rural areas, it was 0.52. Though it has increased over time and during 2008, the national average was 21.20, and in urban areas, it was 56.08 whereas it was only 6.75 in the rural areas. Moreover, it indicates that in the rural areas, the situation has gotten worse than before. Internet usage during 2008 shows that the majority, 70%, were fromSumanjeet Singh the 7 main metropolitan cities whereas other areas and cities had only 30% usage. There was a clear divide in internet usage among the urban and rural areas. In urban India, about 12% of people had internet access whereas, in rural India, only 1.2% of people had internet access. In the case of mobile penetration, there is a huge divide between urban and rural areas. Rural mobile penetration is 4.92% which remains far below 43.88% in the urban areas (Singh, 2010).

Even though the government has made a conscious attempt to improve the infrastructure to support technology development, India is lagging behind in the digital world and also, there exists a huge urban–rural divide. For an easy transition into digital learning, it requires some prerequisites such as access to electricity, internet, compatible devices and parents or family members with the required skill set to guide children through the tech-savvy applications. Key Indicators of Household Social Consumption on Education in India, a report by National statistical office, reveals some vital statistics regarding the availability of electricity, internet and devices in India. The finding of this study shows that only 47% of Indian households receive more than 12 h of electricity, and more than 36% of schools in India operate without electricity. The students currently enrolled in any courses have essential digital infrastructure for education like computers with internet and it is available with only 9% in India. In the urban areas, it is 21% and in the rural areas, it is only 4% of the students who have a computer with internet. As described elsewhere (Sharma, this volume), the urban/rural tech divide had specific implications for public health knowledge dissemination to tribes during the pandemic lockdown. Students using any device to access the internet are only 25%. The divide between urban and rural areas shows that about 44% of urban households have internet access compared to 17% rural households. Only 5% of students in rural areas have access to computers against 24% of students in urban areas. The top income decile (richest 10%) is having the highest (41%) access to computers with internet among students. About 66% of them have access to computers at home and 45% of them have the internet. However, in the case of the bottom income decile (lowest 10%), it is 2% who have a computer with internet, 3% have a computer and 10% have Internet. Among the socio-religious groups, students having computers with internet are 21% from 'others/general' as compared to 4% SC, 4% for ST and 7% for OBC. In the case of internet access, about 45% of Others have it as compared to 13% ST, 17% SC and 23% OBC (Reddy et al., 2020). As described elsewhere (Ziyauddin, this volume), Muslim minorities are suffering from lower tech infrastructural development, alongside lower SES, lack of sanitation facilities, lower rates of higher education and lack of proportionate representation in government jobs.

There is a divide among students in terms of access to digital infrastructure in urban and rural areas. Apart from urban–rural divide, socio-economic condition and the caste are the other two factors that play a crucial role in determining access. The studies have shown that there is a clear link between the caste background of a person and his occupation (Reddy et al., 2020). Ambedkar has very clearly pointed out that the varna system is hierarchical where the person on the top occupies the job which has higher social status and income whereas the people in the lowest hierarchy have to do menial jobs with low social status and income. The status of the individual in society is ascribed rather than achieved and therefore, it does not allow people to take up job other than the job prescribed in the varnashrama dharma. It is not division of labour rather it is division of labourers (Ambedkar, 1968).

Caste is an institutionalized structure of oppression that is part and parcel of the Indian scenario for centuries. Caste is a system where endogamous groups discriminate against each other using an imaginary scale of hereditary purity. It has a rigid structure that blocks people by birth into a hierarchical structure that is arranged in ascending order of privileges and descending order of disabilities. Over the course of history, due to constitutional amendments and natural modernization, the force of caste has been weakened to an extent. However, despite many headways, caste as a unit of social stratification continues to dominate. Cultural stereotypes which glorify the privileged castes and demean those who are not are prevalent in the mainstream media. About 95% of marriages happen on a caste basis strictly and majority of the marriages are arranged. Though it is gradually getting semi-arranged now, still they are happening within their caste (Choudhury, 2020). Dalit atrocities are still common in most places. On the one hand, we can observe the persistence of certain dimensions or characteristics of caste such as endogamy, but on the other hand, we can observe a transformation in the economic domain of caste. Even highly qualified members of lower caste face social and economic discrimination resulting in inequality of outcomes (Thorat et al., 2010). Access to productive resources, particularly education and skills, remains closely associated with caste. Children from lower castes continue to be educationally disadvantaged (Nambissan, 1996). Material resources continue to consolidate in the hands of upper castes. The higher castes are mostly engaged in white-collar jobs, large business and farming. Despite the fact that positive transformation is happening in recent years, which paves way for the low caste to move up in the occupation ladder, however, the progress is very slow. Still, higher castes maintain their edge in the labour market by denying members of other castes similar opportunities (Vaid, 2012).

In the case of the land market, Scheduled Castes (erstwhile untouchable) were traditionally denied from owning land and this led to drastic inequality in land ownership. Historically, lands were owned and controlled by the upper caste dominant groups '*mirasi*', in their lands '*Pariahs*' (SC) were engaged as slaves. Based on

Tremenheere's report, the British government passed the Depressed Class Land Act in 1892, which paved the way to provide land rights to SCs (Rajasekharan, 2017). After independence, the land reformation act was one of the key initiatives that aimed to provide land for the SCs. Only a few states like Kerala and West Bengal are considered as (partially) successful examples of state-mediated land redistribution. However, even in Kerala, which is considered as a successful example, the land that was acquired and given to the Dalits was situated at geographically isolated places like hilltops, wastelands, uncultivable fields, shores of canals, and other such uninhabitable places that were visibly away from the coveted social structures of possession (Pramod, 2020). Infrastructure developments in these dwellings are notably neglected, and houses built inside these overpopulated dwellings are tiny. Essentially, these caste-based dwellings are caste-based ghettos, and the residents are discriminated against in multiple spheres, such as the discrimination induced by caste, geographical isolation and cultural perception towards ghettos (Pramod, 2020).

Historically, in India, the Gurukulam system of education was followed, and it allowed only 10–15% dominant castes to get Sanskrit education. The majority, 85–90%, of the people belonging to OBC, SC and ST were denied education in the gurukulam. This was changed by the British rulers. Lord McCauley introduced Modern English Education for Indians, and this helped the OBC, ST and SC to get English medium education (Jamanadas, 2000). Because of this historical denial of OBC, ST and SC from getting education for more than 2000 years, even now we can observe inequality in the education outcome. The NSSO and Census data shows that there is a disparity between the SC/ST and Others in education attainment. This inequality in education outcome is observed from primary class to professional studies. As the education level increases, the inequality between the SC/ST and Other castes increases, and it is more observed at the higher and professional level of education (Borooah et al., 2015). This divide in education outcome is mainly because of the discrimination faced by the children in school. They face discrimination at 3 level, (i) inside the class, (ii) school premises and (iii) outside the school (Nambissan, 2010).

Government Initiatives and Programmes to Address Digital Divide

At the beginning of the twenty-first century, India struggled with the digital divide issue (Servon, 2008; Singh, 2010), and therefore, the government has initiated several programmes and projects to address the gaps. Some of the programmes initiated by the government were CARD (Computer-Aided Administration of Registration Department) project, Kisan call centres, Lifeline India, Sourkaryan and E-Seva, Bhoomi Project, Gyandoot Project. Similarly, TDIL, FRIENDS (The fast, reliable, instant, efficient network for disbursement of services), E-Chaupals Project, Lokmitra project, Toarahat project etc. are some of the projects initiated by the state and central governments that have existed with the objective of eliminating the digital divide by increasing digital literacy and providing opportunities and skills required to access the digital world (Bansode & Patil, 2011; Panda et al., 2013; Singh, 2007; Sipre & Malik, 2017).

The CARD focuses on the computerization of the land registration process. Kisan Call Centres is a helpline initiative launched by the Ministry of Agriculture to answer the farmers' queries in their dialect. Furthermore, an initiative named Kisan Knowledge Management System (KKMS) was established to facilitate correct, consistent and quick replies to the queries of farmers and capture all the details of their calls (Department of Agriculture & Cooperation and Farmers Welfare, 2021). Lifeline India is a charitable organization working to provide telephone-based information services to cater to the needs of farmers. Gyandoot is a project launched by the Madhya Pradesh government in 2000. The project strives to help the citizens to access government services by establishing rural cybercafes. It won the Stockholm Challenge Award in Best Public Service (IT) category in 2000 (Malhotra, 2018). The Fast, Reliable, Instant Efficient Network for Disbursement of Services (FRIENDS) is a project that has been launched by the state of Kerala to enable the citizens to pay taxes through digital methods. Sourkaryan and E-Seva is a project launched by the Andhra Pradesh government to enable the citizens to shift towards e-governance by promoting digital alternatives. Similarly, Lokamitra/Smart Project is a project launched by Himachal Pradesh to provide the citizens with easy access to government services.

Besides these government initiatives, non-governmental stakeholders like Azim Premji Foundation, Tata, Amul, Ogilvy and Mother India and Hindustan Unilever attempted to create projects that aimed to develop digital literacy at the community level (Singh, 2007). These efforts were successful only to a limited extent. Some of the ambitious projects, such as the Akash tablet project, were colossal failures (Bapna et al., 2020). At the end of the first decade, the internet connectivity rates in metropolitan cities soared to rates comparable to developed countries, while the connectivity rates in rural areas were still worse than some least developed countries (Singh, 2010). The game-changer initiative happened in 2016 with the launch of Jio, a commercial venture by India's biggest private company that used fourth-generation telecommunications technology to provide data services. The launch of Jio, which offered data services at prices hitherto unheard of in the Indian market, created a huge ripple effect that forced all the telecom companies to drop data services prices (Bhatia & Palepu, 2016). Various studies suggest that the launch of Jio had a massive effect in increasing internet access in India (Daga et al., 2018; Gupta et al., 2019; Jasrotia et al., 2016; Singh & Srivastava, 2018).

However, the sudden shift to digital learning because of the COVID-19 lockdown was not foreseen by the Ministry of Human Resource Development (MHRD) and the Department of Education. Even then, they have made several attempts to address the need for digital learning. The imposition of social distancing guidelines and regulations/restrictions in response to the COVID-19 pandemic has forced educational institutions to adopt remote learning strategies. A total of 320 million learners in India, about 250 million school-going students and the remaining higher education students had to depend on online education. Secondly, about 32 million children were out of school even before the pandemic. The pandemic and lockdown have affected 1.4 m migrant workers and others working in the unorganized sector (90% of India's population is engaged in disorganized work). The case study of Ho tribals in Jharkhand (Sharma, this volume) clearly illustrates the plight of tribal migrant workers in cities across India. The majority of them migrated because of high rates of school drop-out, economic distress, the death of primary breadwinners, overbearing medical expenses of ailing kin, and low-wage earnings.

These challenges might have an effect on SDG4: Quality Education. Extended school closures will result in a loss in human capital and diminished economic opportunities in the long run (World Economic Forum). Even the premier institutes like IIT, IIM, NITs, IIIT are facing problems to cope with online education because of lack of facilities. Even students from premier institutions like IIT face inadequate Internet connection and a lack of electronic devices back in their hometowns, which has kept the attendance rates in online classes to as low as 30%. The same problem persists with students of government schools in Delhi, where attendance ranges between 25 and 30% only.

The Ministry of Human Resource Development (MHRD) has taken a few initiatives to address the sudden online education requirements. It has reported a nearly five times rise in access to HRD Ministry's E-Learning platforms between March 23rd and 9 April 2020. The ministry is also promoting television and radio channels to help those who live in areas that do not have internet capabilities (Ministry of Education, 2020). In early April, the University Grants Commission constituted separate committees to examine changes in the academic calendar and promote online learning. The expert committee's recommendations and suggestions were deliberated, and detailed guidelines regarding online learning to the educational institutions were released on April 29th (UGC, 2020). Based on this assessment, the Union government insisted that online education was taking place across schools, colleges and universities despite the lockdown (Nagarajan, 2020).

Apart from these measures, the finance minister, Nirmala Sitharaman, announced the launch of the 'PM eVIDYA programme' in the special economic package in response to the pandemic. The PM eVIDYA project allowed the top 100 universities to start online courses by May 30th automatically. However, it is essential to note that PM eVidya is a rebranded version of the planned expenditure announced in the union budget for 2020–21. Furthermore, the government also launched DIKSHA, a platform set up to aid teachers in developing skills required for the successful delivery of e-learning. Swayam Prabha, a group of 32 channels, was also launched as part of an emergency response to schools' shutdown. Again, Swayam Prabha, even though announced as something new, was also a pre-existing platform. A noteworthy point here is that the government is trying to rebrand the already existing projects as an emergency response.

We can consider, for instance, the government of the state of Chhattisgarh in India's centre-east. It launched the Padhai Tuhar Dwar (Education at Your Doorstep) portal. The launch of the National Broadband Mission to provide broadband service to all villages in India by 2022 is a welcome step towards digital inclusion, but the need is to ensure last-mile connectivity and ownership of digital devices for accessing the content.

Gender and E-learning Accessibility

India has always been a traditionally patriarchal society. In the course of human history, all countries were patriarchal, but some patriarchal elements and practices are uniquely Indian. For example, India is infamous for patriarchal practices such as dowry, female infanticide, domestic violence and low levels of human development. The human development report, released by the United Nations Development Programme, focuses on inequalities and deprivations that go beyond income by measuring loss in human development due to the existing disparities. As per the UN Human Development Index (2019), India occupies the 129th rank among 189 countries surveyed. This is an abysmally low rank for a country that prides itself to be the greatest democracy in the world. However, it is not very surprising if we study the country's cultural history, which shows that the government was always discriminatory.

The aggression towards a woman's identity starts from birth itself. The practices such as sex-selective abortion and female infanticide are indicators of this aggression. The practice of female infanticide was first recorded in India during colonial rule in 1789 (Saravanan, 2002). The British government later enacted the Female Infanticide Prevention Act, 1870 (Act VIII of 1870), in an attempt to put an end to this gruesome practice. Female infanticide happens due to a host of reasons. The lower status of women, the existence of the dowry system, son preference and superstitions all contribute to female infanticide. This has improved with time but has persisted. For example, in the 1980s, new technologies like amniocentesis and ultrasonography, initially designed to detect congenital abnormalities of the foetus, were used to identify the sex of the foetus with the intention of aborting if it was a female foetus (Ansari, 2018). Again, the government had to adopt several legal provisions to prevent infanticide and sex-selective abortions. The Indian Penal Code has defined infanticide as murder. Sections 312–318 of IPC have the provisions required to deal with infanticide (IPC, 1860). Even though governments tried to ban the sex determination tests through a series of government circulars, the attempts were unsuccessful. In response, the Pre-natal Diagnostic Techniques (Regulation and Prevention of Misuse) Act was passed in 1994, making it illegal to conduct sex determination tests (Tandon & Sharma, 2006). Even with all these initiatives, 2011 census data shows the low sex ratio among the 0–6 years, there are only 919 female children for every 1000 male children. The worrying situation is that the female sex ratio is steadily decreasing for the last five decades.

Similarly, spousal violence or 'intimate partner violence' is yet another issue that India has to deal with. Domestic violence is most widely employed as an umbrella term to cover spousal and intimate partner violence. However, terminology-wise, 'domestic violence' is wide because the term can also encompass child, partner, elder, or any household member. International organizations prefer to use the term 'intimate partner violence' to pinpoint the issue. Intimate partner violence is a gendered issue in the sense that it primarily affects women. Although women can also be violent in a relationship, the most common perpetrators of violence against women are male intimate partners (WHO, 2012).

In India, the issue of domestic violence and dowry deaths was widespread in 1980s following the media coverage of dowry deaths and localized protests against these deaths. The wide prevalence of dowry deaths triggered a public chain reaction that acted as a catalyst for the formation of many new women's organizations and led to discovering different forms of violence on women (Gandhi & Shah, 1992). In October 2006, another act named 'Protection of Women from Domestic Violence Act 2005' was enacted by the Parliament of India. This act defines domestic violence and is comprehensive in nature since it is not restricted to physical violence alone. It also includes other forms of violence, including sexual, emotional, verbal and economic abuse. This act is civil and further acknowledges the importance of collaboration between the government and external organizations in protecting women.

Even despite all these laws, domestic violence persists. National Family Health Survey (NFHS-4) statistics show that 30% of women have experienced physical violence from the age of 15. Among them, 6% have even experienced sexual violence in their lifetime. As for spousal violence, 33% experienced sexual violence in their lifetime, with physical violence being the most prevalent. Among all these victims, only 14% sought help to stop the violence (NHFS-4, 2016). However, even now, domestic violence forms the top category of violence committed against women (NCRB, 2018). These dowry deaths, movements against them and their impacts are covered in the case study section of the gender methodology. In 2018, 12,826 cases were registered under the dowry prohibition act alone. Furthermore, 7166 cases of dowry deaths were reported to police in the same year (NCRB, 2018). From the statistics, it is evident that domestic violence and dowry systems are still prevalent in our country.

India is a highly gender unequal society. If we observe the Gender Development Index (GDI), Gender Empowerment Measures and Gender Inequality Index (GII), it becomes very clear. The data shows that in the case of GDI for the male, it is 0.699 whereas, for the female, it is only 0.573. The index clearly shows the mean years of school for females, and the estimated per capita GNI for females are very less compared to male (Dhawan, 2020). Even the GII value for India is only 0.488, and India ranks 123 out of 164 nations. The index shows that the labour participation of female members is only 20.5% compared to 76.1% for males. Even the reproductive indicators also show the deplorable condition of women (Dhawan, 2020).

Even though we claim that the HDI performance of India is low because one-quarter of our population is living below the poverty line. However, the GDI for female, GEM and GII clearly indicated that there is a clear-cut gender differential in the outcomes. This is not only because of poverty, but it is majorly because of the patriarchy and the reduced participation of women in the social, economic, cultural and political spheres. In the social spheres, a girl child is not preferred, which leads to female foeticide and female infanticide (Tandon & Sharma, 2006). If we observe in the areas of education, women's literacy rate is only 65.5% whereas the male literacy rate is 82.2%. This clearly shows a gender gap of 17% points. This is mainly because of the low priority given to female education in the households. The health indicators clearly show that the reproductive health of women is very low. In the case of economic indicators, as I have mentioned above, the female labour participation and their per capita income is very less compared to their male counterparts.

To address these problems, a change in the policymaking and specific measures for their development are required. For this, the participation of women in the political sphere is very much important. In India, women are still not allowed to go outside the home freely, and they have to be always accompanied by a male member. The restriction starts at a very young age, which creates a dependency among them in all aspects which curtails their freedom and participation (Diwakar et al., 2018). This is very much visible even in the women's participation in the parliament. Their participation is only 13.5%. It clearly shows the multiple manifestations of the deprivation and subjugation of women.

Considering the given situation, if a new model of the education system—digital education—comes as an alternative to the regular/conventional method, it will affect the girl children in its way. The implication of digital education on gender can be observed through the 'digital gender divide'. The term 'digital gender divide' is used to denote the types of gender differences in resources and capabilities to access and effectively utilize ICTs within and between countries, regions, sectors and socio-economic groups (Borgonovi et al., 2018). The digital gender divide is caused by several factors such as lack of technological literacy, affordability and hurdles to access arising out of inherent biases and socio-cultural norms (Borgonovi et al., 2018). Denying equal access to technology and internet usage based on one's gender would exacerbate the existing inequalities and lead to the deterioration of advancements we made in the gender category.

As per NSSO (2017–2018) data, within the 37% of urban dwellers who can use the internet, 43.5% are males while only 30.1% are females. Similarly, within the 13% of rural dwellers who can use the internet, 17.1% are males while only 8.5% are females. This shows that besides regional disparity, gender-based disparity also exists within the digital divide.

Globally, girls are less likely to go online in low connectivity countries (UNICEF, 2017). We have to also consider that in households where only one device is available for educational purposes, there may be a chance of prioritizing the male child's education, which will further marginalize girl children.

Even if female students have access to online classes, they may not be able to attend the classes due to the unequal distribution of work at home. Also, we have to consider that women using mobile phones is often viewed with suspicion and is considered taboo (Singh, 2010).

A Framework to Understand the Digital Divide in India

Understanding the digital divide in education and how it affects society's various sections is very much required in this present situation. Willfully or forcefully, all students across the globe have moved towards digital education. There are specific prerequisites required for effective digital education. Considering the class, caste, geographical location and gender divide in the countries, the accessibility and the availability of those prerequisites such as electricity, smartphone, laptop, internet connection and connectivity are not uniform to all the people.

The existing inequality in society directly impacts the accessibility and availability of prerequisites like electricity, smartphone, laptop, internet connection and connectivity. This inequality has resulted in various consequences for the different sections of society. Realizing this inequality and its implications is very crucial to address this issue effectively.

The conceptual framework clearly shows that COVID-19 has further exacerbated the existing inequality in society and access to online education. Some of the issues which were observed in accessing online digital education were lack of infrastructure facilities like internet connectivity to attend the online class without any disruption, lack of technology necessary for attending classes, lack of money for internet connection fees and inability to follow the online classes. Even though these problems persist for most Indian students at varying levels, students from economically and socially backward sections are disproportionately affected. This inequality translates into increased psychological pressure on marginalized students and contributes to the extreme decision, borne out of helplessness, to commit suicide. In those cases, there is a clear relationship between student's suicide and the broader socio-economic disparities. Therefore, administrative and institutional policy measures are required to address this issue.

Methodology

The studies which are available to understand the digital divide and the increasing vulnerability among students during COVID-19 pandemic mainly look at the issues of access and lack of skills to attend online classes. There are no studies available on student suicide and the examination of the correlating factors associated with those suicides. Therefore, this study is exploratory in nature and unveils the factors contributing to the increasing vulnerability among students and its consequences. The study uses the qualitative method, and for this purpose, 11 case studies of the students who committed suicide during COVID-19 are taken for analysis. Content analysis is carried out to analyse the case studies.

Case Studies of Student Suicides

Across India, 11 students have committed suicide. The incident of suicide has taken place even in the most literate states, states with better educational infrastructure facilities and economically well-developed states. Therefore, it becomes pertinent to analyse the factors contributing to these suicides.

Case number	Name, age and gender	Demographic details	Reason for suicide	Occupation and economic status
Case 1	Devika Balakrishnan, a Dalit girl, class X student	Mankeri village near Valanchery, Malappuram district	She was upset that she could not afford to attend the online classes as she was not having smartphone- June 2	Daily wage labour
Case 2	Aishwarya, a student of Lady Shri Ram College for Women in Delhi,	Telangana	Her scholarship was stopped in March. She wanted to purchase the used laptop to attend the online lab class—November 3	Daily wage labour
Case 3	Nityashree Second-year BSc nursing student	Ulundurpet in Tamil Nadu	After having arguments over sharing the single phone between 3 siblings and unable to handle the pressure of not properly continuing the classes	Agriculture labour
Case 4	Shabini Kumari Sau 16-year-old girl, grade 10 student	Nischinda area of Howrah district of West Bengal	Committed suicide on June 18 after failing to attend online classes due to the absence of a computer or a smartphone	Truck Driver
Case 5	Sakshi Abasaheb Pol 15-year-old girl	Karad town in Maharashtra's Satara district	she did not have a smartphone to attend online classes- September 23	Daily wage labourer
Case 6	Jayanti Bauli 20-year-old college-going girl student	West Bengal's Jalpaiguri district	Hung herself	Daily wage labourer

(continued)

(continued)

Case number	Name, age and gender	Demographic details	Reason for suicide	Occupation and economic status
Case 7	Kushi, 12-year-old schoolgirl	Rajkot District, Gujarat	Committed suicide after being frustrated with online classes and homework	Mechanic (daily wage)
Case 8	Vikrapandi Class 11 student	Theni district in Tamil Nadu	Committed suicide after failing to cope with the pressure of online lessons	Not available
Case 9	Harishma 17-year-old student, 12th student	Pudhukottai district in Tamil Nadu	Committed suicide after her NEET entrance exam hall ticket did not arrive September	Daily wage labourer
Case 10	Harendra Singh Gurjar A class 10 male student	Madhya Pradesh	Lack of money to pay school fees	Daily wage labourer
Case 11	Vignesh, male student	Elanthankuzhi in Ariyalur, Tamil Nadu	The Supreme Court dismissed the petition to postpone the NEET exam amid the COVID-19 pandemic	Not available

Analysis of Case Studies

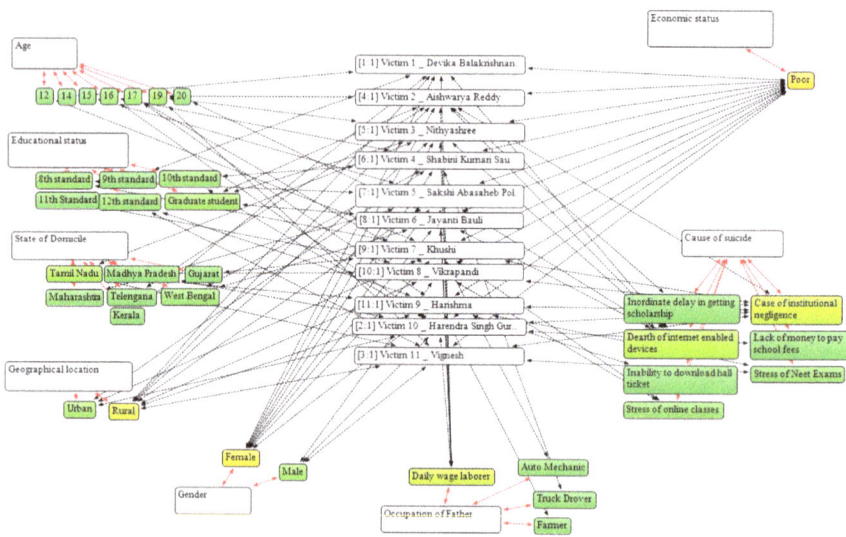

Age

The analysis shows that the age of the victims is between 12 and 20 years. The findings indicate that 8 of the students who have committed suicide are school-going students and only 3 are college-going students. Even among the school-going students, the majority of them (7 students) are in 10th, 11th and 12th, and they have to face public examination this year. Therefore, they are under a lot of psychological pressure to attend classes regularly and perform better. Three students are college-going students and have higher aspirations to do something better in their life.

Gender

About 8 of the students who committed suicide are females and only 3 are male students. The review clearly indicates the girl child has a double burden, as they have to take care of the household chores and do the regular class activities. COVID-19 has increased the household work of the girl child as they are staying at home and attending online classes. They cannot concentrate on studies, which affects their academic performance (Bhattacharya, 2020). The data on rural suicides shows that more females are committing suicide below the age group of 30 years whereas above the age group of 30 years, the suicide is more among males (Rane & Nadkarni, 2014). Even the recent Harvard study shows that increasing educational possibilities for women, matched with the burden of traditional patriarchal expectations, also contribute to higher rates of female suicide in India (Smith, 2018).

Economic Status

The finding shows that among the students who have committed suicide, all of them are from economically and socially backward sections. Because of their poor financial condition, their parents could not afford to purchase a smartphone or laptop, and had no money to spend on internet recharge. Though other infrastructural factors like poor internet connectivity were there, that was a common problem faced by all the students irrespective of their economic condition.

Occupation of Father

Apart from one case where the father's occupation (breadwinner) is not spelt out, all other students' fathers who have committed suicide are daily wage labourers. Mostly, they worked as an auto mechanic, truck driver and agriculture worker. Three of the families did not have any job during that time because of lockdown, and they had encountered a severe financial crisis.

Geographical Location

With regard to the geographical location of these cases, three are from urban settings and seven are from the rural settings. However, the geographical location of one case is unknown. As we all know that the poor economic condition and poor infrastructure is common feature of rural India, the students in rural areas have to face more burden of digital education. The SRS (2019) data shows that the mortality rate is more in rural areas than the urban areas, 5.3 and 6.8 respectively. The major contributing factors for rural suicide are low socio-economic condition, mental illness related to alcoholism and interpersonal difficulties (Rane & Nadkarni, 2014).

State of Domicile

Cases were reported in (one each) Maharashtra, Madhya Pradesh, Gujarat, Kerala, Telangana, two from West Bengal, four from Tamil Nadu.

Causes of Suicide

From the analysis, it is evident that one of the major factors that contributed to the students' suicide is their poor economic condition. However, there are also few contributory factors observed among students who committed suicide. They are cases of intuitional negligence (6), a dearth of internet-enabled devices (5), an inability to pay fees (1), and inordinate delay in getting fellowships (1). Apart from these reasons, online education also forced the students to commit suicide because of educational stress and pressure. The reasons expressed by the family were the Stress of online exams (1) and the Stress of NEET Exams (2).

Cases of Institutional Negligence

Upon studying the case, it can be noticed that some of the victims have tried to seek help before they committed suicide. Victim 1, Devika, tried to communicate and share her distress with her family and some teachers. Although the family and teachers were not harsh to her concern, they could not sufficiently pacify her or give her mental support that would have to give her the courage to go on. Victim 2, Aishwarya, contacted her university and UGC office for seeking information about her fellowship status. She did not receive any help or words of comfort from either party. Victim 7 and victim 8, Kushi and Vikrapandi, both communicated that they were stressed about the online classes but did not get any kind of help from family. Here, families cannot be solely blamed as they were unsure about what they need to do, and we also need to consider that they were also going through their problems amid the COVID-19 crisis. Victim 9, Harishma, sought help from her school authorities to download her misplaced NEET hall ticket, but she got a dissentient response. These cases show that our institutions, both educational and family institutions, could not handle such difficult circumstances. Educational institutions, ideally, should have mechanisms that can help their stakeholders when they are in distress.

Other Observable Patterns

The investigation reveals that the relatives of the victims have noticed that the victims are displaying symptoms of depression because of the difficulties they have faced due to online classes. However, they were unable to do anything to address the problem and they were also not aware of the counselling support required to relieve their psychological stress. A majority of the victims are from socially backward communities. Devika, the child victim from Kerala, belongs to the Dalit community. Kerala has a high human development index and standard of living, yet this case reveals the backwardness of the Dalit community in the state. Similarly, other victims are from socially backward communities. This shows the vulnerability of the students who belong to backward communities.

Discussion

In India, inequality exists on the basis of class (Borooah et al., 2015; Vaid, 2014), caste (Thorat et al., 2010; Nambissan, 1996), gender (Borgonovi et al., 2018; Diwakar et al., 2018) and religion (Ziyauddin, this volume), tribal ethnicity (Sharma, this volume), geographical location (Singh, 2010). Even in the case of education, this has a direct bearing on the accessibility, affordability and utilization of education facilities. The students who are getting better access, and who could afford and utilize the services better have shown better education outcomes. On the other hand, the other students who could not get access and afford the facilities have lagged behind. Individual and group identity of a person has an important role in determining the education outcomes such as literacy rate, retention, completion and higher studies (Diwakar & Neathravathi, 2014).

Considering this given situation, if the country is suddenly shifting to digital education, it will further magnify the existing inequality in the education outcome. Because of the existing digital divide in the country on the basis of urban–rural, male–female, rich–poor, low socio/religious groups–high socio/religious groups, low caste–high caste, it will create differential outcomes. The people who have access to digital resources will reap more benefits and the rest will get sidelined.

To address the issue of the digital divide in India, a multi-pronged approach is required. Firstly, the country needs to address the problem of digital infrastructure. People should have access to the internet with adequate speed and bandwidth. Though it has been achieved to some extent in the metropolitan cities, however, in the smaller cities, towns and rural areas, it is a distant dream. Along with the internet connection, internet-enabled devices to utilize it properly are also very much needed. The NSSO 75th round clearly illustrates the existing gap in internet access and the availability of computers (internet-enabled devices). In a vast country like India, this is easier said than done. The government must realize the importance of addressing the digital divide and the grave complications that it will cause if the country fails to do so.

Keeping this in mind, the government should take steps to ensure that all students have access to an internet-enabled device.

Though there is no programme currently at the national level to provide free or affordable laptops to the economically weaker section. However, states like Tamil Nadu and Kerala are providing free laptops to the students, and it is a way forward to ensure access to the internet and reduce the digital gap. In the case of Tamil Nadu, it is provided to 10th and 12th passed students belonging to Scheduled Caste, Scheduled Tribe and Economically weaker sections (Govt of TN, https://it.tn.gov.in/). In Kerala, the meritorious students of Scheduled Caste, Scheduled Tribe and OBC students who have passed 12th standard or pursuing professional studies get laptops. Similarly, the government of India introduced the project Akash tablet in 2009 and later revived it in 2012, which aimed to put internet-enabled devices in learners' hands from disadvantaged social segments, at a lower price. Because of a lack of clear objective, unreliable software and poor-quality devices (short-lived), the project failed, so it was discontinued in 2015 (Bapna et al., 2020). However, a project of this nature with a much clear objective, good quality and properly targeting the beneficiary at the national level is required to address the digital divide. Ensuring devices is only the first step, but assuring that adequate connection facilities are available at affordable prices is equally important. Ensuring connectivity can be accomplished if the government institutions, both central, state and local, work together with internet providers in the private and public sectors. The affordability of internet plans is also a significant issue among poor households. To counter this, prepaid internet packages should be provided to families. The data allotment should be based on the household members and the expected data usage, it can be addressed by taking account of their nature of work and the education status of the children. Along with this, the tariff of these plans should be subsidized by the government.

Secondly, to address the issues of the digital gender divide, the cultural and social factors which hamper their participation should be addressed. There is a need for attitudinal change among the parents and other family members. Still, they are bound by the patriarchal norms and gender stereotypes which act as barriers to girls and women's full participation in the digital world. The inherent biases that prohibit women from accessing technologies and gender norms and gender roles that limit their usage need to be addressed. The parents and the family members should be sensitized, and girl child/women should get equal opportunity to use smartphones, laptop and internet-enabled devices. Teachers should also be sensitized on the existing gender stereotypes and they should be more considerate towards female students. They should have regular interaction with students and provide required psychosocial support to the students in need, especially to the female students.

Thirdly, the education institutions should be aware of the grave digital divide which exists in society, consciously or unconsciously they should not put further stress on the students who do not have the internet-enabled devices. Not having the means to be part of ICT-enabled education is not the problem of the student. Instead of putting the entire blame on the students, Institutions should, instead, be advised to strive to find solutions. Educational institutions can work with local governments and Parent–Teacher Associations to bridge this digital divide. It is important to create awareness among the parents and teachers not to stress the students who are facing the public examination. Both parents and teachers should regularly observe them, and they should be more responsive and supportive. In addition, if they need any psychological support, it should be immediately provided. Service from professional social workers could also be mobilized for this purpose.

The vital thing to keep in mind is that the COVID-19 crisis is affecting all strata of society, but the most affected ones are those who are the most marginalized. We need to understand that the COVID-19 crisis and the digital divide are affecting the multiple marginalized sections. Only those solutions which realize this intersection of inequalities can make meaningful changes. A bottom-up approach that prioritizes the needs of the marginalized should be the way to move forward.

References

Ambedkar, B. R. (1968). *Annihilation of caste with a reply to Mahatma Gandhi*. Bheem Patrika Publications.

Ansari, S. N. (2018). Born to die. Female infanticide and Feticide: An analysis of India. *International Journal of Social Science and Economic Research*.

Bansode, S., & Patil, S. (2011). Bridging digital divide in India: Some initiatives. *Asia Pacific Journal of Library and Information Science, 1*, 58–68.

Bapna, A., Garg, K., & Mehra, A. (2020). Digital divide and the Aakash tablet: Technology intervention in education. *Economic and Political Weekly, 55*(10), 27–34.

Bhatia, J., & Palepu, A. R. (2016). Reliance jio: Predatory pricing or predatory behaviour? *Economic and Political Weekly*. Retrieved January 12, 2021, from https://www.epw.in/journal/2016/39/web-exclusives/reliance-jio-predatory-pricing-or-predatory-behaviour.html.

Bhattacharya, S. (2020). What is so wrong with online teaching. *Economic and Political Weekly, 55*(23), 19–21.

Borgonovi, F., Centurelli, R., Dernis, H., Grundke, R., Horvát, P., Jamet, S., Keese, M., Liebender, A.-S., Marcolin, L., Rosenfeld, D., & Squicciarini, M. (2018). *Bridging the Digital Gender Divide* (pp. 1–151). Retrieved January 13, 2021, from https://www.oecd.org/digital/bridging-the-digital-gender-divide.pdf.

Borooah, V. K., Diwakar, D., Mishra, V. K., Naik, A. K., & Sabharwal, N. S. (2014). Caste, inequality, and poverty in India: a re-assessment. *Development Studies Research, 1*(1), 279–294. https://doi.org/10.1080/21665095.2014.967877.

National Crime Records Bureau. (2018). *Crime in India*.

IPC. (1860). Chapter XVI (312–318) of IPC—Of the causing of miscarriage, of injuries to unborn children, of the exposure of infants, and of the concealment of births.

Choudhury, D. R. (2020). The evolution of marriage from strictly arranged to semi-arranged. *The Indian Express*. Retrieved May 15, 2021, from https://indianexpress.com/article/lifestyle/feelings/matchmaking-india-semi-arranged-marriage-parents-6533072/.

Compaine, B. M. (2001). *The digital divide: Facing a crisis or creating a myth?* The MIT Press. Retrieved January 12, 2021, from https://doi.org/10.7551/mitpress/2419.001.0001.

Daga, T., Chandra, V., & Malik, A. (2018). Effect of reliance jio on digital India. *International Journal of Advanced Research, 6*(6), 395–401. https://doi.org/10.21474/ijar01/7224

Department of Agriculture & Cooperation and Farmers Welfare, 2021 About KCC. (2021). Department of Agriculture & Cooperation and Farmers Welfare. https://mkisan.gov.in/aboutkcc.aspx

Dhawan. Bulbul (2020). India ranks 131 on human development index 2020: All you need to know. Retrieved February 12, 2021, from https://www.financialexpress.com/lifestyle/health/india-ranks-131-on-human-development-index-2020-all-you-need-to-know/2155827/.

Van Dijk, J. A. G. M., & Hacker, K. (2003). The digital divide as a complex and dynamic phenomenon. *The Information Society, 19*(4), 315–326. Retrieved January 15, 2021, from https://doi.org/10.1080/01972240309487.

Van Dijk, J. A. G. M.(2017). Digital divide: Impact of access. *The international encyclopedia of media effects.* Wiley. https://doi.org/10.1002/9781118783764.wbieme0043.

Van Dijk, J. A. G. M. (2020). *The digital divide.* Wiley. Retrieved January 12, 2021, from https://books.google.co.in/books?id=6DvKDwAAQBAJ.

Diwakar, D. G., & Mishra.V.K., & Acharya S.S. (2018). Reproductive and sexual health education: Addressing challenges of physiological changes among adolescents. *Indian Anthropologist, 48*(1), 13–30.

Diwakar, D. G., & Neathravathi. (2014). Caste and education exclusion among the scheduled caste in India: A case study of Tamil Nadu. In R. Kumar & N. Kumar (Eds.), *Elementary education in India* (pp. 186–200). Atlantic Press.

Enoch, Y., & Soker, Z. (2006). Age, gender, ethnicity and the digital divide: University students' use of web-based instruction. *Open Learning: The Journal of Open, Distance and e-Learning, 21*(2), 99–110. Retrieved January 12, 2021https://doi.org/10.1080/02680510600713045.

National Telecommunications and Information Administration. (1995). *Falling through the net: A survey of the "have nots" in rural and Urban America.* U.S. Department of Commerce. Retrieved January 12, 2021, from https://books.google.co.in/books?id=gvhSvgAACAAJ.

Fletcher, A., Simon, G., & Adele. (2000). *OFT study on e-commerce and competition.* Retrieved May 15, 2021, from http://www.out-law.com/page-954.

Fong, M. W. L. (2009). Digital Divide Between Urban and Rural Regions in China. *The Electronic Journal of Information Systems in Developing Countries, 36*(1), 1–12. https://doi.org/10.1002/j.1681-4835.2009.tb00253.x.

Gandhi, N., & Shah, N. (1992). *The issues at stake: Theory and practice in the contemporary women's movement in India.* South Asia Books

Government of Tamil Nadu (n.d). Student free laptop. *Information technology department.* https://it.tn.gov.in/index.php/en/ELCOT/Student_Free_Laptop.

Gupta, A., Raghav, K., & Dhakad, P. (2019). The effect on the telecom industry and consumers after the introduction of reliance jio. *International Journal of Engineering and Management Research, 9*(3), 118–137. https://doi.org/10.31033/ijemr.9.3.16.

Hanimann, T., & Ruedin, E. (2007). *Digitale Gräben oder Digitale Brücken?—Chancen und Risiken für Schwellenländer.*

ITU (International Telecommunications Union). (2019). Measuring digital development. *Facts and figures 2020.* ITU Publications, 1–15. https://www.itu.int/myitu/-/media/Publications/2020-Publications/Measuring-digital-development-2019.pdf.

Jamanadas, K. (2000). Is gurukulam education suitable for Indians?. Retrieved May 15, 2021, from http://www.ambedkar.org/research/Is_Gurukula_Education_Suitable_For_India.htm.

Jasrotia, S. S., Sharma, R. L., & Mishra, H. G. (2016). Disruptions in Indian telecom sector : A qualitative study on reliance jio. *The Indore Management Journal, 37*–45.

Kos-Łabędowicz, J. (2017). The issue of digital divide in rural areas of the European Union. *Ekonomiczne Problemy Usług, 1*(126/2), 195–204. https://doi.org/10.18276/epu.2017.126/2-20

Lohr, S. (1996). A nation ponders its growing digital divide. *The Newyork Times.* Retrieved Jan 12, 2021, from https://www.nytimes.com/1996/10/21/business/a-nation-ponders-its-growing-digital-divide.html.

Malhotra, R. (2018). Gyandoot: E-Governance Project in India. *Medium.* https://medium.com/%40rridhee/gyandoot-e-governance-project-in-india-9664acf38e9d.

Ministry of Education. (2020). *Digital learning sees a big upsurge during COVID-19 lockdown period. Nearly five times rise in access to HRD Ministry ' s e-learning platforms Union. HRD* minister urges learners to also make use of educational TV channels like SWAYAM PRABHA and GYAN DAR (Issue April).

Nagarajan, A. (2020). Online illusion. *Frontline*. Retrieved Nov 15, 2020, from https://frontline.the hindu.com/cover-story/article31739849.ece.

Nambissan, G. B. (1996). Equity in education: Schooling of dalit children in India. *Economic and Political Weekly* (pp. 1101–24).

Nambissan, G. B. (2010). Exclusion and discrimination in schools: Experiences of dalit children. In S. K. Thorat, & S. N. Katherine (Eds.), *Blocked by caste: Economic discrimination in modern India* (pp. 253–286), Oxford University Press.

National Statistic office. (2020). Household social consumption on education in India. *Government of India, ministry of statistics and programme implementation*. Retrieved November 15, 2020, www.mospi.gov.

National Statistical Office. (2017). *Key Indicators of household social consumption on education in India report*.

Nishida, T., Pick, J. B., & Sarkar, A. (2014). Japan's prefectural digital divide: A multivariate and spatial analysis. *Telecommunications Policy, 38*(11), 992–1010. https://doi.org/10.1016/j.telpol. 2014.05.004.Accessedon15thMay2021

Panda, M. I., Chhatar, D. C., & Mharana, B. (2013). A brief view to digital divide in Indian scenario. *International Journal of Scientific and Research Publications, 3*(12), 1–7.

Perrin, A. (2019). Digital gap between rural and nonrural America persists. *Nonrural*. Retrieved May 15, 2021, from https://www.pewresearch.org/fact-tank/2019/05/31/digital-gap-between-rur aland-america-persists/.

Philip, L., Cottrill, C., Farrington, J., Williams, F., & Ashmore, Fiona. (2017). The digital divide: Patterns, policy and scenarios for connecting the 'final few' in rural communities across Great Britain. *Journal of Rural Studies, 54*, 386–398.https://doi.org/10.1016/j.jrurstud.2016.12.002

Pramod, M. (2020). As a dalit women. *CASTE/A Global Journal on Social Exclusion, 1*(1), 111–124. https://doi.org/10.26812/caste.v1i1.69.

Rajasekharan, I. (2017). How dalit lands were stolen. *Frontline*. Retrieved May 15, 2021, from https://frontline.thehindu.com/social-issues/social-justice/how-dalit-lands-were-stolen/art icle23595691.ece.

Rane, A., & Nadkarni, A. (2014). Suicide in India: A systematic review. *Shanghai Archives of Psychiatry, 26*(2), 69–80.

Reddy, B. A., Jose, S., & Vaidehi, R. (2020). Of access and inclusivity digital divide in online education. *Economic and Political Weekly, 55*(36), 23–26.

Sahni, U. (2020). COVID-19 in India: Education disrupted and lessons learned. *Education plus development*. Retrieved January 12, 2021, from https://www.brookings.edu/blog/education-plus-development/2020/05/14/COVID-19--in-india-education-disrupted-and-lessons-learned/.

Saravanan, S. (2002). Female infanticide in India: A review of literature. *Social Change, 32*(1–2), 58–66. https://doi.org/10.1177/004908570203200205

Servon, L. J. (2002). Bridging the digital divide: Technology, community and public policy. Wiley. https://doi.org/10.1002/9780470773529.

Servon, L. J. (2008). *Bridging the bigital divide: Technology*. Community and Public Policy.

Singh, S. (2010). Digital divide in India: Measurement, determinants and policy for addressing the challenges in bridging the digital divide. *International Journal of Innovation in the Digital Economy, 1*(2), 1–24. https://doi.org/10.4018/jide.2010040101

Singh, R., & Srivastava, A. (2018). Impact of reliance jio on telecom industry of India. *International Journal of Research, 6*(6), 91–95.

Singh, N. (2007). *Bridging the digital divide in India: Some challenges and opportunities*. World Libraries. Retrieved January 11, 2021, from https://worldlibraries.dom.edu/index.php/worldlib/article/view/37/71.

Sipre, Y. S., & Malik, M. (2017). Bridging digital divide in India: Some factors and initiatives. *International Journal of Digital Library Services, 7*(2).

Smith, Dana G. (2018). *More than a third of female suicides are committed by Indian women—Scientific American.*

Srinuan, C., & Bohlin, E. (2011). Understanding the digital divide: A literature surveyand ways forward. In *22nd European Regional Conference of the International Telecommunications Society (ITS): "Innovative ICT Applications—Emerging Regulatory, Economic and Policy Issues."* Retrieved Nov 15, 2020, from http://hdl.handle.net/10419/52191.

SRS (2019). *SRS Bulletin, Office of the Registrar of India, 52*(1), 1–9.Retrieved May 15, 2021, from https://censusindia.gov.in/vital_statistics/SRS_Bulletins/SRS_Bulletin-Rate-2017-_May_2019.pdf.

International institute for population sciences. (2016). *National Family Health Survey (NFHS-4).* Retrieved April 16, 2021, from http://rchiips.org/nfhs/NFHS-4Reports/India.pdf.

Tandon, S., & Sharma, R. (2006). Female foeticide and infanticide in India: An analysis of crimes against girl children. *International Journal of Criminal Justice Sciences, 1*(1), 1–10.

National Telecommunications and Informations Administraion. (1998). *Falling through the net II: New data on the digital divide.*

The World Bank. (2016). *World development report 2016: Digital dividends.* The World Bank.

Thorat, S. K., Katherine, S., & Newman,. (2010). *Blocked by caste: Economic discrimination in Modern India.* Oxford University Press.

National Telecommunications and Information Administration. (1999). *Falling through the net: Defining the digital divide : a report on the telecommunications and information technology gap in America.* U.S. Department of Commerce. Retrieved January 12, 2021, from https://books.goo gle.co.in/books?id=QGO1MQEACAAJ.

UNCTAD. (2019). *Digital Economy Report 2019 : Value creation and capture—implications for developing countries.* United Nations Conference on Trade and Development.

UNICEF. (2017). *State of the Worlds Children 2017 - Children in a Digital World.* In Unicef. https://www.unicef.org/publications/index_101992.html.

UNICEF. (2020). *COVID-19–19: Are children able to continue learning during school closures? Unicef.* Retrieved November 15, 2020, from https://data.unicef.org/resources/remote-learning-reachability-factsheet.

United Nations Development Programme. (2019). *Human development report 2019 beyond income, beyond averages, beyond today .* Retrieved April 16, 2021, from http://hdr.undp.org/sites/default/files/hdr_2019_overview_-_english.pdf.

University Grants Commission. (2020). *Press Release regarding Examinations and Academic Calendar.* Retrieved November 15, 2020, from https://www.google.com/url?sa=t&rct=j&q=&esrc=s&source=web&cd=&ved=2ahUKEwjS2vCOz5LtAhU8_XMBHY3pBAkQFjACegQ IBRAC&url=https%3A%2F%2Fwww.ugc.ac.in%2Fpdfnews%2F6765580_Press-Release-reg arding-Examinations-and-Academic-Calendar-pdf.pdf&usg=AOvVaw1q68meRNdZ6OjMlgTT xjCl.

Vaid, D. (2012). The caste-class association in India: An empirical analysis. *Asian Survey, 52*(2), 395–422.

Vaid, D. (2014). Caste in contemporary India: Flexibility and persistence. *Annual Review of Sociology, 40*, 391–410. https://doi.org/10.1146/annurev-soc-071913-043303.

Van Dijk, J. A. G. M. (2005). *The network society.* In SAGE Publications.F.

Van Dijk, J. A. G. M., & Van Deursen, A. J. A. M. (2014). *Digital skills: Unlocking the information society.* Palgrave Macmillan.

Vicente, M. R., & López, A. J. (2011). Assessing the regional digital divide across the European Union-27. *Telecommunications Policy, 35*(3), 220–237. https://doi.org/10.1016/j.telpol.2010.12.013

Warschauer, M. (2003). Technology and social inclusion: Rethinking the digital divide. MIT Press.

WHO (2012). *Understanding and addressing violence against women.* Retrieved May 19, 2021, from http://apps.who.int/iris/bitstream/handle/10665/77432/WHO_RHR_12.36_eng.pdf; jsessionid=6E61DE1223891C42926503023068FF1F?sequence=1.

Chapter 7
Segregation of Muslims: A Reflection on Urban Living Environments and Infrastructure Conditions in Hyderabad

K. M. Ziyauddin

Abstract The recent decades have seen how Indian Muslims have been pushed to the receiving end, and consequently, they have been referred to as a minority at the margin. The sphere of marginalization is not merely symbolic but also manifested by examining the socio-economic indicators to understand the life of Muslims today. With a few exceptions, Muslims can also perform well if their living environment and infrastructure are improved. The paper examines the multitudes of discrimination being faced in the everyday life of the Muslim community, and the misery increases day by day with the kind of residential segregation that cities witness today. The gravity of the problem is examined by focusing on the availability of basic amenities and infrastructure in Muslim concentrated areas in the city of Hyderabad and Sangareddy Town Telangana. A sizeable Muslim population lives in Hyderabad and Sangareddy towns, comprising around 35–40% of the total population. Both the towns offer interesting cases of 'urban deprivation', and more specifically, 'multiple deprivations'. Given continuous segregation and exclusion of Muslims, the paper also finds an interesting fact that how reservation given to Muslims in the state has proved to be a boon to the Muslim community that has been reflected in the empirical data in the area of employment and educational attainment. This paper also analyses the needs of people and how the outreach of these policies can be further improved and expanded to include vulnerable Muslim groups.

Keywords Muslim minority · Hyderabad · Segregation · Reservation · Discrimination

Introduction

The recent years have seen how the Muslims of Hyderabad are being pushed to extreme marginalization. With a few exceptions, Muslims can also perform well if

K. M. Ziyauddin (✉)
Department of Sociology, School of Arts and Social Sciences, Maulana Azad National Urdu University (MANUU), Hyderabad, Telangana, India

© The Author(s), under exclusive license to Springer Nature Singapore Pte Ltd. 2022   127
S. S. Acharya and S. Christopher (eds.), *Caste, COVID-19, and Inequalities of Care*,
People, Cultures and Societies: Exploring and Documenting Diversities,
https://doi.org/10.1007/978-981-16-6917-0_7

their living conditions are improved. The paper, however, does not examine deeply the multiplicity of discrimination experienced and suffered by Muslims in everyday life of the Muslim community. The gravity of the problem is examined at the back-drop of basic amenities and infrastructure available and accessible to such marginal-ized Muslims inhabiting the aforesaid locale described above. Apart from Srinagar in Kashmir, Hyderabad, the capital of Telangana, has the highest Muslim popula-tion (43.45) amongst other Indian cities, as per the report of the Social Develop-ment Report of Telangana, 2017. Moreover, Sangareddy, the district headquarters of Medak, having the second-highest Muslim population (35%), is also considered for analysis. Hyderabad, particularly the old city, offers an interesting case of urban depri-vation and, especially multiple deprivations, a notion which refers not only to a lack of infrastructure and facilities but also to poor education and training, low income, poor diet and unhygienic conditions leading to poor life chances (Max Weber) and capability approach (Sen, 1999). The fieldwork was based on the survey and subse-quent interviews across the locale, and the survey results powerfully revealed the layers of state-sponsored deprivations concerning Muslims. The available facts and figures concerning basic amenities and facilities available in Muslim communities, the paper presents its perspectives regarding a complex matrix of human development and the theoretical schemes available.

Segregation as Process and Reality

This paper begins with the Sachar Committee Report (2006) observation that the most scientific way of assessing the quality of life and living environment is by examining the access and availability of residential options or choices for any socio-religious communities in a given locale region, or state in general. 'In determining access (or lack of it) to infrastructure, three broad dimensions of social and physical infrastructure have to be taken into account—"presence", "access" and "utilization". Access also depends upon the place of residence. […] Lack of access can emerge either due to the absence of social and/or physical infrastructure or through inacces-sibility to such facilities of SRCs even when they are present' (Sachar Committee Report, 2006: 139–140).

On a few occasions, the same report mentions how the differential existence of living environment and sanitation was reported in various cities of India. Hyderabad is a classic case of deprivation and under-development to the core that the old city shows apathy and negligence of the state machinery. In contrast, the new city Cyberabad competes with any world-class city to attract the multinational companies as their destination of investment. The field observations and interviews demonstrate a sharp division between Hyderabad and Cyberabad (both fall under Greater Hyderabad Municipal Corporation).

Compared to the Muslim majority pockets of Hyderabad, the less Muslim popu-lated areas have better sanitation, tap water supply, improved electrification, and connecting roads to each locality (*mohalla*) and drainage. In terms of economic background also, less Muslim populated areas at least show well-functioning school with a maximum strength of teachers including toilets with water facilities, improved quality of roads, working drainage system, availability of proper sanitation and sewage disposal, etc. whereas these facilities were almost negligible or minimal where Muslims were in the majority. Similar field stories emerge from the observation of slums where a high Muslim population has fewer amenities than the less Muslim populated slums in Hyderabad.

Segregation of Muslim communities also represents similar stories of underdevelopment and dearth of civic amenities in the urban pockets of Sangareddy town. In all focused group discussions, the data tells the ironic face of urban governance. Muslims with low political participation in urban governance, less education, and high dropout in higher education migrate to Gulf countries in search of employment and livelihood. The families and children stay back at home. The absence of good schooling adds to the drop out of children from school at a higher percentage. A contrasting picture emerges at the professional front. Multinational companies look for modern and skilled workers with new knowledge whereas the majority of the Muslim children do not get the education and training solicited and required in such companies which results in further frustration and feeling of deprivation.

Sangareddy is located close to the most developed new town near Hyderabad. Due to the high expansion of real estate and steep rise in the construction business, the cost of living in this town has increased, unlike ten years down the lane. In most FGDs at Muslim majority pockets, the attention of urban local bodies is found to be apathetic and continuous negligence is observed in attending any complaint related to sewerage blockage, improper garbage disposal, and mostly damaged road or no connecting roads for easy commutation. Women find it more difficult to travel to reach hospitals and markets citing that auto-rickshaws do not run into their lanes due to damaged roads or no roads. During emergencies, women have to risk safety and security during late hours in the evening and night to walk for longer distances. Public transport is negligible in Muslim populated areas. Hence, this increasing residential segregation, even in Sangareddy, only adds to the deprivation and exclusion of people living in those pockets (Ziyauddin, 2018). More importantly, impediments to access hospitals and healthcare get reduced in the absence of proper road connectivity and the deficiency of sanitation infrastructure and poor quality of care in government hospitals (Hathi & Srivastava, 2021, this volume) have added to the burden of poor Muslim families.

The priorities of the state government including the Millennium Development Goals (MDGs) have been considered in making infrastructure for water supply, sewerage, solid waste management, traffic and transportation, drainage and urban poverty. These are adversely impacting and affecting the lives of Muslims in Indian cities. The cases of Hyderabad and Sangareddy are the reflections of poor urban life of Muslim communities, having little or no civic amenities, and hence this is perceived as the institutional exclusion of the community (Ziyauddin, 2018; Rao et al., 2012; Srinivas, 2010; Vithal, 2002).

Unlike the studies on Muslims in northern states of India that describe the presence of lower caste groups among Muslims in urban pockets and slums, this social indicator is found invisible in Hyderabad and Sangareddy. Discrimination based on caste-like divisions is not observed in both cities (Hyderabad and Sangareddy) and is non-significant but discrimination due to the religious background and residential segregation is quite high. However, these aspects may not be common when studying cities in the northern and eastern parts of the country. The ways 'Caste act as a unit of social stratification' (Diwakar and Viswambaran) also functions as a social barrier in certain cultural aspects of Muslim life in India. The following reference of occupational groups in Hyderabad does manifest the stratified society within the Muslim though the social interactions and religious ceremonies do not discriminate rigidly as it is in Hindu caste.

Segregation among Dalits is similar in urban India including Mehtarwadi (erstwhile manual scavenging communities) in the old city of Hyderabad. The centuries-old caste scarification has been deeply rooted in segmentation and segregation (Ghurye, 1969) that continues even today. Class and power are closely linked to an individual's caste (Beteile, 1966) that sustained the spatial segregation and discrimination even in twenty-first-century India (Desai, 1994). The proponents of Dalits' development wanted urbanization as a solution to escape caste discrimination (Bharathi et al., 2017). In some studies, the urbanization of Dalits is seen as a way out of segregation and discrimination, whereas Muslims in India, especially in Telangana, have been segregated by various forms of institutional exclusion and marginalization. How far urbanization has helped to overcome caste oppression is not under the scope of this research but a few studies in Delhi (Jamil, 2017) and Hyderabad (Rao et al., 2012) show the continuous process of segregation of Muslim localities filled with the apathy of the state in providing minimum basic amenities to live.

Studies on Indian Muslims have shown that they have been living in deprivation and discrimination, including segregation (Mitra & Ray, 2014; Khan, 2007; Shaban, 2018; Rahman, 2019). Though the Indian social structure allows Muslims to live with other religious communities, there has been an unholy alliance and subsequent sufferings on the part of their socio-economic life. This precarious situation would be worse in the post COVID-19 period to all marginalized communities in India due to the ways the Indian government took few steps to curtail the spread of COVID-19 including nation-wide lockdown and correctly examined in the chapter by Jay Sharma (this volume) while studying the Ho community in Jharkhand.

As Muslims live closely with all other social groups, they should have improved their living conditions. The mixing of the communities taking place over centuries is not merely due to proximity but it is, by and large, the conversion of low caste born Hindus embracing Islam mostly in southern states of Kerala, Tamil Nadu and Andhra Pradesh. In response, some Hindu groups, such as Arya Samaj, have attempted the mass conversion of Muslims, belonging to lower strata, into Hinduism (Sikand & Katju, 1994). The facet of discrimination varies, depending on the agencies of exclusion. The ghettoization of urban Muslims is due to economic deprivation, continued threat of communal violence, discrimination in urban housing, and so on. Muslims are not allowed to have houses in mixed areas. Discrimination is a social fact that is constantly being faced by Muslims as a community. The paper does not try to differentiate between Muslims and Dalits, but it brings out the fact that the Sachar Commission Report has mentioned some sort of comparison. There is a threat to life and property, especially during communal violence which is very common in India. The concentration of the Muslim population has historical bearings. Cities such as Lucknow, Bhopal, Delhi, Patna, Hyderabad, and many more have concentration. Moreover, one should also study how Muslim ghettoization takes place in small towns.

The existence of Hyderabad as one of the most pluralist cities emerged during Nizam's rule. The city was known for the coexistence and cohabitation of multi-cultural social groups. The way several Muslim groups have concentrated in towns in the erstwhile Andhra Pradesh testifies this fact. Nizamabad, Karim Nagar, Sangareddy, Adilabad, etc. are a few names of the Muslim concentrated towns of Telangana, a province of the Indian Union. It has witnessed several communal riots in the recent past. The vulnerability of the urban Muslims has increased manifold despite being considered as the largest minority population in India. The identity of belonging to a religious community in itself poses structural problems to the families living in those areas having Muslim concentration. They are, consciously and unconsciously, deprived of most state-supported benefits that could improve their living conditions. The concentration of Muslim households in the slums of Hyderabad testifies to the miserable socio-economic conditions of the community living without basic amenities. One cannot simply relate backwardness to the culture of poverty (Lewis, 1966). The deliberate attempts of communal forces threaten the very social existence of Muslims. It is a fact that the alienation of Muslims has its roots in colonial India.

Following the recommendation of the Sachar Committee, Telangana is taking up the matter to improve the socio-economic conditions of vulnerable Muslims living in a sad plight. Telangana State has also constituted a committee to study the Socioeconomic and Educational Status of Muslims and a few schemes have been implemented upon the recommendations of the committee. Precisely, for these above-mentioned reasons, the study on living conditions seems to be imperative. The states are constitutionally duty bound to initiate affirmative action and strive to put an end to discrimination. The lack of empirical data has posed serious challenges to those intending to study issues related to Muslims. While collecting qualitative data, it is found that some of the Muslim students are reluctant to pursue research on Muslim issues.

Reasons for Segregation of Muslims

The primary objective of this paper is to see how and why the segregation of Muslims in urban clusters takes place in post-independent India. Are there undercurrents to ignite fear and threat to their life and property? Rajagopal (2010: 529–556) puts this in the context in his paper on Ahmedabad Muslims. This serves as a reference to the study deprivation of Muslims in Hyderabad and other towns Telangana. There has been a slow but steady migration of Muslims to urban settlements. They mostly rely on semi-skilled and self-reliant work. Extreme poverty and illiteracy have deprived Muslims of living in better houses despite available facilities. The paper captures the social construction of violence against Muslims in day-to-day interactions in public places. A key aspect of this process is categorising people by naming and fixing them into categories such as Hindu and/or Muslim. The usage of one against the other in media and popular proverbs further divides the already divided society. Rajagopal (2010) writes how Hindus feel about Muslims in Ahmedabad city: 'Muslims are the unsanitary and criminal-minded population that clearly explains the spatial segregation in ghettos and their economic marginalization along with their political subordination to Hindus'. (3) The stories in other cities are more or less the same.

Segregation is a sociopolitical reality of urban India today. It is injurious to India as a democratic nation. The pattern of segregation mainly revolves around Muslims unlike Blacks in American states. Yasir (2017) in his critical working paper on Delhi gives a few examples which show that the segregation of Muslims in some localities is largely due to sporadic communal violence, lynching and Islamophobia, etc. and consequently, there is visible housing discrimination in Indian cities, including Hyderabad. The IT industry has its dominance in Bangalore, Chennai and Hyderabad. Any urban agglomeration does have an impact on the availability of basic facilities and the cost of living. Hyderabad is not an exception. It is true that 'the Housing issue in India, as in the United States and South Africa, cannot be investigated completely without acknowledging its intersectionality' (Crenshaw, 1989 and 1991; Yasir, 2017). Due to the scarcity and high cost of residential facilities, the poor Muslims fail to buy decent shelter. Above all, the contention of the research is to identify those barriers arising out of Muslim identity rather than affordability to buy a house. The denial of selling property to Muslims leads to the ghettoization and segregation of Indian Muslims in urban areas.

Methods and Research Questions

The study aims to utilize the exploratory research design to examine the living environment of Muslims residing in Telangana. The dearth of research data on Muslims makes it important to explore and examine both available primary and secondary sources. Intensive fieldwork method has been used to study the living environment of Muslims in the newly formed state of Telangana in 2014. Intensive fieldwork has been very crucial and qualitative in the process of studying a less-researched population in India. This is one reason that the sociological method has relied heavily on intensive fieldwork in India and European societies. This study also uses the case study method and would also rely on the data provided and collected from the key informants and the stakeholders of the resources. Factually, many excluded communities and groups have received the attention of policymakers due to reliable qualitative data. Keeping this in mind, the qualitative data is given significant importance in this study and has been examined properly.

The demographic character of Telangana Muslim areas are found to be more urban than rural. It is also true that the urban living problems and infrastructural difficulties are different from rural areas. The historicity of the city, Hyderabad, makes it a classic example of deprivation and segregation that modern India would not have envisioned as it becomes an apt example of tradition in modernity and development with deprivation. The institutional data available with the community and organization is analysed to enhance the reliability of the facts. The Sachar study (2006) and the P. S. Krishnan report are used to assessing the urbanisation and lack of infrastructure among Muslim communities in Telangana.

Why are most Muslim populated localities deprived of basic living infrastructure facilities, including Hyderabad? Like other cities across the country, Muslims in Hyderabad also started moving to the localities where they feel safe and secure, leading to self-segregation or creating Muslim clusters/enclaves, which resulted in the ghettoization of Muslims. At a certain point, ghettoization is not seen as a negative outcome of external factors but a conscious choice of Muslims. Peer (2015), in an article, writes about one of the largest urban ghettos of Muslims in Mumbai—Mumbra when thousands of families, who were uprooted after the 1992–93 riots, found safety in the outskirts of Mumbai, Mumbra and got settled there. In that neglected township area, more than nine lakh people call it their home. Basharat Peer writes, 'On a recent afternoon, after a two-hour drive out of Mumbai, I followed a highway hugging the low hills of Mumbra, northeast of the city, near the Thane creek. As the road forked downhill, hundreds of grimy, teetering buildings stacked like tattered books in a neglected public library were the first glimpse intimation of Mumbra, India's largest Muslim ghetto. Despite the heat, young boys played cricket in a clearing by a graveyard. A chaotic medley of vehicles choked the main street leading into the Kausa area of the ghetto' (Peer, 2015). The aftermath of the demolition of Babri Masjid in Ayodhya resulted in the large scale of massacre of people, largely Muslims, in Mumbai that left a deadly fear not only to the residents of Mumbai but also shook the heart and soul of every Indian Muslim. After the demolition of Babri Masjid, the retaliatory bomb blast by the underworld reconfigured the demography of Bombay Muslims who had to look for safe geographical areas as their home. It was Mumbra, where the Konkani coast already had old Muslim settlements, which became the natural choice of thousands of families resettling here. The rural-urban migration and cheaper houses or flats led to an increase of more than 20 times in population from just 45000 to 900,000 population, reported in the census of 2011. This jump shows the highest growing urban city in India.

Similar reasons are being studied in the case of Hyderabad. Once affected by riots, the families looked for the safety of life and children's future which became a zone of deprivation and extreme backwardness. By narrating the glory of Hyderabad erstwhile Nizam's state cannot bring and provide access to education, health and basic amenities to the people at present. Rather people in the city have memories and stories filled in with the pain of losing their own during the police action and the continuous riots afterwards added another factor to the already Muslim clustered urban pockets. The polarization of urban areas in Telangana state is threatening to the peaceful co-existence of Muslims with their co-residents in all the towns of the state. It is extremely disturbing on one hand whereas the same factor accounts for the high pace of rural–urban migration in Hyderabad. As a result, urban poverty and deprivation of basic amenities in the city is a common narrative to most households. A respondent, Baba Saheb, narrated, 'I worked in the historical Mecca Masjid as a cleaner or sweeper over two decades, but I still struggle to marry grown-up daughters and could never send them to a school, an aspiration I always had throughout my life. Hyderabad is a city of the poor like me! Where are Nawabs now?' (12 April 2017).

The government's continuous neglect of Muslim localities in providing civic amenities and infrastructure facilities resulted in 'inadequacy of infrastructural facilities, shrinking of common spaces where different socio-religious communities (SRCs) can interact and reduction in livelihood options' says a civil society member. The process has been reinforced doubly by the socio-economic marginalization affecting Muslims and thus, creates a substantial economic burden upon the community on health and educational expenses.

Contextualizing Segregation and Muslim Neighbourhoods

Segregation is often understood in two ways; firstly, as a condition that describes the self-isolation of a community, and secondly, more often than not, as an institutional exclusion of a community to the access to state's resources and provisions that are meant to be available to every citizen.

Similarly, it is not only the concept of segregation and the communities, but the writings and studies on segregation are also observed and placed at the marginalized spaces within the disciplinary domain. The studies on Muslims' segregation are not encouraged in Indian sociology at first instance. This group of population is often perceived as a community living in self-isolation by choice, thereby overlooking the institutional exclusions that lead to the process of segregated residential developments almost in all cities and metropolitan spaces in India. A few studies that could give new insights into the living social realities of Muslims in urban spaces have been produced in the last decade (a few are Shaban, 2013; Gayer & Jaffrelot, 2012; Jamil, 2017).

The terminology of exclusion in Indian social sciences finds a new life after European nations found its relevance as an interventionist tool in their policies. Much was written on segregation in American sociological literature to describe a few historical cases. At the same time, African-Americans and Natives asserted their territorial acclamation and settled in those regions to save their culture and autonomy. Therefore, these reflections in the past demonstrate self-isolation as visa-wise segregation of black or Native Americans. However, Muslims' segregation is beyond isolation and is a consequence of institutional segregation.

Indeed, excluding a community is not limited to residential facilities only. However, it takes an institutional form where disempowerment is constituted by using various tools of exclusion. Such a process leads to the exclusion of communities from institutional knowledge formation in the long run. This phenomenon is often termed self-isolation, and all latent exclusionary factors are undermined. Segregation extends its arms to further denial of rights and access to social interactions, social capital and limiting the community within themselves, and considering these factors, the urban densely populated areas of Hyderabad and Sangareddy are to be mentioned here, though the situation is similar across the cities in India (Gayer & Jaffrelott, 2013; Hathi and Srivastava, 2021; Desai, 1994; Beteile, 1966; Ghurye, 1969; Lewis, 1966; Crenshaw, 1991; Shaban, 2013; Sudhir Commission Report, 2016; Saunders, 1986; Sultana, 2016; Moid, 2011; Bhambra, 2014).

At this juncture, it is proposed and discussed in this paper that segregation takes a serious turn and manifests as a new phenomenon in India in the post-Babri Masjid demolition (1992) phase and redefines the understanding of segregation. The segregation of Dalits' ghettos finds a place in recent studies, but there is less research on Muslim pockets. For instance, a working paper on residential segregation in urban India shows 'how intra-ward segregation is a central driver of ghettoisation of the most spatially marginalized groups in urban India—Muslims and Dalits' (Bharathi et al., 2017: 1). This document gives an idea of the ghettoization process in urban India and demonstrates this through census documents of India for both Dalits and Muslims.

Segregation is considered a 'separation of groups of people with differing characteristics, often taken to connote a condition of inequality' (Bhambhra, 2014). However, the scenario in Hyderabad and likewise shows inequality in housing, markets, lack of access to credit by financial institutions, an absolute difference of basic amenities and sanitation between Muslim localities and non-Muslim areas (Sudhir Commission, 2016). In short, segregation of Muslims in India brings a new face of life that Muslims live in urban pockets. The history of the conceptual sketch of segregation does not get translated to Indian Muslims that was studied in the context of African Americans and Native Americans.

Segregation is often grossly understood in the form of housing settlements, but the other consequential forms are not studied. The ghettoized urban pockets, thus, become an easy target in terms of chances of getting killed mercilessly during communal violence, resulting in huge damage to property, houses, business establishment, life, and even the dignity of women. Is it not an institutional exclusion and consequence of segregation? A well-established explanation of 'segregation provided by American sociologists is the well-known assumption of a 'natural' phenomenon' (Park, 1925) that does suit the American social structure at a given time, but how can the expansion of Muslim localities in India be considered as 'natural'. This phenomenon is a conscious outcome of institutional exclusion in most of the pockets in various cities of India including, Hyderabad and Sangareddy. The American sociological analysis on segregation is important to examine racial and ethnic discrimination in a certain time frame. However, they didn't provide any apt analytical model of how the 'natural' phenomenon of segregation is correct. The discussion and analysis of class and racial exclusion and discrimination at the core didn't find important to them about considering religion as a variable.

Studies on the housing market in India have demonstrated discrimination based on religion and caste, but very few studies highlighted the residential segregation of Muslims that results in multiple deprivations to the community at large. Lately, one does find conceptual criticism of the Chicago School's account of segregation on three bases; firstly, ecological fallacy, secondly, the positivist emphasis, and thirdly overlook of political-economic factors (Saunders, 1986). Therefore, segregation is a phenomenon showing subtle and spatial discrimination and an outcome of the circumstances and conditions that bring layers of deprivation and exclusion to Muslims in India. Necessarily, segregation is, conceptually and experientially, different from inequality. A group of people in India would argue that segregation is voluntary and self-imposed. There are a few valid questions, why do Muslims choose to construct, buy and reside more in Muslim pockets than in new cities, in gated communities of Hyderabad and other nearby towns of IT city?

The crux of several interviews for the above question hints at the choice that large Indian Muslims opt for. The everyday life of a Muslim household is much more convenient with the availability of graveyards and food culture, among others. Based on empirical shreds of evidence, it has been observed that these factors have not been considered more than mere perceptions and do not examine the reasons for the occurrence of a vast number of segregated urban pockets even in new cities of India.

Patterns of Discrimination

The various patterns of discrimination in terms of availability and accessibility of basic infrastructure available in concentrated Muslim areas in particular and to all Muslims, in general, are a common sight unlike, the brand image of Hyderabad as a hub of information technology. In particular, the social discrimination regarding the access to education, health, livelihood sources, housing, banking or credit support (whoever looks for), drinking water and sanitation and political participation in general and employment opportunities in public organizations is visibly a living reality, reported in most of the Focused Group Discussions (FGDs) held during 2016–2018.

The meticulously conducted in-depth interviews and narratives obtained during the group discussions and Key Informants interviews bridge the knowledge gap between Muslims as citizens and Muslims as a community. Both conceptions are to be interlinked to demonstrate the living reality of Muslim life in Hyderabad. This reflection of empirical data is also substantiated by the fact that social evils in the name of marrying very young or under-aged girls to Arabs were a familiar story in the 1980s–1990s that gradually got counter-attacked by academic groups and activists working in the old city of Hyderabad. 'I have always dreamed of seeing the daughters of my city getting a higher education and dignified employment in modern industry and companies. This can only free the innocent poor daughters to be sold in the hands of Arabs and all in the name of urban poverty and lack of education. Parents perceive that their daughters will live a dignified life with Arab Shaikh who is three times older than the young girls being forced to marry that never happens' (Sultana, 2016).

Considering the field data, it appears that Muslims live in a high level of segregation. The persistence of poverty since the 1970s and 80s has added misery to the already confined lives of Muslims living in the Old City of Hyderabad. It is found that several localities in Hyderabad's old city remain the most visible and palpable forms of Muslim segregation, which can be conveniently called Muslim ghettos that appear to be on the lines of African-American ghettos in the USA. A Muslim locality is a place today that spatially isolates Muslims of different socio-economic classes. This trend is taking shape in most cities having a concentrated Muslim population. Recent studies observed the role of segregation over time in creating Muslim clusters and made a connection between the isolation of Muslims and the concentration of poverty. It is true to Hyderabad and other cities that religion is the dominant organising principle when it comes to housing and residential patterns. No matter their economic status, social background, or personal characteristics, Muslims continue to be denied full access to Indian housing markets and employment opportunities. Segregation and ghettoization of Muslims in certain localities have led to the deprivation of Income, Employment, Health, Housing Deprivation, Education, Skills and Training, and lack of Geographical Access to Services. These unequal socio-economic conditions have also brought a digital divide to the urban segregated marginalized groups during the COVID-19 pandemic, as discussed in great detail by Dilip Diwakar and Visakh Viswambaran (2021, this volume).

In their edited book, *Muslims in Indian: Trajectories of Marginalisation*, Gayer and Jeffrelot mention that various segregation features are relevant to understanding Muslims' segregation in cities of southern states. Certain social and political constraints affects peoples choices in finding residential construction. Because of these constraints; people from similar socio-economic backgrounds regroup in common localities with similar ascribed status such as religious identities.

It has been highly reported that such localities are highly neglected by the state authorities and administrative machinery that reflects upon the lack of infrastructures, poor environmental conditions, symbolic availability of sanitation and good educational facilities, etc. And, lastly, the 'estrangement of the localities and residents settled there from the rest of the city, due to lack of public transportation and limited job opportunities and restricted access to public spaces beyond the locality. And the experiences and sense of being in a closed locality by the residents relate to an objective pattern of estrangement they have from the rest of the city' (Gayer & Jeffrelot, 2012).

Muslims, Segregation and Ghettoized Pockets

The town of Hyderabad is analysed by studying the living and environmental conditions where more than 40 percent of Muslims live in segregation and experience extreme poverty unlike their friends from Hindu communities.

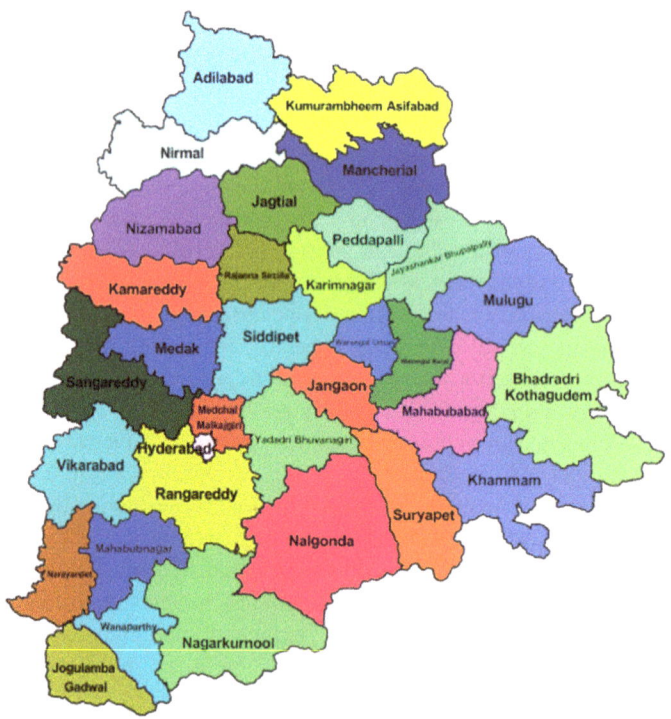

Map 7.1 Telangana state. *Source* telangana.gov.in/about/districts

Political Map 7.1, shown below, has 31 administrative divisions (a district of Telangana in India). Initially, there were 10 when Telangana state was carved out from the erstwhile state of Andhra Pradesh that came into existence on 2 June 2014. As one of the newest carved out states in southern India, bordered by Andhra Pradesh in the southern side, the north and west bordered by Maharashtra and Chhattisgarh in the east, Telangana has great cultural diversity in the urban pockets. The Telugu state, known by different names in the past, 'Telinga', 'Telungalu', 'Tenugulu', refers to the people of Telugu language speakers, that became a popular name during the Telangana youth movement for the separation of the state. Historically, the Telangana region remained a part of the Hyderabad state or under Nizams dominion from 17 September 1948 to 1 November 1956 until it was absorbed in the Andhra State. Later it got renamed Andhra Pradesh.

Another adjoining town to Hyderabad is Sangareddy that has a population of 72,395, comprising 18,427 households with an average size of households at five in the town (DE&S, Government of Telangana, 2016). The town has over 35% Muslim population living in misery and lack of basic sanitation systems. A town located just at a distance of 65 km away from Hyderabad and known as the Industrial capital of the Telangana State due to the increased number of industrial units (national and multinational companies) could not bring basic public facilities to the urban families.

Sangareddy became a municipality in 1953, while this town has 72,395 people living within the municipal limits. The percentage of the urban population in the state of Telangana is 33.36. Whereby newly formed Sangareddy district with a population of 1,861,560, the urban population is 974,309. Sangareddy town has a 24% urban population. This district was carved out as a new district from Medak on 11 October 2016 by Telangana State. After the capital city of Hyderabad, Sangareddy town has the highest percentage of the urban population in the district with a high Muslim concentration which is 35% of the total population. (Akbar, 2020) It is observed that the Muslim population in the town largely depends on small business establishments such as bakeries, hotels, *paan* shops, garment shops, fruit and flower shops, repair shops, and auto and transport business.

It is observed that Sangareddy town has 66.06% tap water from the treated source and 14.82 from the untreated source, whereas 0.23% use covered well and 0.09 use uncovered well. Further, 1.12% have a dependency on hand pump, 15.21% are using tubewell/borewell, 0.4% are sourcing spring, 0.44% are using tank/ pond/ lake and 1.55 reported having some other sources, as per 2011 census reports for the district (Bharathi et al., 2017).

In this overview of the drinking water situation in Sangareddy, it is found in the field study, that mostly urban Muslim localities are deprived of tap water. A large number of people included in the group discussion shared how the local administration has failed to provide the basic minimum facility of safe drinking water and that, in turn, increases the incidence of illness. These outcomes, in the form of illness, are hardly noticed in any government study reports. Comparing both towns, the electricity consumption is high in both towns in general. Sangareddy has 98.55% of the population with electricity, with 1.07% and 0.27 using solar as their source of energy. Hyderabad is in a better situation where mostly all the households have electricity facilities. The reportage of frequent power cuts and at times higher electricity bills are observed in Muslim localities. However, such data is not available in published form except field interviews.

According to the District Census Handbook of 2011, concerning the number and percentage of households by type of drainage connectivity for the waste outlet, Sangareddy urban households had 45.62% closed drainage, 46.68% open drainage, and 7.7% have no drainage at all. It is reported during the field visits to the mohallas[1] (Census of India, 2011) of Sangareddy town that the town does not have an underground drainage system though it is the headquarter of Medak district (now a separate district as Sangareddy). Most of the residents of Muslim localities complained of health problems due to the open drainage system. They pointed out the negligence of their localities by municipal authorities in cleaning the drains and streets.

The Muslims are in sizable numbers especially in a few pockets and localities like Nalsab Gadda, Eidgah Gadda, Osman Pura and Rajampet, etc. As per the field

---

[1] Mohalla, which may originate from the Western Islamic world, is a traditional neighbourhood unit common in North Indian cities. A city was regarded as an aggregation of mohallas, and the establishment of a new mohalla meant an expansion of the city.

data, it is estimated that there is approximately 60–70% population that belongs to the Muslim community in these areas.

The majority of Muslims are engaged in petty business, like pan shop, tea shop, Kirana (grocery), and fruits shop. There is a trend to impart education to children in Urdu and English medium schools. The dropout rate is higher among Muslim boys than girls since boys have to support or take care of the economic activity of the house, and they discontinue education after 8th or 9th class, whereas girls continue their education till graduation. The dropout Muslim boys also engage themselves in mechanical workshops, petty businesses, hotels, and child labour. Given this explanation, it is helpful to briefly examine the below-given table on urban poverty in Sangareddy. The field-level data suggests that Muslims comprise high numbers of households among the slum population of the total 34 slums. However, an actual figure can help in elaborating the population structure among Muslims in Sangareddy town located in slums.

The slum population in Sangareddy town does not identify a community-wise slum population. The field observations correlate to the point that most Muslims live both in notified and non-notified slum areas of the town. Except for a small number of Muslims who live in middle-class locations near the collectorate complex and Mumbai X road—the outskirts of the town, the majority of them are settled within the town. The fieldwork data substantiates the concentrated areas in Sangareddy towns as the most backward and deficient in urban amenities: Maqdoom Nagar, Riksha colony, Nalsab Gadda, Jalal Bagh, Shanti Nagar, Upper Bazar, RahmatPura, Osmania Masjid, and Kalva Kunta Road.

Ironically, it has been observed that concerning political participation of Muslims and political empowerment in Sangareddy, till 2020, all the ten (10) elected ward councillors were Muslim in Sangareddy Municipality but that has never helped to solve the problem in the Municipal areas due to the internal dynamics in the Municipal Council. The apathy of the state and district administration is visibly recorded in the field data.

The Muslim Dilemma and Institutional Exclusions

Hyderabad forms the largest Muslim urban populated city in India with 43.45% of the total population. Among the total population (3,943,323) of Hyderabad district, Hindus are 51.89% (Census of India, 2011). According to the Telangana Social Development Report (2017), it is estimated that the capital city of Hyderabad comprises 30% of the total urban population in Telangana. There is a phenomenal record in the growth of urban population, at the rate of 38%, during the decade of 2001–2011 whereas just 2% growth is witnessed in the rural area. Hyderabad city, the capital of Telangana and Andhra Pradesh states, one of the nation's leading information technology areas, has a population of 7.7 million people according to Census 2011, and it increased from 5.5 million in 2001.

The sporadic expansion of Hyderabad with rapid urban population growth in the state at 21% higher than the national urban population of 18% shows both historical and contemporary developmental processes taking place in the state and mainly in the city of Hyderabad. A higher trend in population has been observed since 1971 (21%) against the national average only at 18%. Since then, the urban population growth kept increasing, in 1981 at 25.3%; and from 2001 to 2011, it jumped from 31.8 to 38.9%. The urban population growth in the state has been much higher than all India levels (2011 census report). The Muslims in the city are largely settled and reside in the localities of the old city of Hyderabad and a few other Muslim segregated areas that developed late after the 1990s. Toli Chowki, Golconda, Mehdipatnam, Shaik Pet, Atta Pur, Asif Nagar, Murad Nagar fall in the new city. There are also a few visible mixed localities in twin city Secunderabad. The problem is similar to Sangareddy and is typical of the state's all-urban Muslim concentrated settlements. The data of Hyderabad, a modern and metropolitan city, also does not reflect any positive picture of the living environment of Muslims.

Poor Water Drainage Facilities and Health Hazards

This sociological study, based on a sample size of 1000 respondents, aims at understanding the exclusionary process of Muslims and their health conditions in Andhra Pradesh and Telangana. It was found that in all concentrated Muslim towns of Andhra Pradesh (Guntur and Kurnool) and Telangana (Hyderabad and Nizamabad), the majority of households lived in poor housing, lack of sanitation, basic amenities, and minimal public health care availability (Ziyauddin, 2018). Muslim pockets are located in congested localities and ghettos having no running water and drainage. The pipelines are non-existent. In case there are pipelines, they do not work. There is leakage of water owing to apathy and neglect of the local government. In many cases, drinking water and drainage water gets mixed up due to damage in the pipeline, and this contaminated water spreads water-borne disease.

Amenities Versus Policing

Table 7.1, below, gives a comparative overview of the provisions and public services available. However, it is difficult to compare the Muslim and non-Muslim populations in terms of the availability of these provisions and public services. The questions related to amenities have taken a back seat whereas extra vigilance in the name of safety and security has taken the centre stage in Muslim populated zones.

Moreover, there is state surveillance, and it reflects the suspicious mindset of the state apparatus towards Muslims living in mohallas. The old city of Hyderabad has 29 police stations for 47% (1,799,030 persons) of the total population whereas the new city (Cyberabad) has only 35 police stations 53% population (2,030,723

Table 7.1 Hyderabad comparative information (old city and new city)

Sl. no	Particulars	Old city	%	New city	%	Total district
1	Population (2001)	1,799,030	47	2,030,723	53	3,829,753
2						
3	Area (m^2)	65.63	33	134.05	67	199.68
4	Density (km^2)	27,411		15,065		19,179
5	Literacy	66%		71.29		68.80
6	Government schools	471	57	351	43	822
7	Government schools in rented buildings	178	91	16	9	194
8	Government junior colleges	5	26	14	74	19
9	Government degree colleges	1	14	6	86	7
10	Hospitals	7	31	15	69	22
11	Urban health centres	27	40	39	60	66
12	Bank branches	138	49	579	51	717
13	Post offices	34	30	78	70	112
14	Parks	34	5	650	95	684
15	Parks total area (Area)	23.80	6	367.04	94	390.84
16	Play grounds	210	43	279	57	489
17	Play grounds total area (Area)	32.99	37	55.99	63	88.78
18	Public toilets	53	32	110	68	163
19	Government buildings (state, central, undertakings)	36	16	187	84	223
20	Electricity connections	473,461	34	914,435	66	1,387,896
21	Electricity transformers	3860	24	11,725	76	15,585
22	Road length (km)	1357	33	2691	67	4048
23	Foot path length (km)	1141	36	2024	64	3165
24	But depots	3	14	18	86	21
25	Setwin buses	0	0	100		100
26	Cinema theatres	13	20	50	80	63
27	Libraries	56	44	70	56	126
28	Anganwadi centres	259	40	380	60	639
29	Pensions (old age, widows, handicapped)	40,713	37	67,668	63	108,381
30	Ration shops	401	46	469	54	870

(continued)

Table 7.1 (continued)

Sl. no	Particulars	Old city	%	New city	%	Total district
31	Police stations	29	45	35	55	64
32	Large and medium scale industries	3	20	12	80	15
33	Factories	0		40		40
34	Small scale industries (SSI Unites)	438	33	851	67	1289
35	Main workers	442,531	40	649,670	60	1,092,201
36	Marginal workers	39,078	35	75,079	65	113,157

Source M. Srinivas, "Hyderabad Old City: A Saga of Discrimination", *People's Democracy*, Vol. XXXIV, No. 15, April 11, 2010; statistics tabulated by COVA organization, under PUCAR Program, Hyderabad

persons). It substantiates the narratives of people that government wants to have more police stations than basic amenities including schools, colleges, and health centres in Muslim settlements. People are very cynical and critical of this move of the government and are extending it to the people living in the old city of Hyderabad. They construct their social reality with the understanding that the state is not going to uplift their living conditions, but will only use them as vote banks. It also transpires from the study that the shabby socio-economic conditions have an impact on the decreasing population growth. Precisely, this is one of the reasons for the declining Muslim population in Hyderabad. Their access to higher education and demand for quality living seems to have convinced them to adopt the family planning methods to reduce giving birth.

Multiple Exclusions and Muslim Urban Poverty

The size of the population in Hyderabad which is living below the poverty line is 23%. It's the second biggest habitation of the poor population after Mumbai having 27%. This tells the story of the exclusion and vulnerability of the Muslims in Indian cities. The exclusion in other metropolitan cities is quite low and these include Delhi (8%), Kolkata (6%), and Chennai (20%). A recent survey conducted to study the socio-economic conditions of Hyderabadi Muslims found that less than 2% of families in the city belong to elite groups having a net wealth of over one crore. The glaring contrast is that about 63% of Muslim households fall under the BPL and are miserably dependent on government schemes to survive (Akbar, 2020).

Economic Deprivations

The city has a huge percentage (37%) of the population living in slums. The average (piped) water supply per day is for 2 h in Hyderabad, and 81% of households have access to water. There is the degradation of living conditions owing to the absence or nonfunctioning of drainage. In 2001, towns were provided with only 41% sewerage connections (UA). There is little improvement even after a gap of two decades.

Life Without Potable Water Sources

In Hyderabad city, the drinking water facility has been made available to 881,512 households. Out of them, 846,470 households are receiving tap water from treated sources; 15,584 households receive from untreated sources; 1,108 households receive from covered water, and the remaining 913 households rely on uncovered sources. There are 6,139 households having tube wells/borewells, 84 households remain dependent on springs and 1,196 on tanks/ponds/lakes, etc. and finally, only 6,777 are dependent on other sources of drinking water (2011 census report). Households having bathing facilities within premises have been taken into consideration. Hyderabad has about 881,512 households of which 863,553 have a bathroom; 9,546 have a bathroom without a roof and 8,413 have no bathroom facility.

Wastewater outlets connected to houses with closed drainage are 850,570, the open drainage houses are 20,810, and 10,132 are having no drainage in Hyderabad. The fact is that there are still many houses without basic amenities of water, drainage, drinking water and waste disposal systems. This makes the situation alarming. The Muslim areas in the towns are highly congested and full of filth in the surroundings of mohallas and colonies. The living conditions of Muslims are pathetic in urban areas where it could have been otherwise better. There is a gradual decline in the status of Muslim houses. Similarly, Sangareddy too has a large number of Muslim households. They do not have drainage and toilets without a roof. There are 8,413 households that do not have bathrooms on the premises, and 197,199 households don't have drainage at all. The living condition of women is pathetic in Muslim households owing to the socio-cultural practices as they do not prefer to bathe in an open area. It amounts to their trouble.

The data provided by Census Houses by Predominant Material of Roof is analysed and shows another form of existing institutional exclusion in urban Hyderabad. If we examine the houses by kind of roofs, there are 1,021,234 houses, and of them, 10,098 are made of bamboo/grass/ wood/mud, etc. The houses made of polythene/plastic are 8,183 in number. The houses with handmade tiles are 10,452; machine-made tiles are fitted in 10,403 houses; the burnt brick houses are 6,656, and stone/slate-based houses are 25,948. Another 239,059 houses have asbestos sheets etc.; the concrete houses are 706,543, and the remaining houses numbering 3,892 are made up of any other items.

Households by Availability of Electricity and Latrines

Out of a total 881,512 households, there are 859,576 houses having latrine; another 10,145 don't have a latrine. However, all the houses have electricity connections. Moreover, 8,610 houses have latrines without electricity, and 3,181 houses reported latrines are not available and without electricity. The facility of transportation is minimal in the Muslim concentrated areas. People reported that autos and taxis do not prefer to ply in certain Muslim concentrated localities, and the same was experienced by the researcher while in the fieldwork. This is an alarming situation. Why is the prejudice prevailing that Muslims do not pay travel fares?

Size of Households and the Mean Household Size

The mean household size in Hyderabad is 9.2, whereas Medak has 14.4 for the entire district including Sangareddy. The undivided state had 12.1 mean households, which is higher in number. The research on Muslims as a religious community faces crucial challenges. There is no separate data based on religious groups. Therefore, the primary data can be relied upon to understand the gravity of Muslim problems in urban areas. In this context, the life of Muslims is not very different from that of other social groups. It's since the poor living conditions have added to their vulnerability and marginalization. The densely populated areas in both cities are marked with declining living conditions.

The Hyderabad City Development Plan also illustrates urban development as well as the conditions of the poor Muslims. As per the available data, the number of people living below the poverty line (BPL) is 540,000 of which about 430,000 people live in the MCH area and the rest in the surrounding municipalities. The population living below the poverty line constitutes around 13% of the total population. There are wide variations in the number of people living below the poverty line across the municipalities. For example, the percentage of BPL population is very high in Quthbullahpur and Rajendranagar constituting about 37% and 24%, respectively, and very low in Serilingampally, Uppal, and LB Nagar constituting around 3–4%. The latter pockets are having less Muslim concentration. Further, slum settlements have multiplied over decades, and the living conditions of the poor have not improved. This also reflects the grown-up Muslim slum dwellers. Murshidabad, First Lancer, Gachibwoli (Anjaiah Nagar), Hafizpet, and Hafiz Baba Nagar are among a few slums that have a higher concentration of urban poor Muslim households.

Apathy of QQUDA

The Quli Qutub Shah Urban Development Authority (QQUDA) was constituted in August 1981 to make the old city a planned settlement with better civic amenities including communication, electricity, water supply, drainage, housing, education, recreational, and marketing facilities. The condition would have improved had this authority got good financial allocation. This demonstrates visible neglect towards Muslim localities, adding to the irony of the segregation of Muslims.

At the grassroots level, MIM plays an important role in the life of Muslims living in the slums of Hyderabad. The Majlis party headquarter is at Darussalam, Hyderabad where people from the constituency of Hyderabad can visit and lodge complaints. The complaints lodged are followed up by the MIM members at the respective levels. There are honest efforts to solve the problems. It is a way to stay connected to the people in the city that gives a return at the time of elections. Muslims from the old city want to have proper birth, death, income, residential certificates, voter ID, ration card, Aadhar card, licenses and other documents. He said that 'In the new city, some of the other VIPs reside in some of the other localities, many governments and business offices are there, so the municipal authorities take up all kinds of work without any representation. On the other hand, making them work for the old city requires hard work, especially making them work in the interiors of the old city- which is the priority of Majlis, and it is a very uphill task'. He believes that despite these difficulties, the old city's condition has improved with the constant efforts of Majlis (Moid, 2011; Civic Activism of MIM).

Multiple Deprivations of Urban Muslims

Today, the old city area can best be described not only as a congested area but also as a case of 'multiple deprivations' in sociological terms. Ratna Naidu in her study noted that 'The problem of the old city was identified as one of widening the roads, laying new sewage lines along narrow lanes and renovating buildings. These are not only expensive in terms of compensatory payments but also require sensitivity to the emotional and cultural needs of the local people as well as the need to conserve historical-cultural styles' (Naidu, 1990: 13).

In the social science literature, the term 'vicious cycle of Multiple Deprivation of, (for instance, poor education and training, low income, poor diet and poor hygienic conditions leading to low efficiency and ability to enhance incomes), is analytically applied to understand poverty at the individual, community and class levels: (Naidu, 1990: 15–16). Several research reports also indicated that the Muslim localities in urban areas do not have the infrastructure needed to support urban living with economic, social and cultural needs. The erstwhile abode of the elite, the symbol of pride, the old city area today is largely inhabited by Muslims and has been reduced to ghettos. These references are already analysed in this paper. Muslim mohallas have low-rise densely packed houses. The mixed and intense land-use patterns create problems of congestion. Some houses are built in a small area having 10–15 square yards, accommodating around 5–6 persons. The new generations, who are not so well educated, also find it difficult to move to newer areas for not having income-generating skills; nor can they afford housing in developed colonies outside of the Muslim mohallas due to their poor savings.

Being deprived of civic and economic opportunities, the Muslim mohallas in both the towns languish in multiple deprivations. To the economic and civic deprivations, the deprivation which accrues from the alienation of communities from each other must also be added, resulting in further exclusion, mutual distrust, and discrimination. Thus, a classic syndrome is observed in the Muslim localities wherein the 'different types of deprivation mesh into one another to create, for those who must endure them, a total situation shot through and through by one level of deprivation after another.

Concluding Observations

Urban Muslims face multiple interlocking problems in Hyderabad and Sangareddy town, making the situation worse. One can easily see the disposal of rubbish, debris, rank vegetation on roadsides, cleaning of drains, overflow of drains, filling up of potholes and road cuttings, repairs, replacement of streetlights, repairs of roads, drains, street lighting, maintenance of sewerage, repairs to public taps, leakage of water and pipelines and water supply and so on in the old city areas. Muslim mohallas remain a Case of Multiple Exclusions. The situation of Muslims living in mohallas is an example of the inter-linkage of the four dimensions of the division of urban areas in the city.

Among the Muslim residents, most of them live in a hand-to-mouth situation and are impoverished, which means that they cannot afford or have access to quality housing, health, and education. As most of the houses located in these areas do not have proper municipal land layouts and approvals for constructing houses, most of them are not in a position to get loans from the formal banking sector. Consequently, the banks do not issue credit cards and personal loans to the residents of these areas, marked as 'red zones', which forces most Muslims to fall prey to private money lenders or make them feel excluded from the formal economy. 'The lack of adequate social and physical infrastructure for the people living in a particular area can also lead to congestion. When physical infrastructural facilities like sewerage, water and condition of roads, and social infrastructural facilities like schools, colleges, hospitals, parks and playgrounds are overloaded, because their demands are greater than they are designed to cater for, they function at a lower level of efficiency.'

The lack of proper documents, quality housing, and access to resources, health, education and employment make them vulnerable to shocks and helplessness. In India, a person without a proper address cannot get a voter card, and therefore, it leads to the feeling of being excluded from formal political participation. This political non-identity translates into social and political exclusion; for example, a person without proper identities such as ration card, voter card or Aadhar card cannot obtain food ration cards and cannot utilize the 'Arogyasree' programme for hospitalization.

Cultural exclusion takes hold as the label of being 'others' is reinforced in different ways. The state plans to supply drinking water to every village in Telangana. The state has a plan to supply drinking water to every village in Telangana. It is frequently reported that the old city is a criminal zone where most crimes take place. The labelling of the area is also a part of the process of discrimination and exclusion. Therefore, the severe infrastructure shortage is identified during the field visits, which needs to be addressed by the state, not a party. The conclusions also recall what Muslims want and whether there are good representations of people in the Urban Local Bodies (ULBs). It is also important to note that JNNURM was launched in December 2005 with a target to initiate reforms and complete the planned development of cities within seven years (2005–12) with the help of residents and Urban Local Bodies (ULBs). The inclusions of Muslims in the programme of civic amenities have not been addressed, and they lag far behind the required development of the modern hi-tech city of Hyderabad.

The average standard of living of urban Muslims has improved over the years. The Muslims in old cities are still neglected and marginalized due to the extreme discrimination prevailing in the old city of the town. A classic case of segregation is the old city of Hyderabad, including a few other towns in the state. The recent development activities should include Muslims and create trust among them. The benefits of the metro track have not reached the old city, whereas another most congested locality in Delhi could find metro crossing quite easily. The question seems to have no answer. Further, the prevalence of stereotype narratives against Muslims is assumed to be one of the underlying causes of socio-spatial exclusion of the Muslim community.

Being poor and marginalized, Muslims find it difficult to get the education that can lift them from poverty and exclusion. Social mobility is only possible with opportunities for education and work that can be made available in the areas where marginalized Muslims live. Residents of these localities demand good quality schooling right from the nursery to higher education. The Telangana Rashtra Samithi (TRS) government has to implement the programme from 'KG to PG'. Most of them want to send their wards to English medium schools, with a subject of their mother tongue, i.e. Urdu. They do not want to sacrifice their mother tongue, primarily opting for English education. It is indeed a complex question to address. However, the minority residential school scheme would be a means to overcome educational deprivation at the school level.

Therefore, the Telangana Minorities Residential Educational Institutions Society (TMREIS) initiative, having residential infrastructure, is a step forward to stop the segregation process, a unique experiment in India. With 204 Minority Residential Schools, the state has addressed the questions of infrastructure and governance in the school systems. The segregation and deprivation led to the inaccessibility of public policies that the state of Telangana implemented to target minorities. A well-built argument developed among the deprived Muslims that the government can minimize the segregation and ghettoization by allocating 12% of the houses under

State Housing Schemes to Muslims in Muslim-dominated areas under the ongoing 'two-bedroom flat' scheme. An immediate and prompt response has been given to the drainage problems, polluted water supply, repairs to street lighting, and water supply lines which are partially available in Muslim populated localities in Hyderabad. The question is why such civic amenities have not been provided in Muslim localities. It's a matter of deliberate negligence reflecting institutional discrimination. Moreover, access to modern amenities is one of the fundamental rights in modern life. The construction of parks, playgrounds, community halls, hospitals and schools in Muslim-dominated areas can provide a better ambiance. These amenities help build a healthy population with a greater sense of civil life.

Financial inclusion acts as a soft tool of social inclusion in society if concerns like opening up banks to facilitate easy loans to be self-reliant and overcome financial backwardness can be addressed. There is an easy way to blame the community for its backwardness. However, state has to formulate policy for the upliftment of the Muslim community and provide them credit facilities. This will break the myth that Muslims do not wish to avail themselves of credit and financial support from the formal banking system. Some studies have shown ways of improving the economic conditions of Muslims through financial inclusion. The Telangana Government has allocated more than 1100 crores to develop of minorities. Instead of dispersing at the state level, all the district collectorates should be made as nodal centres for processing and disbursement of benefits.

Above all, there has to be some initiative for deconstructing the myth of naming Muslim areas as red areas/zones. It creates a barrier to their socio-economic inclusion. These terms need to be deleted from the rule book or unwritten norms in the banking system. Such nomenclature is at the root of the institutional exclusion of Muslims. These have already been mentioned about how stereotype narratives damage the trust between the state and its people. Herefore, segregation is simply a complex phenomenon generated from various reasons and multiple factors in any society.

Acknowledgements It is a great pleasure to acknowledge the contribution of all the respondents of this study. My sincere thanks to Sudhir Commission members Prof. Amirullah Khan and Prof. Abdul Shaban for initially encouraging me and contributing as a working paper that helped bring out this research paper. I also acknowledge my thanks to Dr. Abdul Thaha for his contribution and giving initial comments and suggestions while writing a working paper for the Sudhir Commission Report. Lastly, I must thank Dr. Subhankar Basu, Dr. Mudassir Nazar and Dr. Hena Kauser for their comments and meaningful discussion. I cannot miss the opportunity to place my gratitude to the editors of this volume, Prof. Sanghmitra Acharya and Dr. Stephen Christopher, for their well-argued suggestions and comments in finalizing this paper.

References

Akbar, S. (2020). 63% Hyderabad muslims are poor: Helping hand foundation. *Times of India.*
Bharathi, N. Deepak, M. & Andaleeb, R. (2017). Village in the city: Residential segregation in Urbanizing India. *IIMB-WP,* (588).

Beteile, A. (1966). Caste, class and power: Changing patterns of stratification in a tanjore village. Oxford University Press,

Census of India (2011). District census handbook, Medak district, series-29 part XII-B. *Directorate of census operations.*

Crenshaw, K. (1991). Mapping the margins: Intersectionality, identity politics, and violence against women of color. *Stanford Law Review, 43*(6), 1241–1299.

Gayer, L., & Christophe, J. (Eds.). (2012). *Muslims in Indian cities: Trajectories of marginalisation.* Hurst.

Ghurye, GS (1969). Caste and race in India. Bombay, Popular Prakashan.

Jamil, G. (2017). *Accumulation and segregation: Muslim localities in Delhi.* New Delhi.

Khan, S. (2007). Negotiating the Mohalla: Exclusion, identity and muslim women in Mumbai. *Economic and Political Weekly, 42*(17), 1527–1533.

Mitra. Anirban, and Debraj Ray,. (2014). Implications of an economic theory of conflict: Hindu-muslim violence in India. *Journal of Political Economy, 122*(4), 719–765.

Lewis, O (1996) [1966]. The Culture of Poverty. In G. Gmelch; W. Zenner (eds.). Urban Life. Waveland Press.

Naidu, R. (1990). *Old city, new predicament: A study of hyderabad.* Sage.

Park. R.E. 1925. The growth of the city: An introduction to a research project. In R. E. Park, E. W. Burgess, D. M. Roderick & W. Luis (Eds.), *The city.* University of Chicago Press.

Peer, B. (2015). In India's largest muslim ghetto. *The Hindu.*

Rahman, A. (2019). *Denial and deprivation: Indian muslims after the sachar committee and Rangnath Mishra commission reports.* Manohar Publishers & Distributors.

Rajagopal, A. (2010). Special political zone: Urban planning, spatial segregation and the infrastructure of violence in Ahmedabad. *South Asian History and Culture, 1*(4), 529–556.

Rao, N. A., Abdul, S., & Thaha,. (2012). Muslims of Hyderabad: Land locked in the Walled City. In L. Gayer & C. Jaffrelot (Eds.), *Muslims in Indian cities: Trajectories of marginalisation* (pp. 189–212). Hurst.

Report of the Commission of Inquiry on Socio-Economic and Educational Conditions of Muslims Government of Telangana. (2016). Government of Telangana.

Sachar, R. (2006). *Sachar committee report: Social, economic and educational status of the muslim community of India.*

Saunders, P. (1986). The ideology of the new right. 20(3):477–479

Sen, A. (1999). *Development as Freedom.* Alfred Knopf.

Shaban, A. (2018). *Lives of Muslims in India: Politics, Exclusion and Violence.* Routledge.

Sikand, Y., & Manjari, K. (1994). Mass conversions to hinduism among Indian muslims. *Economic and Political Weekly, 29*(34), 2214–2219.

Srinivas, M. (2010). Hyderabad old city: A saga of discrimination. *People's Democracy, XXXIV*(15).

Sudhir, G. (2016). Report of the commission of inquiry on socio-economic and educational conditions of muslims, Government of Telangana.

Vithal, B. P. R. (2002). Muslims of Hyderabad. *Economic and Political Weekly, 37*(28), 2883–2886.

Yaseer, H. (2017). Master plans and patterns of segregation among muslims in Delhi. *Critical Planning, 23*(0). Retrieved April 15, 2021, from https://escholarship.org/uc/item/5jd9d353.

Ziyauddin, K. M. (2018). *Exploring the exclusionary perspective of muslim community and their health condition: A case of selected pockets of Andhra Pradesh.* A Major Research Project Study (unpublished) Report. ICSSR.

Chapter 8
Experiences of and Responses to COVID-19 in a Ho Tribal Village in Jharkhand

Jay Prakash Sharma

Abstract The COVID-19 pandemic has caused an unprecedented impact upon human society across the globe. Evidently, it is going to have far-reaching consequences touching upon almost every single aspect of our lives, yet the magnitude and severity of sufferings will remain as differentiated as our societies and people are around us. The horrific suffering endured by migrant workers during their mass exodus from Indian cities in the wake of the government-imposed lockdown leading to a humanitarian crisis is a telling example. Through this chapter, I explore how a pandemic of this scale was perceived, experienced and responded to in a small village in the West Singbhum district of Jharkhand inhabited predominantly by the Ho tribe. To that end I will be discussing different phases of the pandemic—initial infection spread, economic lockdown and restriction upon people's movement; arrival of the migrants; staggered unlocking and everyday life—from a perspective informed by the Ho community. I argue that although the narratives around the pandemic made their way into the village through mainstream, popular and social media, the Ho community's response to it was mediated by local socio-cultural and political contexts. The pandemic, indeed, elicited varying feelings ranging from anxiety and hopelessness to indifference and factitious reactions; however, their responses during each phase mentioned above were expressed through idioms that sit uncomfortably with the mainstream narratives. These inconsistencies in the narrative must also be seen from the backdrop of a history checkered with practices of exploitation, oppression and alienation.

Keywords Tribal inequality · Ho · Jharkhand · Colonial exploitation · Rural studies

J. P. Sharma (✉)
Department of Anthropology, Syracuse University, New York, USA
e-mail: jasharma@syr.edu

Introduction

We will die from hunger and desperation, anyway, why fear this disease one cannot even see.

These words spoken by Dugru,[1] a disabled man in his early 30 s, came in a quick reply—with a wistful smile as he glanced towards the ground—when I asked whether villagers are scared of the COVID-19 virus. For Dugru and his fellow villagers, the more immediate, tangible concerns deserve more attention than this 'foreign' disease that no one from the village has heard of or encountered. Born out of state apathy and a long history of exploitation, oppression and alienation, these concerns form sediments in everyday tribal memories (Christopher, this volume).

On 24 March 2020, the Prime Minister of India made a sudden televised announcement appealing to the public to observe *Janata Curfew*, the People's Curfew—a three-week lockdown—in a bid to contain the spread of COVID-19 in India. The announcement came with just a four-hour notice, and the Prime Minister emphatically urged people not to step out of their homes. Before people could grapple with the uncertainties and suddenness of the unprecedented Janata Curfew, the lockdown, amended with much more stringent guidelines, was extended on April 14 for three more weeks, this time with no advance notice. The immediate implications of this lockdown were a complete shutdown of economic activities and compulsory confinement of people in their homes or temporary shelters; this would have long-lasting consequences. A study on housing conditions of urban poor suggests that there are around five million casual labourers temporarily staying in cities and living in adverse housing arrangements (Majid, 2020: 186–88). A complete economic shutdown, which eventually led to a state of joblessness with no food or rations and adverse accommodation arrangements, pushed many migrant workers onto the streets. They had no option left but to journey home by any means necessary. The media in the two months following the lockdown were rife with reports showing inhuman suffering and hardships that the migrant workers went through while making their way back home (Mander, 2020: 145–157; Sriraman & Vasudevan, 2020).

The Indian lockdown, ranked as the most severe in the world,[2] was imposed with a blanket approach without any second thought to how it could exacerbate existing vulnerabilities and sufferings of millions of people in a country marked by steep social and economic inequalities. The pandemic and resulting lockdown have variously impacted Indian citizens and continue to do so on a scale that we have only begun to fathom. However, the horrific experiences of stranded migrant workers made it clear that the worst hit are those already living on the margins.

This chapter aims to bring forth the experiences and responses of the Ho tribe, a historically marginalized community living in Nakahasa, a remote village nestled in the hills of West Singhbhum district of Jharkhand. The main source of livelihood in

---

[1] All the names in this chapter have been changed to keep the identity of the respondents anonymous.

[2] See 'COVID-19: Government Response Stringency Index', Our World in Data, available at https://ourworldindata.org/grapher/covid-stringency-index?tab=chart.

the village is subsistence farming, horticulture, daily wage labour in MGNREGA[3] and agriculture and construction work in neighbouring villages and towns. Out-migration for better wages and employment opportunities is quite high as 30% of households have some family member(s) who have migrated to the cities for work. While the discourse around this global pandemic is bound to be dominated by urban-centred, mainstream media and society, the variegated experiences and responses of the rural tribal communities are fated to be homogenized, just like the blanket lockdown.

In this chapter I discuss different phases of the pandemic—initial infection spread, economic lockdown and restrictions on people's mobility; arrival of the migrants; staggered unlocking and everyday life—from a perspective informed by the Ho community. The narratives around the pandemic that made their way into the village were mediated by local socio-cultural and political contexts—a marginalized tribal community with a long history of resistance against intrusion from 'outsiders' in order to save their land, forest and water. Such forcible intrusions preceded coercion, violence, deceits and betrayals to enable incessant exploitation of natural resources and socio-cultural subordination. The outsiders, historically, have ranged from Hindu traders, moneylenders, land grabbers and rent collectors under different regimes—the British and later the post-colonial state consistently engaged in continued economic exploitation on the pretext of bringing development to the region and civilizing the 'wild' people (Munda & Bosu Mullick, 2003).

Dugru's statement that begins the chapter comes from one of my first interactions during fieldwork in the Ho community that I began just prior to the imposed lock-down in anticipation of the COVID-19 pandemic outbreak. In the community, the pandemic indeed elicited varied feelings ranging from anxiety and hopelessness to indifference and factitious reactions. During each new phase of restrictions in the name of safety protocols, respondents expressed a sense of disbelief and mistrust that emanated from their long historical experience, one checkered with practices of exploitation, alienation and betrayal that continues to exist in various forms today. Precisely because of this history, the Ho community saw the impending pandemic as a hoax and conspiracy by the state and outsiders to further the process of exploiting the 'wild' people.

Historical Background

Although Jharkhand is one of the youngest states in India, the 'Jharkhand Movement' that led to its formation was the oldest movement for autonomy in post-independence India. The political mobilization to carve out a separate state began in 1938, the year

---

[3] 'Mahatma Gandhi National Rural Employment Guarantee Act', MGNREGA, is an Indian labour law and social security measure that aims to guarantee the 'right to work'. It does so by enhancing livelihood security in rural areas by providing at least 100 days of wage employment in a financial year to every household whose adult members volunteer to do unskilled manual work.

that the Adivasi Mahasabha (The Great Council of the Indigenous people) was formed (Munda & Bosu Mullick, 2003: x). This movement is seen as a direct result of the ruthless processes to dispossess and exploit the people of Jharkhand of their natural resources, first by the British and later by the Indian state in the guise of development (Parajuli, 1996; Stuligross, 2001). The process of internal colonial exploitation of the region began in 1774 when mining formally started with the first lease granted to the East India Company by the colonial government for coal mining (George, 2009: 161–62). The British not only crushed tribal insurgencies in the region but also prepared fertile ground for its internal colonization, a condition that continued to flourish in post-Independence India. Since the early 1900s, the colonial government established new acts and mining rules to encourage private capital investments in mining, thereby facilitating large-scale mineral exploitation and establishing a monopoly over timber and non-timber produce from the dense forest cover in the region (Rath, 2006). After independence, the situation further deteriorated. The Jharkhand region emerged as a key supplier for mines, which in turn actualized more ruthless dispossession of the people. Furthermore, almost four decades later, the neo-liberal reforms of the 1990s paved a way for unchecked exploitation of minerals and ores by private companies (George 2009: 161–62). The protracted resistance of Jharkhand's people against this continuous dispossession of their land and natural resources since colonial times gave birth to the Jharkhand movement.

Driving forces for both the Jharkhand movement for the formation of a separate state and contemporary Adivasi (indigenous) politics have included constant resistance against exploitation by the Dikus[4] and the British; a protracted struggle for water (jal), forest (jangal) and land (jameen) and a different way of life. However, the notion of distinct ethnic identity, a rallying point for political mobilizations, has time and again been contested and thus variously interpreted by scholars. Left scholars argue that besides shared cultural traits, the subjection of people to the same kind of economic exploitation that gave them a sense of class oppression has been a major force in their mobilization (Alam, 2003; Nathan, 2003; Rana, 2003; Roy, 2003). The movement has also been seen as a socio-political expression for a pan-ethnic identity that is based upon a shared Jhakhandi (tribal) culture (Bosu Mullick, 2003; Keshari & Munda, 2003). Others view it as a transformation from demands based on ethnicity to assertions based on regionalism (Alloysius, 2003; Singh, 2003). However, the reduction of ethnicity to regionalism has been criticized for betraying tribal political reality (Sharma, 2003) because the movement was never aimed at just demanding more resources and special privileges for the region (Alam, 2003). Thus, notions around Jharkhandi identity or tribal culture have never remained static and have morphed with changing political conditions (Hebbar, 2003; Prakash, 1999).

As highlighted by Subaltern Studies scholars, mainstream historiography has largely portrayed Indian nationalism as a middle-class response led by caste Hindus

---

[4] Diku etymologically means other people; however, in this context it refers to the Hindu moneylenders, merchants and outsiders whose arrival in the region marked the beginning of exploitative, feudal practices leading to land alienation of resource usurpation of the adivasis (see Roy, 1946; Hoffman, 1961; Sinha et al., 1969; Sachidananda, 1970).

and Muslims to British colonialism. Consequently, many of the tribal insurrections and resistance movements were either subsumed under Indian nationalism or rendered invisible. The 'subaltern groups' were considered too primitive to have developed a political consciousness. Post-independence, both the state and mainstream socio-political classes have consistently made an effort to integrate tribal communities into mainstream society by bringing them back into the Hindu fold through social and economic upliftment (Sundar, 1997: 180). However, neither tribal communities nor the Other Backward Caste groups and Dalits who remained integrated with tribal society in the region, ever associated with Hindu nationalism. The intention of the overarching nationalism of the Indian state was to forcefully integrate tribals into the mainstream rather than accommodating their own aspirations in the political system after independence (Bosu Mullick, 2003: xv). The rejection by the State Reorganization Commission in 1956 of the demand for the formation of Jharkhand as a separate state clearly reflects this nationalist intention since the Jharkhand Party—a party with its origin in the Jharkhand movement for statehood—had registered a landslide victory in the first general election of Independent India. Even so, the movement went on for almost four decades, witnessing vicissitudes of mass support as well as state repression. Eventually, after undergoing a protracted struggle by the people, the state of Jharkhand was carved out of Bihar in 2000.

The formation of a separate state inaugurated a formal incorporation of a distinct ethnic and cultural identity of the region in the mainstream political discourse; however, the political gains did not translate into socio-economic upliftment of the people. On the contrary, the state projected processes of privatization, globalization and sanskritization as harbingers of sustainable development in the region (Mullick, 2003: xvi). The state government, through its industrial policies, embarked on a path of neo-liberal, market-oriented development and deliberately pushed aside the long tradition of protest over control and access to natural resources (Jewitt, 2008). A prominent human rights organization, Bindrai Institute for Research Study and Action (BIRSA), soon after the formation of the state, flagged apprehensions about the state's control:

> We have finally got the Jharkhand state, but what we have got is only a physical layout of the same. If we ask ourselves the question as to *who* controls the lives of people within this physical area, then in order to give an honest answer we would have to admit that the controls are not in the hands of the Jharkhandi people. At the economic level, outsiders and non-tribes, industrialists, merchants, traders, mine-owners, government employees and contractors own our waters, forests and lands as well as our mineral resources. (BIRSA, 2000)

The status of statehood proved to have little impact on fulfilling the original aspirations of the people for autonomous control over natural resources, vis-a-vis land, forest and water, in the region. Nakahasa presents a microcosm of the larger Jharkhandi movement. In Nakahasa, a movement against limestone mining led by the villagers for five years eventually succeeded in stalling the mining operation. Based on my fieldwork and interviews with those involved in the movement, it was clear that the state police and local administration sided with the mining company—a pattern easily observed at the state level and across India.

Foucault defined the pervasive dualism of power through his dictum, 'Where there is power, there is resistance, and yet or rather consequently, this resistance is never in a position of exteriority in relations to power' (Foucault, 1978: 95). The portrayal of tribal resistance in India has been mostly seen as an oppositional response directed against the exploitative state practices and structures of power—notably Guha's (1982) thesis of subaltern political consciousness as a sphere separate and distinct from political cultures of elite politics, later reformulated as 'political society' by Chatterjee (2004). However, there has also emerged a body of work that brings forth a dialectical relation of the subaltern class with the structures of power. This body of work has demonstrated the multiple ways through which subaltern groups engage with state institutions, governmental technologies and democratic discourses while simultaneously resisting them.[5]

Drawing on Foucault's dictum, however, Abu-Lughod cautions us not to romanticize resistance by implying 'power as always and essentially repressive' (Abu-Lughod, 1990: 42). She rather proposes an inversion of Foucault's dictum—'where there is resistance, there is power'—and suggests to use 'resistance as a diagnostic of power' in order to investigate 'not about the status of resistance itself but about what the forms of resistance indicate about the forms of power that they are up against' (Ibid: 42–47). Yet, while investigating the forms of resistance, 'we respect everyday resistance not just by arguing for the dignity or the heroism of the resistors but by letting their practices teach us about the complex interworkings of historically changing structures of power' (Ibid: 53). Following Abu-Lughod, I argue in this chapter that the Adivasi resistance and mistrust towards state health advisory and medical establishments in general is diagnostic of new forms of (exclusionary and alienating) power at play with ever-increasing pervasiveness of the state and its governmental technologies including public health matrices (Thakur, this volume). The residents of Nakahasa, in claiming COVID-19 news as false and conspiratorial, are resisting a probable claim that the state can take over their bodies through biomedical interventions on the pretext of a pandemic outbreak.

Nakahasa: A Placid Reception of an 'Unseen Pandemic'

The tribal village of Nakahasa comes under the most backward, according to the state's socio-economic parameters, Tonto block in West Singhbhum District that forms the southern part of the newly created state of Jharkhand. The geographical topography of the district is characterized by multiple hills alternating with valleys and deep forests along with 38 rivers and rivulets passing through it. The district also has three major watersheds covering an area over 6,941 km^2. The total population of West Singhbhum district is 1.5 million, of which about 49.8% is male and 50% is

---

[5] See (Heller, 1999, 2000; Fuller & Harriss, 2001; Corbridge et al., 2005; Gupta, 1995; Subramanian, 2009; Shah, 2010; Corbridge & Harriss, 2000; Guha, 1999; Sinha, 2003; Sivaramakrishnan & Agrawal, 2003; and Sundar, 1997).

female. A majority of the population, around 85%, live concentrated in rural areas, and the primary source of livelihood is based in agriculture, forest produce and daily wage labour.

While the reality in Indian cities and towns showed hasty, panicked preparation to battle COVID-19, another reality existed in the villages, where a sense of equanimity and life-as-usual persisted. I was in Nakahasa conducting fieldwork when the lockdown was announced. I interacted with the local community and observed everyday life with the backdrop of an impending pandemic. Village life in Nakahasa indeed experienced the initial effects of the panic and anxiety that emerged in the cities, but these were registered and manifested in quite a different fashion. On 14 April 2020, three weeks after the announcement of the first lockdown, I made my way to meet Sidiu. He was busy cooking rice and vegetables on a hearth outside his thatched roof kutcha house; his friend Kanai helped him with the cooking that day. Soon we were joined by Bamai, who retired a few years ago from a government job and had stayed in the village since, and Dungru, a casual labourer who mostly sought employment within the village.

Sidiu informed me that Jharkhand State Livelihood Promotion Society (JSLPS) had given him 1,000 rupees to run a community kitchen in order to feed the poorest of the poor in the village. He declined initially, citing the paltry amount as insufficient to feed the needy people for a month, but the JSLPS staff insisted that he take the money and told him that he was free to feed people as long as the money lasted—feeding the needy for a week or two would be better than nothing. With annoyance at the memory, he told me that, 'Rs. 1000 is not enough for buying rice, lentils and vegetables, forget about oil, spices, and salt'. Due to insufficient funds, Sidiu used his own stock of lentils from this year's harvest, took vegetables from his own backyard and relied on his own household supplies for salt, oil and spices. He did all of this even in the absence of government compensation, just to receive divine blessings and be of service to the needy.

I asked the men about the impact of the pandemic on the people in the village. Sidiu responded that:

> There is not much impact, we have everything available in the village to eat, we grow rice, lentils and vegetables, and there are wild vegetables, various kinds of edible tree leaves are available as well. However, the only adverse impact we are having from it is in terms of access to Haats (local markets), as many people are not able to sell vegetables, fruits, agricultural produce and livestock. One more problem is commuting to Chaibasa to buy household supplies. Many of us fear going to Chaibasa because policemen are beating them with cane sticks. Otherwise, we have everything in our village, we have just harvested lentils and have sufficient stock of rice from last year.

This kind of response was quite common among other villagers as well in the early days of the pandemic. I asked them about those who do not own land and are entirely dependent on daily wage labour, as they would not get any employment due to lockdown. Sidiu replied that people are getting free rations, even those without a ration card, and living off whatever savings they had. Then Sidiu and Bamai went on to talk about the online process, which restricts the access of people involved in applying for free rations and a free cooking gas cylinder (on the Digital Divide see Diwakar

G and Viswambaran, this volume). There are only a handful of individuals who own smartphones in the village and can navigate through the online government websites to avail these benefits. Sidiu came to know about the free ration from newspapers and social media that he accessed online on his smartphone.

Most of the respondents in the village had no idea about COVID-19 except from village gossip. Neither the village headman (Munda) nor the local administration had begun any initiative to spread awareness about the disease. There was a complete lack of credible information, except rumours and gossip, on 'what is this disease', how does it spread or what precautions one should take if someone falls sick with COVID-19. There were a few exceptions, as mentioned those who owned smartphones and had access to online news and social media; however, it increasingly became difficult to distinguish reliable news from rumour and propaganda once media got swamped by the pandemic—it is a city disease; it is conspiracy against the Adivasis; it is nothing but just like cold and flu but the government is spreading fear to benefit businessmen (pharmaceutical companies); if it is so deadly it should also affect the animals as they also breathe air through nose; it can also spread through urine and stool, it is a contagious (*chuachut*)[6] disease; it is similar to the disease that happened to chickens; and so on. The only person with some credible information I came across was Bamai, who told me that he learned from YouTube videos that we should maintain distance, should not touch our nose and mouth, should use hand wash and drink boiled water. He further added that cold, coughing, fever, breathing difficulties are symptoms of COVID-19. Soma, a daily wage labourer who works at a stone quarry near the village, complained, 'There is no information about the disease in our language [Ho], how can you be sure whether it is malaria or some other disease?' Many other respondents echoed a similar concern regarding the lack of any information in the Ho language on this disease. Despite the fact that 'Ho' is a widely spoken language in the region and a rallying point for the Ho tribe's distinct linguistic identity in Jharkhand (Sen, 2003: 4–5), the official language for local administration, banks and other services has remained Hindi.

I witnessed a contrasting picture when I visited Chaibasa, an urbanized locality that also houses the district headquarters. Local health department officials distributed pamphlets and e-rikshaw driven carts accessorized with loudspeakers travelled the streets announcing COVID-19 guidelines and precautionary measures for residents to follow. Needless to say, most of the households in this urban locality have access to television, smartphones or newspapers. I noticed people coming outdoors, although in small numbers, and there were police personnel deployed at almost every major square. The overwhelming presence of police reminded me of an oft-repeated response from the villagers that they really fear going to Chaibasa because the police chase and beat people with cane sticks. The inability to commute to Chaibasa was indeed a matter of concern for the villagers as it served as a nodal point for various essential services and supplies, as well as a source of daily wage and salaried jobs in

---

[6] A literal translation of Chuachut will be contagious, but it also carries along the connotation attached to untouchability, a hallmark of caste-based discrimination based upon purity and pollution, a status ascribed by birth.

the informal sector. However, what deterred the villagers from travelling to Chaibasa was not fear of contracting the disease, but the threat of brute force applied by the police.

On being asked whether they feared the novel coronavirus, villagers usually responded, 'Why fear something that you cannot see'. Some of the respondents stressed that since they had not come across any corona patients, why should they trust that this disease even exists. They believed that it must be a rumour spread to destabilize a government led by an Adivasi party and an Adivasi leader, unlike earlier regimes dominated by an outsiders' party (BJP). I also came across advice, such as if a person drinks Hadiya/Rasi, a traditional alcoholic drink made of fermenting rice, it will kill the coronavirus. Many suggested that since Adivasis are so hardworking and used to toiling their land under scorching sun and heat, they have too much immunity to get infected by this disease. Some argued that it is just a common cold and cough that we have had for centuries, and people are just blowing it out of proportion and spreading rumours to benefit the state and industrialists. Asked if she knew anything about corona, Guari, a middle-aged woman, replied with a smile, 'I only know that it is a disease, it has never happened in my family. Look at my kids, they are healthy and growing fine'. Manaki, a middle-aged man who works as a mason in Chaibasa, remarked that:

> We are not afraid of corona; we have not witnessed it yet. Madam (a local school teacher) was saying one day it is like this, other day it is like that on WhatsApp (chuckles as he says it), I do not believe. Also, how are we supposed to maintain social distance in villages, and we were asked to live separately. Look, we live in a small house, where will we leave our kids? They can't live without us. I told Madam that yes, maybe it is spreading in other places but let it come here first. There are cows, goats, sheep living with us, who also have mouths and they breathe as well, why don't they get the disease too. You have stayed here for so long, has anything happened so far? It is just like the common cold, cough that has been around us since ages. We never trusted that the corona disease even exists.

Fortunately, until mid-February 2021, no one from the village reported positive with COVID-19. West Singbhum District remained in a green zone even when the national figure hit its peak. However, reports of positive cases in the district started to emerge once the migrant labourers returned to their home states during mid-May 2020.

The French anthropologist Didier Fassin, while writing on heuristics of conspiracy theories, points out that 'instead of decrying or mocking them, we need to examine them from a dual perspective: for what they are and for what they tell us about our world in general and about specific situations in a given national or local context' (Fassin, 2021: 136). Within anthropology, scholars have always treated conspiracy theories, gossip and rumours as 'social facts', constitutive of 'social relations, political tensions, cultural disquietude, and moral uneasiness' (Ibid: 128–130).[7]

It will be impetuous to treat the disbelief among Hos towards the COVID-19 news and state advisories as just an overt act of complacency and ignorance. Rather, the

---

[7] See (Coplan 1994; Max Gluckman 1963; Stephen Ellis 1993; Robert Dingwall 2001; George Marcus 1999), cited in Fassin (2021).

mistrust towards state health advisories and the medical establishments among the Ho and many other tribes in Jharkhand is also rooted in a long history of exclusionary practices of the public health system and medical establishments (Poddar, 2021). A similar response was seen among many other marginalized communities across the globe, for instance, indigenous communities in North and South America. As widely reported in news articles in the wake of the COVID-19 pandemic, the distrust by people of colour and indigenous communities towards the medical establishment is rooted in a long history of injustice, mistreatment, discrimination and exploitation at the hands of the health system. The dehumanized bodies of enslaved black people had long been treated as guinea pigs for medical experiments by the establishment and continued to experience this treatment even after the abolition of slavery, one of the most infamous examples in the Tuskegee study. Similarly, a long history of unjust and exploitative relations with medical establishments made indigenous communities in Canada suspicious of the virus and the vaccine, eliciting deep-rooted mistrust towards health care facilities.

Return of Migrants: Longing, Anxiety and Reunion

> They were assured, of course, of the inerrable equality of death, but nobody wanted that kind of equality. Poor people who were feeling the pinch thought still more nostalgically of towns and villages in the nearby countryside, where bread was cheap and life without restrictions. Indeed, they had a natural if illogical feeling that they should have been permitted to move out to these happier places … (Albert Camus, *The Plague*).

In the beginning of April 2020, Sunita and Kaira had sent 10,000 rupees from their savings to their son Lankesh, a migrant semi-skilled labourer stuck in Tamil Nadu, so that he could pay for his living expenses and arrange his journey back home. Sunita and Kaira once worked as migrant workers in the neighbouring state of Orissa. They returned to live in Nakahasa ten years ago. They are dependent on agriculture and vegetable farming to meet their household expenses and receive a monthly remittance from Lankesh. After imposition of the nationwide lockdown, their most immediate concern was not the pandemic but the suspension of public transports that made it difficult for their son to get back to the village. Many other youths, including Sidiu, got constant calls from migrant workers for assistance in applying for tickets under Shramik Special trains. Sidiu once called me late in the evening, asking if I could write an application letter on behalf of five migrants from the village who were stuck in Tamil Nadu. The letter would be submitted at a local police station. Soon after their return from the cities, while recounting their experiences after the lockdown, nearly all my respondents remembered just looking forward to getting home after companies and factories shut down. There was an assurance of safety, food, care, independence, a familiar place and people back at home, while in cities they were overwhelmed with uncertainties, hardship, loneliness and vulnerabilities. The most immediate concern, more than losing their job, was falling sick in a city with strangers and no one to take care of them and dying in a foreign land. For Ho people, having the last rites done in their ancestral village and laid down at the family burial site are prerequisites for a meaningful death and afterlife—once a Ho person is laid down at the family burial site, her spirit is summoned by family members to find a permanent place in a sacred sanctum, called Aadding, already inhabited by the spirits of other deceased family members and ancestors.

The haphazard decision to force everyone to stay in their homes without considering the crude reality that a large share of the urban population lives in densely populated, cramped spaces soon created the 'greatest man-made tragedy' and 'worst migrant crisis'. A sense of acute anxiety and hopelessness arose from the sudden joblessness, lack of rations, money and shelter, along with the fear of contracting a deadly virus. The labourers were forced to journey back home on foot. The electronic and print media was soon flooded with moving images and disturbing reports of swollen feet wrapped in blisters after covering hundreds of miles under scorching sun and heat; mothers carrying babies; a woman pulling her child half asleep on a suitcase; a toddler trying to wake up her dead mother on a railway platform and the list goes on.[8] The horrific ordeal that the migrants and their families went through continued for almost two months until May 1 when the central government finally allowed state governments to arrange for migrants' journeys back home. The same day Jharkhand CM Hemant Soren announced that his government would make all the arrangements to ensure a safe return of the migrant workers hailing from Jharkhand. In the following days, displaying a sensible approach towards the pandemic, the state government introduced various social safety net schemes and initiatives; these included direct cash transfer to all the state's migrant workers, special trains arranged to transport migrants stuck in other states back to Jharkhand, and free food and shelter for stranded migrants in the state.

These arrangements made a substantial difference in mitigating the suffering of migrant labourers from Jharkhand in the early days of the pandemic. Nevertheless, their return also signalled a sense of anxiety among people. This sense of anxiety rose from the fact that they might carry the coronavirus and infect others along the way and in their native villages. By May 13, the total number of cases in Jharkhand numbered 174, still quite low in proportion to the national figure of 74,281 COVID-19 cases, but it was feared that the return of the migrants from highly affected states would push the number up radically. The number of returning migrant workers rose to over three lakhs by May 22; only 6.6%, or 19,686 workers, were tested for COVID-19. The number of workers who tested positive for the virus was quite low, at only one per cent of the total workers tested. Nevertheless, the share of migrant workers in the total number of active cases in Jharkhand was as high as 80%. A heightened sense of anxiety was evident at the time in the media, the local administration and the general population due to the mass exodus of the migrant workers. A similar anxiety, subtler and less diffuse, was also felt by the villagers in Nakahasa.

---

[8] A story of swollen feet: The physical toll of walking home during lockdown, 14 June 2020, Scroll. See https://scroll.in/article/963641/a-story-of-swollen-feet-the-physical-toll-of-walking-home-during-lockdown.

With the arrival of migrant labourers, people in Jharkhand grew increasingly anxious, just like in other parts of India, and anticipated that the number of COVID-19 cases would drastically shoot up. The apathetic response that the public and government showed towards the migrants exposed the reality that their bodies and lives were being subsumed under a 'stigmatizing label' where they were just seen as 'transmitter(s) of disease and someone who can flood us with biological and/or psychological vulnerability' (Vahali 2020: 275). A similar anxiety persisted among the villagers, but something else superseded the fear caused by the pathogen. There was talk making the rounds in the village every now and then that some migrant worker in some village had tested positive. The police were sealing the village. This issue was raised during a village council meeting (Gram Sabha). Bamai Godsora expressed his apprehensions from such news, 'If there is even a single positive case, the police are sealing the entire village, no one is being allowed to go out. I am afraid if our village gets sealed how will we tend to our field. It has to be ploughed for rice cultivation. We buy fertilizers and urea from the market in Chaibasa, how will we get it?' This anxiety was rooted in the possible suspension of agricultural activity if the village is sealed because that could adversely impact paddy cultivation. Rice is not just the principal crop grown in Jharkhand, but the entire process of paddy cultivation and harvesting is intricately enmeshed with Adivasi culture. On the one hand, rice constitutes the staple grain in their daily food, while on the other hand, the traditional drinks Hadiya and Rasi made from fermented rice are indispensable for almost all Adivasi rituals. Neighbours and relatives offer free labour during the whole cycle, from cultivation and harvesting to threshing and storage. In return neighbours are served Hadiya or Rasi, snacks and sometimes full meals.

The villagers who seemed to have remained aloof from the pandemic were now feeling anxious as COVID-19 cases were reported from neighbouring villages. I learned from a respondent that the village chief (Munda)[9] and some village elders had decided not to allow any strangers or outsiders to enter the village as they might spread the disease here. A Gram Sabha was finally called by the Munda on the 24th of May 2020, the first since the lockdown was imposed, in order to discuss what to do in the wake of the return of migrant workers belonging to Nakahasa. The meeting was held under a banyan tree at a square in the middle of the village and attended by 60 residents, comprising around 20 men, 30 women and 10 kids. The age group varied from adolescents and youth to middle- and old-aged folks. As the people settled down the village Sahiya[10] stood up and spoke:

> Almost half of the households in the village have someone who has migrated to cities in search of work. If we leave them on their own, eventually the virus will spread to everyone and we will go to hell. All the people returning from other states are going through health check-ups and are not just being allowed to enter. Those being allowed to come are healthy. Nevertheless, people are saying that it spreads through air and they might get infected while traveling in trains or buses. That is why we will keep them in the school for 14 days and if

---

[9] Munda is a traditional village head in the Singhbhum region of Jharkhand.

[10] Sahiyas are Accredited Social Health Activists (ASHA) appointed under the ambitious National Rural Health Mission and work as community level health activists providing primary treatment, spreading awareness about various diseases, mapping child births, etc.

they still are healthy, we will allow them to shift to their homes. If someone is not feeling well, they will inform us about it and we will arrange an ambulance/conveyance to take them to hospital.

After about half an hour of continuous discussion and deliberations, it was decided that all those returning back to the village would go through a compulsory 14-day quarantine in the school building. Their family members were given the responsibility of cooking food for them, to be served on plates made of tendu leaves[11] while maintaining a proper distance. The ward member's husband Lalit suggested that separate arrangements should be made for people coming from different zones, i.e. red, orange and green zones. It was unanimously agreed upon that everyone would cooperate to strictly follow the quarantine guidelines to avoid a failed situation in which people would contract the disease and the entire village would be sealed. This would jeopardize their health as well as agricultural activities.

The migrants eventually arrived on May 27 and stayed in the primary school building of the village. The building was flooded by the villagers on the first day, exchanging words and asking about their relatives' health while maintaining a proper distance from the boundary walls of the school. Many faces were lit up with smiles and wet eyes after seeing their loved ones back in the village and living in close proximity. Sunita gleefully looked at her son, who had returned after almost a year, trying to strike a conversation with him amidst the cacophony of exuberant voices. She told me, 'That is my son Lankesh, he was healthy, but it seems he has lost some weight'. The sight of their relatives instilled a sense of joy among the villagers, even in this unforeseen and unpredictable moment. They stood right across from them, but an impending threat of the coronavirus made their own kin untouchables. Later, while I was interviewing Lankesh about his recent experiences, he remarked with a chuckle, 'When we were in quarantine our family was giving food like dogs, passing it over in a plate from a distance'. The migrant workers stayed there for just seven days and then went on to their homes. Fortunately, no one in the village fell sick from COVID-19.

Narratives from Migrant Workers: The Pandemic and Beyond

On being asked how he decided to migrate to Tamil Nadu, Lankesh, a youth in his mid-20 s who always wore a composed look, replied with a smiling face:

I decided it on my own, there was financial constraint in the family, and I am the eldest sibling. I went to Tamilnadu and started working as a helper to the welder, on a 12-hours of daily shift earning 315 rupees. I started as a helper but soon, in a month, learnt the work of welder. However, the company did not increase my wage on par with a welder for almost a year. I had to change 5 companies over the last four years before finally receiving a rightful wage that a welder should be paid. I will work there for another 3–4 years, save some money

---

[11] Tendu leaves are traditionally used here to make disposable plates, bowls and cups.

and get back to the village and open a photo studio. I have already learnt online how to use photoshop and edit photos.

I asked if he would like to do farming upon his final return from the city. Lankesh pauses for a moment and says, 'No I don't want to grow vegetables but this crop (paddy) is so essential for us to grow, so that I will have to'. His parents have been growing vegetables that they sell in weekly village Haats (local bazaars) apart from occasionally working as daily wage labourers in the village and Chaibasa.

Ravi lost his father when he was in high school and was struggling to balance his studies with the overwhelming responsibility of taking care of household expenses and his ailing mother. He used to borrow books and money to buy stationary items from his friend. He narrates his story of how he navigated through this economic hardship as follows,

> I worked as *reja* (unskilled casual labor) in Chaibasa at a construction site for three weeks on a daily wage of 120 rupees. I gave some money to my mother at home and then booked a train ticket and left. I went with my friends, those who had failed in inter (high school) and wanted to discontinue study and leave for work. My friends were going out of state to work and asked me to come along. I thought about what I would do here, I had no money, who would take care of my studies and school expenses. My mother was not keeping well, we needed money for her treatment as well. Also, I was the eldest in my siblings, so the responsibility came over me. When we boarded the train and it was about to leave when someone was playing a sad Bollywood song, I felt like crying.

Ravi stayed back in Karnataka for a month after the lockdown, and his company refused to make any payment. Before he left for Nakahasa by a Shramik train, he helped other folks from Jharkhand who could not write applications or navigate through the online application procedures.

Short-term migration has increased rapidly in India post-liberalization (Breman, 1994; Deshingkar & Farrington, 2009; Gidwani & Sivaramakrishnan, 2003; Rogaly & Coppard, 2003); nevertheless, the availability of quantitative as well as qualitative data has remained scarce (Chandrashekar & Deshingkar & Bird, 2009; Ghosh, 2007; Government of India, 2017). Existing studies indicate low economic, educational and social status as the major factors inducing seasonal migration from rural to urban areas (Deshingkar & Start, 2003; Deshingkar et al., 2008; Keshri & Bhagat, 2012). Evidently, temporary migration remains highest among Scheduled Tribes, with the poor and illiterate found to be more prone to migrate (Keshri & Bhagat,). I interviewed around 35 migrant workers in Nakahasa, all of them belonging to an age group ranging from 17 to 30 years. The reasons they cited for their migration included school drop out, economic distress, bearing medical expenses of an ailing kin and lack of jobs as well as low wages in Jharkhand. Most of my respondents had to drop out of high school due to poor performance. Upon further interrogation I discovered that the state of primary school in Nakahasa is so bad that most of the students who pass out and get promoted to high schools elsewhere find it challenging to get through and thus drop out. These unskilled youth with low education work in the nearby town of Chaibasa for some time before deciding to migrate out to other states in search of better jobs and wages.

Many of them were underage when they went to other states for work but were never asked to produce any ID or age proof. Almost all of them faced the same ordeal of getting low wages, doing extra hours of arduous work and having zero bargaining power with their employers in the first few years of their work. Once they reached their destination using informal networks of friends, relatives and local contractors, they spent the next couple of years working at a much lower wage than statutorily prescribed by the states even after they became skilled labourers. Even though they worked extra hours to learn skills like welding, operating heavy machineries and masonry, the hiring companies continued to pay them the wage fixed for a helper, much lower than what they rightfully deserve and are statutorily entitled to. It usually takes around three to four years for them to get familiar with and settle into a complex web of channels through which casual employment in the informal sector is organized and get a decent wage. A vicious cycle has been formed where every year a fresh batch of youth from Jharkhand arrives in cities, with no experience or knowledge of the highly unstable, precarious and exploitative work environment of the Indian informal sector.

Conclusion

Following Abu-Lughod's 'diagnostic use of resistance', this chapter bypasses a straightforward analysis of the status of resistance but rather explores resistance reveals about the forms of power that they are pitted against. Such an approach illuminates the complex ways through which historically changing structures of power operate in a given socio-political context. Drawing on the body of work done by anthropologists on conspiracy theories and rumours, the mistrust around COVID-19 among the Hos cannot be simply discarded as delusional. Rather, by registering their social practices of disbelief, Ho people are resisting exclusionary practices of state institutions. Indeed, as the state practices and its institutions have aggressively extended its outreach and have become almost pervasive, some basic services, such as public health and education, have miserably failed in both providing resources to tribal communities and earning their trust. This is the broader context in which we must analyse Ho distrust towards medical establishments—establishments which have failed to acknowledge, incorporate or adjust to the indigenous ways of perceiving and healing diseases.

Interestingly, more than the pandemic, it was the fear of state violence that the villagers were preoccupied with—fear of the police sealing the village or beating commuters to Chaibasa with cane sticks. However, this time the villagers anticipated state intrusion and violence by responding with self-sufficiency and life as normal—a way of life that is different from Dikus yet sustainable—even during a devastating global pandemic. As Bamai wittily pointed out, 'In Italy you have Rome and Pope, then why Italy is suffering, they should have easily done away with it. Hindus have crores of God/Goddesses, why are they not protecting Hindus from this pandemic. The United States is the strongest nation but people are helpless and dying there'.

This was a fitting response to the dominant narrative of yesteryears, continuing today, that the forceful intrusion of the British and then the Indian state was to bring development, prosperity and civilization to this land.

The state provisioning of food and rations for the villagers in the wake of the pandemic was indeed a thoughtful initiative to ensure and prioritize food security among the tribal community. However, a continued lack of any initiative to facilitate dissemination of credible information among the rural populace further deepened the existing chasm of trust between people and the medical establishments widespread across India (Kane & Calnan, 2017). This lack of trust is further aggravated by the pervasive suspicion among Adivasis towards the state, which has mostly allied with the exploitative Dikus and mining companies. The local administration remained aloof of what kind of (mis)information regarding COVID-19 was increasingly circulated among the Hos through social media and gossip. The village Sahiya could have easily disseminated information on COVID-19, but she was instructed to do so much later when the national figure for positive cases was at its peak and a migrant crisis threatened to exacerbate the situation. Also, a more localized approach, using vernacular language and modes of information dissemination, while also accounting for cultural variations, was imperative for a diverse country like India. For instance, in Nakahasa, a Dakua[12] and Sahiya could have easily disseminated information on COVID-19 in Ho language if the local administration would have demonstrated a strong will.

Almost four months later, around mid-March 2021, India was hit by a much more severe and deadly second wave of COVID-19 pandemic. As I conclude this chapter, by 19 May 2021, Indian cities struggle with shortages of hospital beds, oxygen, medicines and testing facilities. Horrific pictures of around 2,000 dead bodies dumped along the banks of Ganga and in as many as 27 districts across the states of Uttar Pradesh and Bihar are making rounds in the media. What makes the situation more dreadful is the aggressive spread of multiple variants of the novel coronavirus in India's countryside, where people have limited medical access and medical institutions have acute resource shortages. The existing situation in rural areas is further aggravated by people's lack of trust in the vaccine and medical establishments. I recently learned from phone conversations with informants that many villagers fear getting vaccinated, as they have heard that people are dying after taking the vaccine. The mistrust towards the vaccine gets further deepened by the actual side effects that people may experience post-vaccination, considered as a sign of adverse impact on the body that can be lethal. Many are scared of visiting hospitals for treatment or testing since they believe the hospital staff would forcibly institutionalize them and they would drop off the radar. All these doubts and suspicions might eventually become a major obstacle in prophylactic measures including vaccination drives and medical treatment for COVID-19. These doubts could have been easily minimized if credible information was disseminated right in the beginning of the pandemic, a step

---

[12] Dakua is a postman, traditionally appointed at a village level. When a Gram Sabha has to be called or some information has to be passed on to the village folks, he goes around the village playing a drum and makes the announcement or spreads the information.

that many countries took well in advance specifically targeting their marginalized communities.

References

Abu-Lughod, L. (1990). The romance of resistance: Tracing transformations of power through bedouin women. *American Ethnologist, 17*(1), 41–55.

Alam, Javed. (2003). The category of non-historic nations and tribal identity in Jharkhand. In R. D. Munda & S. Bosu Mullick (Eds.), *The Jharkhand movement: Indigenous people's struggle for autonomy in India* (pp. 194–205). International Work Group for Indigenous Affairs.

Alloysius, G. (2003). Ideologies and hegemony in Jharkhand movement. In R. D. Munda & S. Bosu Mullick (Eds.), *The Jharkhand movement: Indigenous people's struggle for autonomy in India*, 206–215. International Work Group for Indigenous Affairs.

BIRSA. (2000). *Jharkhand ko Jharkhandi Banaye* (People's Agenda): Chaibasa.

Breman, J. (1994). *Wage hunters and gatherers: Search for work in the urban and rural economy of South Gujarat.* Oxford University Press.

Chandrasekhar, C P., & Ghosh, J. (2007). Dealing with short term migration. *Business Line.*

Chatterjee, P. (2004). *Politics of the governed: Reflections on popular politics in most of the world.* Columbia University Press.

Coplan, D. B. (1994). *In the time of cannibals: The word music of South Africa's Basotho migrants.* University of Chicago Press.

Corbridge, S., et al. (2005). *Seeing the state: Governance and governmentality in India.* Cambridge University Press.

Corbridge, S., & Harriss, J. (2000). *Reinventing India: Liberalization, Hindu nationalism and popular democracy.* Polity Press.

Deshingkar, P., & Farrington, J. (Eds.). (2009). *Circular migration and multilocational livelihood strategies in rural India.* Oxford University Press.

Deshingkar, P., & Bird, K. (2009). Circular migration in India. *Policy Brief, 4.*

Deshingkar, P., & Start, D. (2003). *Seasonal migration for livelihoods in India: Coping, accumulation and exclusion* (Vol. 111). Overseas Development Institute.

Deshingkar, P., Sharma, P., Kumar, S., Akter, S., & Farrington, J. (2008). Circular migration in Madhya Pradesh: Changing patterns and social protection needs. *The European Journal of Development Research, 20*(4), 612–628.

Dingwall, R. (2001). Contemporary legends, rumors and collective behaviour some neglected resources for medical sociology? *Sociology of Health and Illness, 23*(2), 180–202.

Ellis, S. (1993). Rumour and power in Togo. *Africa, 63*(4), 462–476.

Fassin, D. (2021). Of plots and men: The heuristics of conspiracy theories. *Current Anthropology., 61*(2), 128–137.

Foucault, M. (1978). *The history of sexuality. Vol. 1: An introduction.* Random House.

Fuller, C. J., & John H. (2001). For an anthropology of the modern Indian state. In C. J. Fuller & V. Bénéï, (Eds.), *The everyday state and society in modern India.* Hurst and Company.

George, A. S. (2009). The paradox of mining and development. In S. Nandini (Ed.), *Legal grounds: Natural resources, identity, and the law in Jharkhand* (pp. 157–189). Oxford University Press.

Gidwani, V., & Sivaramakrishnan, K. (2003). Circular migration and rural cosmopolitanism in India. *Contributions to Indian Sociology, 37*(1–2), 339–367.

Gluckman, M. (1963). Gossip and scandal. *Current Anthropology, 4*(3), 307–316.

Government of India. (2017). *Economic Survey 2016–17.* Department of Economic Affairs, Ministry of Finance, Government of India.

Gupta, A. (1995). Blurred boundaries: The discourse of corruption, the culture of politics, and the imagined state. *American Ethnologist, 22*(2), 375–402.

Guha, Ranajit. (1982). On some aspects of the historiography of colonial India. In G. Ranajit (Ed.), *Subaltern studies I: Writings on Indian history and society*. Oxford University Press.

Guha, S. (1999). *Environment and ethnicity in India, 1200–1991*. Cambridge University Press.

Hebbar, R. (2003). From resistance to governance. *Seminar, 524*, 45–50.

Heller, P. (1999). *The labor of development: Workers and the transformation of capitalism in Kerala, India*. Cornell University Press.

Heller, P. (2000). Degrees of democracy: Some comparative lessons from India. *World Politics, 52*(4), 484–519.

Hoffman, J. S. J. (1961). Principles of succession and inheritance among the Mundas. *Man in India, 41*(4), 324–338.

Jewitt, S. (2008). Political ecology of Jharkhand conflicts. *Asia Pacific Viewpoint, 49*(1), 68–82.

Kane, S. & Calnan, M. (2017). Erosion of trust in the medical profession in India: Time for doctors to act. *International Journal of Health Policy and Management, 6*(1), 5–8.

Keshri, K., & Bhagat, R. B. (2012). Temporary and seasonal migration: Regional pattern, characteristics and associated factors. *Economic and Political Weekly, 47*(4), 81–88.

Keshri, K., & Ram, B. B. (2010). Temporary and seasonal migration in India. *Genus*, 66(3), 25–45.

Kumar, S. (2018). Adivasis and the state politics in Jharkhand. *Studies in Indian Politics, 6*(1), 103–116.

Keshri, K., & Bhagat, R. B. (2010). Temporary and seasonal migration in India. *Genus, 66*(3), 25–45.

Majid, N. (2020). How many casual workers in the cities have sought to go home. In *India and the pandemic: The first year, essays from the Indian Forum* (pp. 182–193). Orient BlackSwan.

Mander, H. (2020). Migrant workers, the lockdown and the judiciary. In *India and the pandemic: the first year, essays from the Indian forum* (pp. 145-157). Orient BlackSwan.

Marcus, G. (1999). The paranoid style now: Introduction. In G. Marcus (Ed.), *Paranoia within reason: A casebook on conspiracy as explanation* (pp. 1–11). University of Chicago Press.

Mullick, B. S. (2003). The Jharkhand movement: A historical analysis. In R. D. Munda & S. Bosu Mullick (Eds.), *The Jharkhand movement: Indigenous people's struggle for autonomy in India* (pp. 244–271). International Work Group for Indigenous Affairs.

Munda, R. D. & Bosu Mullick, S. (2003). *The Jharkhand movement: Indigenous people's struggle for autonomy in India*. International Work Group for Indigenous Affairs.

Nathan, D. (2003). Jharkhand: Factors and future. In R. D. Munda & S. Bosu Mullick (Eds.), *The Jharkhand movement: Indigenous people's struggle for autonomy in India* (pp. 119–130). Copenhagen: International Work Group for Indigenous Affairs.

Parajuli, P. (1996). No nature apart: adivasi cosmovision and ecological discourses in Jharkhand, India. *Paper presented during the '2nd conference on the reconstruction of Jharkhand'*. Cambridge, UK.

Prakash, A. (1999). Contested discourses: Politics of ethnic identity and autonomy in the Jharkhand region of India. *Alternatives, 24*(4), 461–496.

Poddar, V. (2021). An old mistrust of government keeps Jharkhand's Adivasis away from COVID-19 vaccines. *The Caravan*. https://caravanmagazine.in/health/an-old-mistrust-of-government-keeps-jharkhands-adivasis-away-from-covid19-vaccines.

Rana, S. (2003). Jharkhand movement. In R. D. Munda & S. Bosu Mullick (Eds.), *The Jharkhand movement: indigenous people's struggle for autonomy in India* (pp. 110–118). International Work Group for Indigenous Affairs.

Rath, G. C. (Ed). (2006). *Tribal development in India: The contemporary debate*. Sage.

Rogaly, B., & Coppard, D. (2003). 'They used to go to eat, now they go to earn': The changing meanings of seasonal migration from Puruliya District in West Bengal, India. *Journal of Agrarian Change, 3*(3), 395–433.

Roy, A. K. (2003). Jharkhand: Internal colonialism. In R. D. Munda & S. Bosu Mullick (Eds.), *The Jharkhand movement: Indigenous people's struggle for autonomy in India* (pp. 78–85). International Work Group for Indigenous Affairs.

Roy, S. C. (1946). The aborigines of Chota Nagpur. Their proper status in the reformed constitution of India. *Man in India, 26*(2), 120–136.

Sachidananda, S. (1970). *The changing Munda.* Concept Publishing Company.

Sen, Ashok. (2003). Conceptualization of the Hos of Singhbhum as a tribe. In S. Padmaja (Ed.), *Changing tribal life: A socio-philosophical perspective* (pp. 1–14). Concept Publishing Company.

Shah, A. (2010). *In the shadows of the state: Indigenous politics, environmentalism and insurgency in Jharkhand, India.* Duke University Press.

Sharma, K. L. (2003). The Question of Identity and Sub-nationality. In R. D. Munda & S. Bosu Mullick (Eds.), *The Jharkhand movement: Indigenous people's struggle for autonomy in India* (pp. 232-242). International Work Group for Indigenous Affairs.

Singh, K. S. (2003). Tribal autonomy movements in Chota Nagpur. In R. D. Munda & S. Bosu Mullick (Eds.), *The Jharkhand movement: Indigenous people's struggle for autonomy in India* (pp. 88–109). International Work Group for Indigenous Affairs.

Sinha, S. C., Sen, J., & Panchbhai, S. (1969). The concept of diku amongst the tribes of Chota Nagpur. *Man in India, 49*(2), 121–138.

Sinha, Subir. (2003). Development counter-narratives: Taking social movements seriously. In K. Sivaramakrishnan & A. Agrawal (Eds.), *Regional modernities: The cultural politics of development in India.* Stanford University Press.

Sivaramakrishnan, K., & Agrawal, A. (2003). *Regional modernities: The cultural politics of development in India.* Stanford University Press.

Sriraman, T., & Vasudevan, N. (2020). Bearing witness to the covid-19 lockdown migrant workers in proof regimes. *The India forum: A journal-magazine on contemporary issues.* Issue: November 6, 2020.

Stuligross, D. (2001). *A piece of land to call one's own: Multicultural federalism and institutional innovation in India.* Unpublished Ph.D. Dissertation, University of California, December 2001.

Subramanian, A. (2009). *Shorelines: Space and rights in south India.* Stanford University Press.

Sundar, N. (1997). *Subalterns and sovereigns: An anthropological history of Bastar, 1854–2006.* Oxford University Press.

Part II
COVID-19 Disparities

During the pandemic, increased social precarity and fumbling public policy have translated into a slumping economy, fractured education, locked-down industries, and heightened social anxiety. These interlocking factors directly and indirectly impacts health. As chapters explore, migrant workers in the informal sector, differently abled people, people suffering from non-COVID-19 comorbidities, women, students, religious minorities, and others, have been particularly affected. It is imperative to critically investigate the effectiveness of public policies to address the current crisis and future pandemics. In the chapters that follow, a variety of social science and public health methods are utilized to paint the most detailed picture of pandemic response in South Asia. Each chapter drives home the central theme of how existing social inequalities exacerbated the impact of the pandemic on subaltern segments of society. We see the varied response from subaltern actors and the state. Compared to Section One, this section is more expressly directed towards understanding public health practice and offering policy recommendations.

Nilika Mehrotra and Mahima Nayar use an intersectional analysis to understand how disability impacted food access during the pandemic. They tease apart the complex interworking of food security and disability. Simply put, food insecurity is driven by poor living conditions, malnutrition, and anaemic health services. Disability also restricts access to food because of its correlation to poor education, employment opportunities, and access to social services and assistive technologies. Disabled people are over-represented in poor communities where food insecurity is prevalent. The devastation of COVID-19 has exacerbated food insecurity and malnutrition, and highlighted the pre-existing inequities in the reach of health care and food systems. Additionally, the pandemic further drove marginalization by stripping many precarious labourers of their sources of income. Mehrotra and Nayar provide an important contribution about how disabled people, among the most socially obscured population in South Asia, were impacted by the pandemic.

Continuing the theme of disability access, **Anwara Begum** examines health care access in Bangladesh during the pandemic. She argues that persons with disabilities are facing double exposure compared to the 'abled' population. Stigma attached to disability has increased their vulnerability. She observes that physical distancing is not possible for people with disabilities, especially those using assistive technologies and requiring personal support. This situation compounds the problems of having limited access to assistive resources in the first place. Through detailed qualitative methods—based on interviews with 65 care providers to persons with disabilities—she examines the severity of constraints placed upon peoples with disability. She analyzes nursing skills, preparedness, and the experiences of patients. As she unpacks the problem, she offers sensitive and empathic policy recommendations. Taken collectively, Nilika Mehrotra, Mahima Nayar and Anwara Begum raise important questions about how to safeguard the most vulnerable during a public health crisis.

Firdaus Fatima Rizvi highlights the plight of the women and children during lockdowns. Based on fieldwork in Allahabad, we see how when urban labourers lost their jobs and got locked down in cities, their absence drastically impacted their families. During this period, women were left at home managing food for the family, school fees for children, online classes and health care issues. Rizvi details how households faced sudden educational closures, increased dependence on the Public Distribution System (PDS) for food, increased household debt, and loss of income to pay rent and basic household needs. Her data closely matches with research from all around the world about the precarity of women and children during the pandemic—either because of absent husbands and lack of income or because husbands, normally working outside the home, were now constantly at home, increasing domestic abuse.

Sobin George, Aditi Paranjpe and Prajwal Nagesh analyzed the intermeshing fates of COVID-19 interventions and the National TB Elimination Programme in Bengaluru, India. When almost all the health care infrastructure was diverted towards COVID-19 care, health care providers and users faced challenges addressing non-pandemic illnesses. Sobin et al. analyzed the tuberculosis (TB) literature to illustrate the point that reallocation of funds to the pandemic response adversely affected several national health programmes in India. The National Tuberculosis Elimination Programme (NTEP) is one such important health programme that faced serious setbacks. TB interventions require constant following-up of patients by frontline workers. Through in-depth interviews with TB health visitors (TBHV), they show that several core functions were impaired, including active case findings, follow-up sputum examinations, distributions of medicine, and monitoring of patients with side effects. Such core functions were either slowed or temporarily suspended, weakening the critical frontline interventions of NTEP. They call for a broader assessment of health care delivery systems so that public health crises, like pandemics, do not disrupt future medical administration.

Trisha Mukhopadhyay and Sumanta Roy focus on violence against women in India. Through a critical analysis of print media and available scholarship, they argue that the pandemic has led to a global increase in gender inequality and gender discrimination, and has disproportionately impacted women and girls (UN Women 2020). They triangulate into this position by reviewing the manifold increase of SOS calls to police stations and helpline numbers and the increasing incidents of rape and sexual assault against women in quarantine centres (Acharya et al., 2020). The authors explore the false promises of the much-hyped notion of 'family time spent in togeth-erness' as part of the 'stay home' protocols. Women were confined to stay at home, often with the abusive, depressed and 'workless' partners. Joblessness, over-crowded households, financial dependency, and role expectations triggered violence against women (Vranda, 2020). This led to increased anxiety and feelings of powerlessness, which in turn drove another cycle of abusive behaviour. Men vented frustrations on women, and recently unemployed women were forced into greater dependency on their abusive partners. Mukhopadhyay and Roy bring out very intelligibly how the lockdown also obstructed abused women from seeking help. They illustrate these arguments with visual representations of data from the National Commission for Women (NCW), focussing on complaints that reflect crimes against women, and from media stories about the impact on women and strategies to empower women. Their chapter merits special notice for the seamless ways in which they brought together media and academic strands into a synthetic analysis.

Chapter 9
Disability, Access to Food and COVID-19: An Intersectional Analysis

Mahima Nayar and Nilika Mehrotra

Abstract People who live on the 'margins' face multiple vulnerabilities because of their social position—a prominent one being food insecurity. Food insecurity has been linked to various physical and mental health problems leading to poor general health. Disability, caste, gender and ethnicity all intersect to impact access to food. Linkages between food security and disability are complex—poor living conditions, malnutrition and poor health services can all lead to food insecurity. Alternatively, disability can restrict access to food because of poor access to education, employment opportunities as well as lack of access to social services and assistive technologies. Increased disability costs related to healthcare, personal care, equipment and/or other accommodations can drive households into poverty as a whole. Poverty is one of the leading causes of poor diet and malnutrition among people with disabilities in the global south. The advent of COVID-19 has exacerbated food security and nutrition crises highlighting the inequalities and inequities of the health and food systems. People with chronic illnesses or disabilities are more vulnerable to food insecurity. The pandemic has endangered their livelihoods and income generation capacities leading to further marginalization. The response of the State in India in recognizing the needs of the disabled has been delayed and largely ineffective. In this paper, we will explore the manner in which disability impacts access to food in general and how COVID-19 has impacted access to food. It also looks at/analyses/examines the role of the State in addressing the food security needs of the disabled especially in the time of COVID-19.

Keywords Disability · Food security · Malnutrition · COVID-19 · Marginalization · Chronic illness

M. Nayar (✉)
Independent Researcher, New Delhi, India

N. Mehrotra
Centre for the Study of Social Systems, School of Social Sciences, Jawaharlal Nehru University, New Delhi, India

© The Author(s), under exclusive license to Springer Nature Singapore Pte Ltd. 2022   175
S. S. Acharya and S. Christopher (eds.), *Caste, COVID-19, and Inequalities of Care*,
People, Cultures and Societies: Exploring and Documenting Diversities,
https://doi.org/10.1007/978-981-16-6917-0_9

Introduction

We see them and yet we don't—the invisibility of disabled people has been discussed in many spaces and yet this invisibility continues. Kafer (2013: 3) points out, disability is continually rendered invisible and undesirable, 'a perspective coloured by histories of ableism and disability oppression'. One of the main reasons for invisibility of the disabled people has been because of the manner in which it is understood. For decades, it was seen as the problem within and of an individual. Though there have been vast changes in the way disability is viewed and understood across centuries; the advent of COVID-19 exposed the continuing invisibility and vulnerability of the disabled across the world. In this chapter, we chose to focus on one of the basic necessities of life 'food' and how people with disabilities accessed it during the lockdowns resulting from COVID-19.

Food incorporates questions of economy, state, society relations and environment, as well as intimate issues of personal, social, cultural and bodily status and identity (Leach et al., 2020: 2). It is a political matter and access to it is influenced by power relations in society (ibid.). Since it is important for human survival and impacted by multiple social situations it has been incorporated into several international treaties. The Right to Food has been enshrined in international policies as a human rights issue, Article 25 of the Universal Declaration of Human Rights and Article 11 of the International Covenant on Economic, Social and Cultural Rights (Hospes & van der Meulen, 2009), UN Food and Agriculture Organisation (FAO Council, 2004) as well as in the Article 28 of the UN Convention on the Rights of Persons with Disabilities (UN CRPD, c.f. Waltz et al., 2018). COVID-19 and its related restrictions brought 'food' into prominence once again. Food access and insecurity were highlighted during the lockdowns –procuring (quantity and quality), storing and making food were some of the main discussion points. Absence of different types of food, restricted timings of markets and permission for only one member of the family to go out for essentials created many food discourses. In the challenges faced, the disabled population faced often insurmountable challenges as their carefully organized lives were disrupted. COVID-19 related restrictions also highlighted the existing inequalities and brought out the manner in which one's social position impacted coping with the pandemic. This chapter explores the manner in which disability, the social position of the person with disabilities affected their access to food in 'COVID times'. We begin with exploring the concepts of disability and food insecurity and their inter-relationships. And then move on to explore how COVID-19 related restrictions impacted this relationship.

COVID-19 not only created new vulnerabilities but also exacerbated the existing ones. The social position of people impacted the manner in which they could cope with the uncertainties of this pandemic. Therefore, it is important to discuss the historical understanding of disability as these understandings had an impact on how persons with disabilities were viewed in the social set up of those times. In this chapter, we begin with discussions around the various models of disability and how this impacts the everyday lives of persons with disabilities. The understanding of disability informs the social and economic positioning of people, which makes it important to explore the relationship between disability and poverty. Poverty is considered both a cause and result of disability and also determines a person's access to food.

Disability Through theTimes

The experience of disability has been seen through a medical lens—any physical or psychological anomaly within an individual without any acknowledgement to the structural issues. The viewpoint that people with disabilities are sick or unhealthy led to the development of a larger medical point of view regarding people with disabilities (Smeltzer et al., 2017). Historically it has been considered as a punishment from God for one's sin or misbehaviour or that of one's ancestors, work of the devil or a failure, deformity or defect of the individual. This has resulted in people with disabilities being feared or ridiculed (used for entertainment, e.g. court jesters, or oddities in circuses). Religious beliefs relating to disabilities range from disability being viewed as a sin to showing care and concern for persons with disabilities (Ingstad, 2001, 775; Miles, 1999). This led to them being hidden, isolated and viewed negatively. These are some of the reasons because of which an understanding of disability based on the 'charity model' continued for a long time. In this model of disability, bodily anomalies are ranked alongside other forms of tragedy and, as such, identify pity and donation of alms as appropriate responses (Clare, 2001). Lumped into a more general 'bundle of misery' (Stiker, 1982: 95) alongside poverty and other types of distress, disability had not yet been differentiated as a category, one that could be relocated, as it was during the enlightenment, within new medical discourses. It is in eighteenth-century Europe that religious discourse receded and the domain of the anatomist, the pathologist and the doctor became more prominent than that of the clergyman or the philanthropist. Disabilities became redefined as flaws measurable by positivist, objective science (Foucault, 1989: 167). It was associated with problems due to disease, trauma or other health conditions leading to the development of a medical model of disability (Smeltzer et al., 2017). The medical model was concerned with the 'cure' or 'modification' of behaviour of the individual with a disability and viewed physicians as the expert. Responses to disability have changed since the 1970s, prompted largely by the self-organization of people with disabilities (Campbell & Oliver, 1996; Charlton, 1998) and by the growing tendency to see disability as a human rights issue (Degener & Quinn, 2002). The transition from an individual, medical perspective to a structural, social perspective has been described as the shift from a 'medical model' to a 'social model' in which people are viewed as being disabled by society rather than by their bodies (Oliver, 1990). According to the social model, it is society 'which disables people with impairments, and therefore any meaningful solution must be directed at societal change rather than individual adjustment and rehabilitation' (Barnes et al., 2010: 163). In this model, disability has been viewed as a result of environmental and societal factors that serve as barriers to the ability of persons with disabilities to participate fully in their communities or families or to obtain the care and services they need. Individuals with a disability, their families and advocacy groups have viewed disability as a consequence of an inaccessible environment and rejected the medical model in favour of other models, such as the social and biopsychosocial models of disability that address barriers to health care from different perspectives (Smeltzer et al., 2017).

The cultural model on the other hand focusses on cosmological, practical and attitudinal issues specific to communities. Within the Indian context, Mehrotra (2008) argues that disability has to be understood as culturally constructed and socially negotiated as it is often shaped by people's cultural and cosmological beliefs. Therefore, apart from the health conditions of the individual or the social structures present in the community—the cultural understanding of disability may influence the experience of disability itself. In India and much of south Asia, disability is largely seen as a product of cultural impediments such as beliefs and stereotypes as well as structural impediments like poverty, lack of development, illiteracy, unemployment and caste, class and gender barriers. Persons with disabilities (PWD) are marginalized in education, employment, mobility and other significant life areas. The meaning of disability in India is embedded in this basic struggle for survival and cultural understanding (Mehrotra, 2013: 66).

Staples (2020) argues the need to move beyond only the medical and social models by drawing from regionally specific experiences. He highlights the need to acknowledge the struggles and experiences related to colonialism, caste, gender as well as neoliberal rationalities that have impacted the South Asian region. The agency of disabled people was shaped and, ultimately, limited by their material impoverishment. It was also shaped by the kind of charity on which they were dependent (ibid.: 148). He explains how begging involving short relationships with random individual donors often gave more agency to the disabled people. This was because in this kind of relationship there was no obligation on them to accept particular rules of behaviour as might be laid down by state or NGO donor agencies (ibid.: 148, 2018). These arguments reveal the discomfort with the binaries created by medical or social models. The medical viewpoint gives excessive emphasis on the individual ignoring the social-structural 'disabling' conditions. Whereas the social model inadvertently fails to acknowledge the vulnerabilities that persons with disabilities can often experience problems arising from their health condition (Thomas, 1999).

The International Classification of Functioning's (ICF) definition attempts to combine both the approaches as it understands functioning and disability as the dynamic interaction between health conditions and contextual, both personal and environmental. According to Shakespeare (2006), ICF is an attempt to establish a 'biopsychosocial' model that can be said, to some extent at least, to integrate two previously conflicting models of disability, that is, the medical and the social models. A more balanced approach comes from the Human rights model. This model looks at PWD as right-holders. The signing and ratification of the CRPD in 2007 brought the discussions around disability into the mainstream and led to changes in laws and policies. This was an extremely important step for the rights of the disabled across countries as it brought about a change in the attitude of the countries across the world. For example, the attitude of the Indian state appeared to be more informed by the medical, charity and religious model. Disabled persons were construed as dependents and beneficiaries of state provisions. They were not seen as capable of formal employment and responsibility for them was invested with families and communities. The failure of the Indian state to perceive PWD as productive members of society was parallel to the invisibility of women's work and non-enumeration of it towards GDP. The theory of karma, family ideologies, attitudes of charity and pity marked the attitudes of society towards the PWD and clearly informed state policies towards them (Mehrotra, 2013). It is pertinent to note here that in international DRM, the definition of disability took away from the focus on the impaired body and its medical construction (medical model) to a matter of social oppression where social-structural arrangements and cultural values were seen as creating a disabling environment for persons with physical or mental impairments and socially engendering and undermining their psycho-emotional well-being (social model).

Disability and Food Insecurity

UNCRPD recognized the importance of access to adequate food as it is necessary for human survival. Worldwide, people with disabilities are more likely than people without disabilities to encounter barriers to adequate food (Conference of States Parties to the Convention on the Rights of Persons with Disabilities, 2015). The quantity and quality of food that disabled people can access may be limited by these barriers, even in developed Western countries (Webber et al., 2007). Food insecurity has increased in recent years, new estimates indicate that global food insecurity and malnutrition persist and remain stubbornly high, with almost 822 million people continuing to suffer from hunger and nearly two billion people experiencing some form of malnutrition (Leach et al., 2020: 2).

The scenario of rising production, the upper classes eating better, declining per capita availability and increasing buffer stocks portrays three main things—the food grains are not reaching those most in need, the gap between those eating less and those eating more is widening and the income of the poor and the price of food are not synchronized. All these reveal a violation of human rights, especially the right to food, as it is available in plenty but a number of people are still food insecure and hungry (Shakeel, 2017). Despite the fact that there has been sufficient food to feed every person in the world for decades (Simon, 2012), approximately one in every nine people worldwide has inadequate food to support a healthy, active life (FAO et al., 2014). This means a large population of the world remains food insecure.

Food security is defined as the circumstance in which all people, at all times, have physical, social and economic access to sufficient, safe and nutritious food that meets their dietary needs and food preferences for an active and healthy life (IFPRI, 2021). This definition introduces four main dimensions of food security: physical availability of sufficient food of appropriate quality; economic and physical access to food, influenced by market factors, the price of food, and individual purchasing power; food utilization determined by general hygiene and sanitation, water quality, and food safety; and stability to ensure that the first three dimensions are not affected negatively by sudden natural, economic or political shocks over time (African Population and Health Research Centre, 2019). This shows that insecurity related to food can stem from many factors related to the health and environment of the individual. Gaur and Patnaik (2011) argue that ideas of health are embedded in social, economic, and emotional conditions of existence. They explain this through their research with the displaced Korwa[1] who fear falling ill because of eating unfamiliar food, crossing the path of spirits, or stepping on their dwelling areas, implying that 'misrecognition' of space becomes detrimental to their existence. Health, therefore, implies harmony and orderliness in the surrounding 'three worlds' that include natural, social, and supernatural components of the living space. Therefore, changes in the living space can also lead to food insecurity as preferred and nutritious food may become unavailable. It may also result in severe social, psychological and behavioural consequences. Food insecure individuals may manifest feelings of alienation, powerlessness, stress and anxiety, may experience reduced productivity, reduced work and income earnings. All these may lead to anger, pessimism and irritability. Food insecure children may also show signs like higher levels of aggressive or destructive behaviour, hyperactivity, anxiety, difficulty with social interactions, increased passivity, poorer overall school performance, increased school absences, depression, suicidal behaviour etc. (Behera & Penthoi, 2017). The detrimental effects of food insecurity are worse for people with existing vulnerabilities.

Most people living with disabilities are at the 'margins' of society and households with disabled persons were found to be more food insecure. Several studies reported that the prevalence of HFI (household food insecurity) among households with PWDs was well above that for the general population (Meishenheimer, 2015; Schwartz et al., 2019). Households with PWDs are more likely to face unemployment, reduced earnings, and significant additional expenses resulting from their disability (Kim et al., 2011). Moreover, the health of individuals with disabilities is often compromised by food insecurity and the negative health consequences of insufficient food or a low-quality diet (e.g. overweight/obesity, and physical and mental health problems) may be greater for PWDs (Darlington et al., 2017). Household food insecurity (HFI) extends beyond measures of hunger, with common measures surveying household conditions from anxiety over having enough money for food to going for days without eating because of financial constraints (Bickel et al., 2000). HFI is associated with a number of adverse health outcomes from poor mental health, to nutritional deficiencies, and chronic illnesses like diabetes and heart disease (Kirkpatrick & Tarasuk, 2011). Erb and Harriss-White's (2001) study of disability in three villages in Tamil Nadu, South India, shows that there were three categories of costs associated with disability at the household level. First, direct costs are attributed to such factors as the need for medical treatment, including travel costs. Second, the opportunity cost related to income is forfeited as a direct result of this disability. Third, indirect costs are associated with the provision of 'care', either provided by family members or

---

[1] An indigenous community in Central India.

from members of the local community. Similar conditions can be seen in examples from across the world wherein disability leads people to be trapped in circles of poverty (see Groce et al., 2013 for details).

Disability, nutrition and food security are interconnected and these issues may be affected at a spectrum of levels ranging from the household and organization levels to government and international levels. However, despite this intersection, the current understanding of food security fails to acknowledge disability-specific access issues, such as feeding or swallowing disorders, further impairing access to food and therefore food security for this vulnerable group of people (Quarmby & Pillay, 2018). In further research with humanitarian aid workers and health care professionals, the authors found that people living with disabilities may not be representatively included in food distribution efforts and that the responsibility for the nutrition and food security of people living with disabilities may be heavily skewed towards caregivers and family, those individuals who are likely in the least favourable position to take on such responsibility (ibid.: 8). These conclusions were based on their findings that apart from physical access, people living with disabilities may have difficulty accessing information about planned food distribution because of a communication disorder or visual impairment (Muurinen et al., 2014).

Disability is commonly defined according to activity limitations (e.g. ADL), including food access-related activities such as food shopping and preparation. Inability to engage in these activities is itself 'disabling' and part of social under-standing of who comes to be defined as disabled (Webber et al., 2007). Most people with disabilities who are dependent on others can feel as if they are a burden on others or they feel restricted in making their food choices thus highlighting the recursive nature of the relationship between food access and disability. Alternatively, social isolation reduced food access, with effects on motivation to shop for, prepare, and eat food (Locher et al., 1997). Relying on others was sometimes problematic as some reported losing control over stores visited and the healthfulness of foods purchased and prepared (Cuesta-Briand et al., 2011). Individuals reported difficul-ties as they were subject to time constraints of others, reducing ability to engage in time-consuming cost-management strategies like bargain-hunting or couponing (Wolfe et al., 1996). Institutional policies represent a key influence on food access. In many places, disability benefits are greater than general welfare. However, this differ-ence may be offset by higher costs, particularly when medical expenses, mobility equipment and other aids are insufficient or unsubsidized (She & Livermore, 2007). The next section explores the interlinkages between food insecurity and disability through the concepts of poverty and malnutrition.

Disability and Poverty

Poverty causes disability through malnutrition, poor healthcare and dangerous living conditions. Disability can cause poverty by preventing the full participation of disabled people in the economic and social life of their communities, especially if the proper supports and accommodations are not available. The United Nations (2018) estimates that at least 10% of the poor in developing countries are people with disabilities. In both developed and developing countries, people with disabilities experience social exclusion and poverty. Globally, people with disabilities make up about 15% of the world's population (WHO and World Bank, 2011). Although there is no consensus on how many people with disabilities live in poverty around the world, 80% of people with disabilities worldwide live in developing countries (United Nations Development Group, 2011).

Poverty is now seen as an inability to achieve certain standards of living, poor people lack adequate food, shelter, education and health care and 'they are poorly served by institutions of the state and society' (Wolfensohn & Bourguignon, 2004: 4). Studies in Norway have shown a gap in living conditions between disabled and non-disabled individuals and that the disadvantaged position of those with a disability is also maintained in times of continuously increasing prosperity among the general population (Hem & Eide, 1998). According to Yeo and Moore (2003) most people living with disabilities in developing nations are the poorest of the poor. Sonpal and Kumar (2012) have also documented poverty as the main basis for a disability which leads to lack of accessibility to all kinds of resources which results from illness, malnutrition, lack of education, joblessness and pathetic living conditions. People with disabilities continue to be 'invisible' to planners and administrators even in countries where there are national strategies for poverty reduction (Eide & Ingstad, 2013). Poor nutrition, dangerous living conditions, limited access to vaccination programmes, and health and maternity care, poor hygiene, bad sanitation, inadequate information about the causes of impairments, politics and natural disasters all cause disability. In turn, disability exacerbates poverty by increasing isolation and economic strain, not just for the individual but often for the affected family as well and this cycle often continues intergenerationally. Relationship between disability and poverty is probably undercounted in most figures because income-based poverty measures do not account for all of the material and social costs of living with disability (Emerson & Hatton, 2007).

Disability is a development issue, because of its bidirectional link to poverty: disability may increase the risk of poverty, and poverty may increase the risk of disability (Sen, 2009). They face what Sen called the 'conversion handicap' wherein people with disabilities may have extra costs resulting from disability—such as costs associated with medical care or assistive devices, need for personal support and assistance—requiring more resources to achieve the same outcomes as non-disabled people (Zaidi & Burchardt, 2005). Because of higher costs, people with disabilities and their households are likely to be poorer than non-disabled people with similar incomes (Zaidi & Burchardt, 2005; Braithwaite & Mont, 2009; Cullinan et al., 2011). Households with disabled people face more challenges including food insecurity, poor housing, lack of access to safe water and sanitation, and inadequate access to health care (Van-Brackel, 2006; Eide & Loeb, 2006); Beresford & Rhodes, 2008). This highlights the need to address disability in all programming rather than as a stand-alone thematic issue (World Report on Disability, 2011). Lack of universally agreed definitions and robust data regarding the social and economic status of people with disabilities results in the existence of policies and programmes on paper unsupported by adequate infrastructure on the ground.

Poverty, Malnutrition and Disability

Most literature on food security has lacked a disability perspective. The health science perspective is inadequate in addressing the existing socio-economic disparities. Acknowledging the linkage between nutrition and disability is important as this association has intergenerational and life-course implications. Risk factors leading to malnutrition and disability are multifaceted and encompass biological, physical, environmental and social factors (Groce et al., 2014). Countries with high levels of malnutrition and nutrient deficiency also often report higher rates of disability and developmental delay (WHO, 2012). There are several important areas of overlap and influence: malnutrition can cause or contribute to a variety of different disabilities; disabilities can cause or contribute to malnutrition. One billion people, including 95 million children, are estimated to have a disability, and 80% of all persons with disabilities live in LMICs (UNICEF, n.d). The link between disability and malnutrition is likely to be strongest where public health systems are weakest (Hume-Nixon & Kuper, 2018). Children with disabilities living in LMICs may be more vulnerable to malnutrition (Khan et al., 1998; Adams et al., 2012), due to failure of public health systems, as the underlying risk of malnutrition is higher in these contexts, and there are fewer services available to provide nutritional support for children with feeding difficulties (e.g. percutaneous endoscopic gastrostomy feeding). Furthermore, qualitative studies have suggested that children with disabilities in LMICs are at a high risk of hunger associated with poverty, particularly as these children may require a large burden of care limiting household productivity. Caregivers who are required to go to work may not have enough time for adequate care for these children, and their skills in feeding the children may be low (Gona et al., 2011; Alavi et al., 2012; Paget et al., 2016).

Girls with disabilities may more often be underweight than boys with disabilities (Tuzun et al., 2013). In disadvantaged communities experiencing limited resources and food shortages, families following culturally determined gender preferences may choose to prioritize the nutritional needs of a disabled boy over that of a disabled girl. Children with disabilities are less likely than non-disabled ones to attend school at all ages (UNICEF, 2013). This results in children with disabilities not only lagging behind their peers in educational attainment but also not benefiting from school-based nutrition initiatives. In extreme cases, some families or communities may place a lower status on a disabled child and prioritize nutrition and health services for their non-disabled siblings. Social stigma attached to the disabled condition leads to various forms of discrimination and exclusion. Various forms of institutionalized discriminations result in deprivation of opportunities for self-development and exclusion from mainstream society (Pal, 2011). The neglect of persons with disabilities from state-sponsored empowerment policies is evident in the limited enabling legis-lations with delayed enactment as well as lack of realistic official estimation of the magnitude of disability and lack of visibility in mainstream academic engagement (ibid.).

The suffering can be even more severe for women and rural habitats as they are subject to other social, cultural and economic disadvantages due to other forms of discriminations. In the discourse of social exclusion, while caste has been a dominant dimension, the intersection of disability with caste and ethnicity can lead to depriva-tion and exclusion in multiple realms of society, resulting in many social handicaps (Pal, 2011). Environmental factors play an important role in disability even before birth. In view of the impact of living conditions on incidence of disability, it can be expected that Dalits with poor living conditions will be more prone to disability by birth or at an early stage of life. The vicious cycle of poverty and disability includes impact of factors such as lack of ownership of key assets like land, poor living conditions, vulnerability to ill-health, denial of opportunities for human devel-opment and economic work participation, engagement in low-paid activities, lower access to nutritious food during early childhood, social discrimination, lack of access to essential public support services and denial of basic human rights (ibid.: 173). The lack of access to basic requirements of living is often a result of the prevailing political and economic discourses which are further discussed in the next section.

Neoliberalism: Disability and Access to Food

Disability and poverty do not exist as a priori condition—rather, it signifies socio-political and economic processes in the development agenda, which emanate from the hegemony of neo-liberal ideology that believes in unfettered economic growth (Hiranandani, 2009: 75). Neoliberalism believes that state intervention is an obstacle to economic growth because it creates inefficiency and market distortions. There-fore, government expenditures should be reduced, allowing provision of services through the private sector that is more efficient due to profit incentives (Gershman & Irwin, 2000). These principles have led to privatization of health and social services, education, transport and, increasingly, water and food provision in many parts of the world. Within the paradigm of market economy food is a commodity rather than a right (Hiranandani, 2009). Food sovereignty is in stark contrast to the neoliberal approach that argues the best way to achieve food security in 'developing countries' is to import cheap food from 'developed countries', rather than producing locally. This philosophy has major implications for PWD. The restructuring of social security benefits for disabled people has become a dominant theme in international policy circles. Across many OECD countries, policies which focus on moving PWD from a world of social security benefits to the world of work, are visible (OECD, 2007). Yates (2015) argues that despite supportive programmes, employment of disabled persons remains low. The expectation that disabled people will find work in a more lightly regulated labour market and the withdrawal of disability benefits led to many disabled persons entering poverty and relying on food banks for daily subsistence. Yeo (2005) cites the example of Chile that has been called the 'social laboratory' of neo-liberal policies of free market economy and cutbacks to government expenditures. In Chile, for 25 years disabled children have been portrayed in pathetic ways to appeal for donations in annual telethon media shows (ibid.). Multinational corporations, such as Nestle and McDonalds, sponsor the telethons that are viewed as the country's most important effort for disabled children. While this boosts the image and sales of corporations, it reinforces the pity/charity model and does nothing to improve the rights of disabled people Disabled people face the dangers that, under current conditions of thought and debate, they could end up caught between two unpalatable alternatives: live a life with increasing poverty and economic disempowerment or cast oneself 'back into the role of tragic victims of […] impairments' and undertake special pleading for ameliorative treatment on this basis (Oliver, 2013, c.f. Yates, 2015).

For people living with disabilities, a global environment dominated by neo-liberal ideology creates many hurdles. They become increasingly vulnerable with many social protection measures being reduced. In times of disasters like the pandemic, already vulnerable positions get further threatened and increase the distress faced by people living with disabilities.

Disability, COVID-19 and Food Insecurity

Disabled persons often face barriers in meeting their basic needs. Access barriers include physical barriers, attitudinal barriers, differential treatment, and inadequate information. Impaired capacity, lack of support to prepare food or eat, lack of adequate income, lack of transportation or other help to obtain food, being unable to enter and use public eating establishments, or feeling unwelcome in public situations involving food (cafés, restaurants, public celebrations and events) can also impact access (Webber et al., 2007). Access to grocery shopping may also be affected by sensory or physical disabilities or sensory perceptual issues experienced by people with autism (Waltz et al., 2018). These access barriers which exist in 'normal times' became even more prominent during the pandemic. People with disabilities had to face many challenges in accessing health care as well as everyday necessities.

Various states announced different measures for relief and mitigation, as did the central government. None of these announcements was made in accessible formats, and many of them remained mere announcements. The DePWD[2] came up with an excellent set of guidelines, but left it to the discretion of state and district authorities to act upon them. Meanwhile, people with disabilities, particularly those from economically deprived sections, continued to suffer severe hardship. Without access to food or money, many were faced with starvation. Caregivers have been unable (and

---

[2] Department of Empowerment of Persons with Disabilities, Ministry of Social Justice and Empowerment, India.

sometimes unwilling) to reach those who need their critical support. Many have lost access to vital medical attention and peer support systems (NCPEDP, 2020). Access to essentials often requires the physical presence of the person with disability, and the commute has been made extremely difficult during the lockdown. Since no financial security has been provided, access to basic essentials is a challenge. Aiyar (2021) reported that the government ration did not find its way to the slum communities. Therefore, food insecurity was one of the major challenges that the families faced as is evident from the manner in which they have reduced their food consumption. The frequent mentioning of food–lack, and the manner in which they were getting it, implies that it was a constant concern for all.

The COVID-19 lockdowns decreased access to food and essentials, especially among the PWD (Kohli, 2020). Approximately 84.7% had to borrow or request for support for food to cope with financial crisis (Murthy et al., 2020). Prolonged lockdown, loss of jobs and fear and anxiety about catching the virus alongside inaccessibility to regular health care services, put PWDs into a seriously compromised situation. They became totally dependent on the State's provisioning of rations and charity of philanthropists (Mehrotra, 2021). A one-time ex gratia amount of Rs. 1,000 (US$14) to be given to disabled persons through direct transfer in two instalments spread over three months was slammed as being too meagre. NPRD also pointed out that this was also limited to those with more than 80% of disability and who came from BPL families, hence excluding everyone else. Although the central and state governments issued guidelines related to the availability of food and other essential supplies, these directives were not relevant to PWD. None of the directives had any specific provisions to ensure access for persons with disabilities. This happened despite the Disability Inclusive Guidelines notifying disability commissioners regarding reasonable accommodation measures such as reserving dedicated timings in supermarkets and other essential stores specifically for persons with disabilities to ensure the ease of access to food and daily essentials (Rising Flame and Sightsavers, 2020). In surveys with DPO activists it was found that across states there were persons with disability who had no access to food and had trouble procuring supplies from the public distribution system due to issues of access (ibid.). This included lack of accessible information about the relief distribution in their areas. There were reports of people being unaware of relief distribution in their local areas, not having required disability or ration cards to access the food being distributed (Gurung, 2021; Nayar et al., 2021).

Research related to access to food across the world has found that vulnerable groups suffer in the quest to access food from the markets and have to rely on others for assistance (African Population and Health Research Centre, 2019). People living with disabilities may have difficulty accessing information about planned food distribution because of a communication disorder or visual impairment (Muurinen et al., 2014). With restrictions related to COVID-19 coming in, the vulnerable populations faced further distress. A major group impacted during the lockdown in India was that of the migrant workers who went through an extremely difficult time trying to reach back home. Among the migrant workers, those with disabilities faced even more adversity as they were unable to access the free food which was being distributed (Varughese,

2020). Among the disabled population, women with disabilities constitute another vulnerable group who faced difficulties across the world. Gurung (2021) describes the case of a woman with a severe spinal cord injury who lives alone in Nepal. She lives alone and is left without information. She can't have access to relief as she doesn't have citizenship/another card, cannot walk to the place where relief is distributed and speaks only her local language; the distributor does not come to her house. She needs food and regular medicines and there is no one to help and she needs continual personal assistance to take care of her needs. She fills her stomach with water brought by one of her far relatives (ibid.).

For women with disabilities who already face high levels of poverty, poor health conditions, lower incomes, lower education and a patriarchal system COVID-19 caused further distress. A report by Rising Flame and Sightsavers (2020) indicates that 75 out of the 82 women who participated in the study had struggled with accessing either information, physical spaces, communication, digital spaces, health services, food and other essentials. Women dependent on the Public Distribution System (PDS) for their rations had a harder time. While the Central and State governments had directives mandating assured access to food and essentials and dedicated supermarket times, women with disabilities in states had to physically go to PDS shops to buy ration as far as five kilometres away and were often not prioritized (Rising Flame and Sightsavers, 2020). While urban women with disabilities could manage somewhat due to online ordering, this is still not an effective solution. In Sri Lanka, the curfew and the resulting limitations on freedom of movement compelled people to rely on the delivery of essential services within their homes. However, the country's online infrastructure to maintain access to food, pharmaceutical and medical care alongside banking and finance were overwhelmed by the sudden skyrocketing of public demand (de Silva 2020, c.f. Kandasamya et al., 2021). Such conditions were seen in India as well. In a survey conducted by the National Centre for Promotion of Employment for Disabled People (NCPEDP), it was found that 67% of people with disabilities reported to have no access to doorstep delivery by the government. Difficulties in ordering food/food items online included problems in communication with delivery boys because of masks (acting as barriers to lip reading). This increased their dependency on other family members.

Under the UNCRPD, accessible information is understood as information provided in formats that allow every user to access content on an equal basis with others. In cases of disaster warnings and messaging, the importance of conveying these in accessible formats cannot be overemphasized. In fact, it can be the difference between life and death. Some governments ensure that communication was done in a disabled friendly manner—for example, in Nagaland daily briefings were done with the help of Indian sign language interpreters and the government of Kerala also ensured that information was available in accessible formats. For most of the states, these facilities were not available.

Governments in Tamil Nadu and Kerala made attempts to ensure that adequate food provisions were available to disabled people. Kerala established common kitchens where cooked food is served. Dry rations are provided to those who cannot reach these common kitchens. They also prepared lists of persons with disabilities at the municipal/panchayat ward level. Such a meticulous approach enabled the disabled to get cooked food, advance pension payments, financial support, smartphones and internet packages to students with disabilities during this pandemic, unlike other states which continue to struggle to reach out to persons with disabilities with aid packages (Ghai, 2021). Such measures ensured that there were no complaints about access to food in Kerala state (NCPEDP, 2020).

Conclusion

This paper attempts to explore the situation of people living with disabilities who faced challenges in accessing basic services during the pandemic. Food, which is a necessity, became difficult to access leading to extreme hardships. Here, we attempt to trace how the historical position of disabled persons contributed to the present situation by exploring the various understandings of disability. According to Hiranandani (2009) food security, poverty and disability are inherently political issues. While individual experiences of living with pain, illness or impairment cannot be discounted, disability is much more than a question of health or illness—it is primarily a social construction, where people with bodily variations live under certain social arrangements that are exclusionary in nature (ibid.: 80). This is further supported by Taylor's arguments who explains how the pandemic clearly showed that our individual health is interconnected—to each other, to our political and economic systems, to the broader ecology and the other species we share the planet with. Disabled ecologies, the trails of disability that are created, spatially, temporally and across species boundaries, when ecosystems are contaminated, depleted and profoundly altered. While disabled ecologies are all around us, emerging from the climate crisis, from long contaminated Superfund sites, from deforestation and fossil fuel extraction, the pandemic's disabled ecology is forcing a response from a global system that has thus far failed to act on environmental catastrophe (Taylor, 2020).

Taylor's explanation about disabled ecologies and interconnectedness of all systems emphasizes how existing marginalization, inequality and vulnerabilities play out in disaster situations. Any response to ensuring accessibility to food for disabled cannot be limited to just responding to the current situation. There has to be an understanding of the historical and macro factors that have led to the current crises. This makes it imperative that future nutrition policy and programming, maternal and child health, disability policy and broader public health initiatives recognize and plan for the malnutrition–disability link. By doing so, many current problems can be transformed into opportunities to benefit both areas of healthcare. For this to happen, resources are needed and effective action planning is required. Issues of disability should be fully integrated into nutrition programmes, policies and services so that malnutrition and disability can be addressed jointly in daily life or during emergency food security crises.

To address widespread poverty, food insecurity and vulnerability, the government of India has since independence implemented multiple initiatives such as the integrated child development services (ICDS) programme, the national health programme, NREGS, national plan of action on nutrition, public distribution system, mid-day meal and *anganwadi*. The government of India provides subsidized food grain under its public distribution system which is among the largest food security programmes in the world. The national food security act 2013 (also the right to food act) is an act of the parliament of India which aims to provide subsidized food grains to approximately two-thirds of India's 1.2 billion people (Behera & Penthoi, 2017: 39). However, these interventions have ignored people living with disabilities to a large extent. Even when guidelines are given by the DePWD, these are expressed to be measures suggested which 'need to be acted upon by various State/District authorities to give focussed attention to protection and safety of persons with disabilities during COVID-19'. When guidelines are not mandatory and they are not seen as urgent and therefore this led to situations where critical directions came almost a full month late (NCPEDP, 2020: 33). Social protection policies and programmes need to be designed keeping in mind the idea of disabled ecologies. If there are efficient services in 'normal' times, ensuring a planned and effective response during disaster situations would be possible. This has been seen in the examples from some of the states within the country (detailed above). This would ensure that the everyday lives of people living with disabilities are impacted to a minimal degree and they continue to have access to the basic essentials of life such as 'Food'.

References

Adams, M. S., Khan, N. Z., Begum, S. A., Wirz, S. L., Hesketh, T., & Pring, T. R. (2012). Feeding difficulties in children with cerebral palsy: Low-cost caregiver training in Dhaka, Bangladesh. *Child Care Health.*

African Population and Health Research Center. (2019). *Annual report*. African Population and Health Research Center, 2020. Retrieved April 1, 2021, from http://www.jstor.org/stable/resrep 26374

Alavi, Y., Jumbe, V., Hartley, S., et al. (2012). Indignity, exclusion, pain and hunger: The impact of musculoskeletal impairments in the lives of children in Malawi. *Disability and Rehabilitation, 34*, 1736–1746.

Aiyar, Y. (May 27, 2021). Covid-19 and the disease of inequality. Hindustan Times. Retrieved 23 December, 2021 from https://www.hindustantimes.com/opinion/covid19-and-the-disease-of-ine quality-101622117390142.html.

Barnes, C., Mercer, G., & Shakespeare, T. (2010). 'The social model of disability'. In A. Giddens & P. Sutton (Eds.), Sociology: Introductory readings, 3rd edn., pp. 161–166, Polity Press, Cambridge.

Behera, S., & Penthoi, G. C. (2017). Food insecurity and government intervention for sustainable food access in Odisha. *International Journal of Latest Technology in Engineering, Management & Applied Science (IJLTEMAS), VI*(II), 38–46.

Beresford, B., & Rhodes, D. (2008). *Housing and disabled children*. Joseph Rowntree Foundation.

Bickel, G., Nord, M., Price, C., Hamilton, W., Cook, J. (2000). Guide to measuring household food security. United States Department of Agriculture, Alexandria, VA. https://fnsprod.azureedge. net/sites/default/files/FSGuide_0.pdf, Accessed date: 27 March 2018

Braithwaite, J., & Mont, D. (2009). Disability and poverty: A survey of World Bank poverty assessments and implications. *Revue Européenne de Recherche sur le Handicap [ALTER—European Journal of Disability Research], 3*, 219–232. https://doi.org/10.1016/j.alter.2008.10.002

Campbell, J., & Oliver, M. (1996). *Disability politics: Understanding our past, changing our future*. Routledge.

Charlton, J. (1998). *Nothing about us without us: Disability, oppression and empowerment*. University of California Press.

Conference of States Parties to the Convention on the Rights of Persons with Disabilities. (2015). Report of the Eighth Session. New York: United Nations. Retrieved from: http://www.un.org/disabilities/documents/COP/cosp8_report_e.pdf

Clare, E. (2001). Stolen bodies, reclaimed bodies: Disability and queerness. *Public Culture, 13*(3), 359–365.

Cuesta-Briand, B., Saggers, S., & McManus, A. (2011). 'You get the quickest and the cheapest stuff you can': Food security issues among low-income earners living with diabetes. *Australasian Medical Journal, 4*(12), 683–691.

Cullinan, J., Gannon, B., & Lyons, S. (2011). Estimating the extra cost of living for people with disabilities. *Health Economics.* https://doi.org/10.1002/hec.1619 (PMID:20535832).

Darling, K. E., Fahrenkamp, A. J., Wilson, S. M., D'Auria, A. L., & Sato, A. F. (2017). Physical and mental health outcomes associated with prior food insecurity among young adults. *Journal of Health Psychology, 22*, 572–581.

Degener, T., & Quinn, G. (2002). A survey of international, comparative and regional disability law reform. In M. L. Breslin & S. Lee (Eds.), *Disability rights law and policy international and national perspectives* (pp. 3–125). Transnational Publishers.

Eide, A. H., & Ingstad, B. (2013). Disability and poverty—Reflections on research experiences in Africa and beyond. *African Journal of Disability, 2*(1), 31. https://doi.org/10.4102/ajod.v2i1.31

Eide, A. H., & Loeb, M. E. (2006). Reflections on disability data and statistics in developing countries. In B. Albert (Ed.), *In or out of the mainstream? Lessons from research on disability and development cooperation* (pp. 89–104). The Disability Press, University of Leeds.

Emerson, E., & Hatton, C. (2007). The socio-economic circumstances of children at risk of disability in Britain. *Disability & Society, 22*, 563–580. https://doi.org/10.1080/09687590701560154

Erb, S., & Harriss-White, B. (2001, September 11 & 12). The economic impact and developmental implications of disability and incapacity in adulthood—A village study from south India. Paper presented at the *Welfare, Demography and Development Conference*. Downing College.

FAO, IFAD, & WFP. (2014). *The State of Food Insecurity in the World 2014. Strengthening the enabling environment for food security and nutrition*. FAO.

Foucault, M. (1989). *The birth of the clinic*. Routledge.

Gaur, M., & Patnaik, S. (2011). Who is healthy among the Korwa? Liminality in the experiential health of the displaced Korwa of Central India. *Medical Anthropology Quarterly, 25*(1), 85–102.

Gershman, J., & Irwin, A. (2000). Getting a grip on the global economy. In J. Y. Kim, J. V. Millen, & A. Irwin (Eds.), *Dying for growth: Global inequality and the health of the poor* (pp. 11–43). Monroe, Maine: Common Courage Press.

Ghai, A. (2021). *A rendering of disability and gender in the COVID-19 era*. Retrieved April 13, 2021, from https://www.epw.in/engage/article/rendering-disability-and-gender-covid-19-era

Gona, J. K., Mung'ala-Odera, V., Newton, C. R., & Hartley, S. (2011). Caring for children with disabilities in Kilifi, Kenya: What is the carer's experience? *Child: Care, Health and Development, 37*, 175–183

Groce, N., Tuzun, E. H., Guven, D. K., Eker, L., Elbasan, B., & Bulbul, S. F. (2013). Nutritional status of children with cerebral palsy in Turkey. *Disability Rehabilitation, 35*, 413–417.

Grocel, N., Challenger, E., Berman-Bieler, R., Farkas, A., Yilmaz, N., Schultink, W., Clark, D., Kaplan, C., & Kerac, M. (2014). Malnutrition and disability: Unexplored opportunities for collaboration. *Paediatrics and International Child Health, 34*(4), 308–314.

Gurung, P. (2021). COVID19 in Nepal: The impact on indigenous peoples and persons with disabilities. *Disability and the Global South, 8*(1), 1910–1922.

Hem, K. G., & Eide, A. H. (1998). Lagging behind, despite improvements. *Social Diary, 2*, 20–25.

Hiranandani, V. (2009). Disability, poverty and food sovereignty: Advancing the human security agenda. *Review of Disability Studies: An International Journal, 5*(3), 74–84.

Hospes, O., & van der Meulen, B. (Eds.). (2009). *Fedup with the right to food? The Nether-lands' policies and practices regarding the human right to adequate food*. Wageningen Academic Publishers.

Ingstad, B. (2001). Disability in the developing world. In G. L. Albrecht, K. D. Seelman, & M. Bury (Eds.), *Handbook of disability studies* (pp. 772–792). Sage Publications.

International Food Policy Research Institute. (2021). Retrieved January 20, 2021, from https://www.ifpri.org/topic/foodsecurity#:~:text=Food%20security%2C%20as%20defined%20by,an%20active%20and%20healthy%20life

Kafer, A. (2013). *Feminist, queer, crip*. Indiana University Press.

Kandasamya, N., Pererab, B., & Soldatic, K. (2021). COVID-19 from the margins: Gendered-disability experiences in Sri Lanka. *Disability and the Global South, 8*(1), 1923–1934.

Khan, N. Z., Ferdous, S., Munir, S., Huq, S., & McConachie, H. (1998). Mortality of urban and rural young children with cerebral palsy in Bangladesh. *Developmental Medicine & Child Neurology, 40*, 749–753.

Kim, K., Kim, M. K., Shin, Y. J., & Lee, S. S. (2011). Factors related to household food insecurity in the Republic of Korea. *Public Health Nutrition, 14*, 1080–1087.

Kirkpatrick, I., & Tarasuk, V. (2011). Housing circumstances are associated with household food access among low-income urban families. *Journal of Urban Health, 88*(2), 284–296.

Kohli, R. (2020). A starved Nation. *The Telegraph*. Retrieved April 12, 2021, from https://www.telegraphindia.com/opinion/coronavirus-for-india-the-covid-19-pandemic-has-brought-about-generalstarvation/cid/1774030

Leach, M., Nisbett, N., Cabral, L., Harris, J., Hossain, N., & Thompson, J. (2020). Food politics and development. *World Development, 134*. https://www.sciencedirect.com/science/article/pii/S0305750X20301509

Locher, J. L., Burgio, K. L., Yoels, W. C., & Ritchie, C. S. (1997). The social significance of food and eating in the lives of older recipients of meals on wheels. *Journal of Nutrition for the Elderly, 17*(2), 15–33.

Mehrotra, N. (2008). Women and disability management in rural Haryana, India. *Asia Pacific Disability Rehabilitation Journal, 19*, 38–49.

Mehrotra, N. (2013). *Disability, gender and state policy: Exploring margins*. Rawat Publications.

Mehrotra, N. (2021). Emergent disability voices on social media during COVID-19 times. *Disability and the Global South, 8*(1), 1993–2006.

Meisenheimer, M. (2015). *SNAP matters for people with disabilities; food research and action center*. Washington, DC, USA

Murthy, G. V. S., Kamalakannan, S., Lewis, M. G., Sadanand, S., Tetali, S. (2020). A strategic analysis of impact of COVID-19 on persons with disabilities in India. Hyderabad, India. Funded by CBM India Trust, and Humanity & Inclusion (HI)

Muurinen, S. M., Soini, H. H., Suominen, M. H., Saarela, R. K., Savikko, N. M., & Pitkälä, K. H. (2014). 'Vision impairment and nutritional status among older assisted living residents', *Archives of Gerontology and Geriatrics, 58*(3), 384–387. https://doi.org/10.1016/j.archger.2013.12.002

National Centre for Promotion of Employment for Disabled People (NCPEDP). (2020). *LOCKED DOWN and LEFT BEHIND—A report on the status of persons with disabilities in India during the COVID-19 crisis*. Retrieved January 8, 2021, from https://www.ncpedp.org/sites/all/themes/marinelli/documents/Report-locked_down_left_behind.pdf

Nayar, M., Juvva, S., & Lakshman, C. (2021). Psychosocial consequences of COVID-19 on persons with visual impairments. *Disability and the Global South, 8*(1), 1958–1971.

News Bureau. (2020, Dec 4). *84.7% Indians with disability had to borrow food to cope with financial crisis during lockdown: Study*. Retrieved April 13, 2021, from https://www.expresshealthcare.in/news/84-7-indians-with-disability-had-to-borrow-food-to-cope-with-financial-crisis-during-lockdown-study/426139/

Nixon, M. H., & Kuper, H. (2018). The association between malnutrition and childhood disability in low- and middle-income countries: Systematic review and meta-analysis of observational studies. *Tropical Medicine and International Health, 23*(11), 1158–1175.

OECD. (2007). *Sickness and disability schemes in the Netherlands*. Organisation for Economic Co-Operation and Development. Retrieved January 26, 2021, from http://www.oecd.org/social/soc/41429917.pdf

Oliver, M. (1990). *The politics of disablement*. Macmillan and St Martin's Press.

Paget, A., Mallewa, M., Chinguo, D., Mahebere-Chirambo, C., & Gladstone, M. (2016). "It means you are grounded"—Caregivers' perspectives on the rehabilitation of children with neurodisability in Malawi. *Disability Rehabilitation, 38*, 223–234.

Pal, G. C. (2011). Disability, intersectionality and deprivation: An excluded agenda. *Psychology and Developing Societies, 23*(2), 159–176.

Quarmby, C., & Pillay, M. (2018). The intersection of disability and food security: Perspectives of health and humanitarian aid workers. *African Journal of Disability, 7*, a322. https://doi.org/10.4102/ajod.v7i0.322

Rising Flame and Sight Savers. (2020). *Neglected and forgotten: Women with disabilities during the COVID crisis in India*. Retrieved January 15, 2021, from https://risingflame.org/wp-content/uploads/2020/07/NeglectedAndForgotten_RFandSS.pdf

Schwartz, N., Buliung, R., & Wilson, K. (2019). Disability and food access and insecurity: A scoping review of the literature. *Health & Place, 57*, 107–121.

Sen, A. (2009). *The idea of justice*. The Belknap Press of Harvard University Press.

Shakeel, A. (2017). The Déjà-vu of food security and the right to food in India. *World Affairs: THe Journal of International Issues, 21*(4), 82–97.

Shakespeare, T. (2006). *Disability rights and wrongs*. Routledge.

She, P., & Livermore, G. A. (2007). Material hardship, poverty, and disability among working-age adults. *Social Science Quarterly, 88*(4), 970–989.

Smeltzer, S., Mariani, B., & Meakim, C. (2017). *Brief historical view of disability and related legislation*. Retrieved February 10, 2021, from http://www.nln.org/docs/default-source/professional-development-programs/ace-series/brief-history-of-disability.pdf?sfvrsn=6

Sonpal, D., & Kumar, A. (2012). 'Whose reality counts?': Notes on disability, development and participation. *Indian Anthropologist, 42*(1), 71–90. Retrieved April 14, 2021, from http://www.jstor.org/stable/41922009

Staples, J. (2020). Decolonising disability studies? Developing South Asia-specific approaches to understanding disability. In N. Mehrotra (Ed.), *Disability studies in India: Interdisciplinary perspectives* (pp. 25–42). Springer.

Stiker, H.-J. (1982). *Corps infirmes et sociétés*. Aubier Montaigne.

Taylor, S. (2020). *What would health security look like?* Retrieved March 11, 2021, from http://bostonreview.net/class-inequality-science-nature/sunaura-taylor-what-would-health-security-look

Thomas, C. (1999). *Female forms: Experiencing and understanding disability*. Open University Press.

Tuzun, E. H., Guven, D. K., Eker, L., Elbasan, B., Bulbul, S. F. (2013). Nutritional status of children with cerebral palsy in Turkey. *Disability and Rehabilitation, 35*(5):413–17.

UNICEF. (2013). *Children and young people with disabilities fact sheet*. Retrieved December 4, 2020, from http://www.unicef.org/disabilities/files/Factsheet_A5__Web_NEW.pdf.2013

United Nations Development Group. (2011). *Including the rights of persons with disabilities in United Nations programming at country level: A guidance note for UN country teams and implementing partners*. United Nations.

United Nations. (2018). *Disability and development report*. Retrieved February 25, 2021, from https://www.un.org/development/desa/disabilities/wp-content/uploads/sites/15/2019/07/disabilityreport-chapter2.pdf

Van Brakel, W. H. (2006). Measuring health-related stigma–a literature review. *Psychology, Health & Medicine, 11*, 307–334. https://doi.org/10.1080/13548500600595160 (PMID:17130068).

Varughese, S. (2020). Response of a non-governmental organization to COVID 19. Nov 2020. *Christian Journal for Global Health, 7*(4), 14–19.

Wolfe, W. S., Olson, C. M., Kendall, A., & Frongillo, E. A. (1996). Understanding food insecurity in the elderly: A conceptual framework. *Journal of Nutrition Education, 28*(2), 92–100.

Waltz, M., Mol, T., Gittins, E., & Schippers, A. (2018). Disability, access to food and the UN CRPD: Navigating discourses of human rights in the Netherlands. *Social Inclusion,* 2183–2803. https://doi.org/10.17645/si.v6i1.1160

Webber, C. B., Sobal, J., & Dollahite, J. S. (2007). Physical disabilities and food access among limited resource households. *Disability Studies Quarterly, 27*(3). https://doi.org/10.18061/dsq.v27i3.20

WHO. (2012). *Social protection: shared interests in vulnerability reduction and development.* Social Determinants of Health Sectoral Briefing Series No. 4. Geneva, Switzerland.

Wolfensohn, J. D. & Bourguignon, F. (2004). *Development and poverty reduction. Looking back, looking ahead.* World Bank.

World Health Organization and World Bank. (2011). *World report on disability.* World Health Organization.

Yates, S. (2015). Neoliberalism and disability: The possibilities and limitations of a Foucauldian critique. *Foucault Studies, 19,* 84–107. Retrieved April 7, 2021.

Yeo, R. (2005). *Disability, poverty, and the new development agenda.* Retrieved March 3, 2021, from https://disabilitystudies.leeds.ac.uk/wp-content/uploads/sites/40/library/yeo-Disability-poverty-and-the-newdevelopment-agenda.-Final-draft-12th-september.pdf

Yeo, R., & Moore, K. (2003). Including disabled people in poverty reduction work: "Nothing about us, without us." *World Development, 31*(3), 571–590.

Zaidi, A., & Burchardt, T. (2005). Comparing incomes when needs differ: Equivalization for the extra costs of disability in the UK. *Review of Income and Wealth, 51,* 89–114. https://doi.org/10.1111/j.1475-4991.2005.00146.x

Chapter 10
Inequality in Access to Healthcare for Persons with Disability During COVID-19: An Illustration from Bangladesh

Anwara Begum

Abstract The world is ill-prepared for COVID-19. Bangladesh too is caught off-guard. Corona infected persons suffer, and for many, it is severe and debilitating, while high treatment costs ensue for patients with complications. If persons with disability are compared to persons without any form of disability, the woe increases manifold, especially for women. Persons with disability are braving the risks of this pandemic, at double the level of risk compared to the general people. Men, women and children with disabilities often operate under a shadow of social stigma and experience financial and social dependency and require caregivers, sighted guides and interpreters. Even during this pandemic, physical distancing is not possible for people with disabilities. Moreover, travelling and manoeuvring patients with wheelchairs require more resources, manpower and structural designing, not to mention empathy, especially in nursing and care that is in short supply. Lack of appropriate vehicle services, preponderance of tertiary healthcare in primate cities, absence of training and awareness among nurses on specific needs of these vulnerable people; physically impaired, neo developmental children, all add up to creating challenges. The primary objective of this study is to understand the severity of constraints, and inequality in access to healthcare of persons with disability, who coped with COVID-19 during this pandemic. In this study, the situation of the hospitals is reviewed and nurses who are at the forefront of this detrimental situation, and persons with disability are interviewed to gauge nursing skills, preparedness, reaction and experiences of patients, through 65 Stakeholder and Key Informant Interviews. Unbundling the issues could inform more sensitive policy formulation in favour of men, women and children with disability, who are inadvertently left out in the arena of COVID-19.

Keywords Pandemic response · Physical distancing · Physically impaired · Tertiary health care · Public policy

A. Begum (✉)
Senior Research Fellow, Human Resource Development Division, Bangladesh Institute of Development Studies (BIDS), Dhaka, Bangladesh

© The Author(s), under exclusive license to Springer Nature Singapore Pte Ltd. 2022
S. S. Acharya and S. Christopher (eds.), *Caste, COVID-19, and Inequalities of Care*,
People, Cultures and Societies: Exploring and Documenting Diversities,
https://doi.org/10.1007/978-981-16-6917-0_10

Introduction

The sudden and catastrophic COVID-19 pandemic has created an unprecedented worldwide crisis, exacerbating the prevailing low access to healthcare, employment and income, quality education and also intensified existing disparity in society. However, this cloud might still have a silver lining as it has brought us face to face with focussing on more inclusive and sustainable solutions to entrenched inequalities in society. This lends credence to discussions in the literature review of this chapter. According to various census data (BBS, 2001, 2011) there are almost ten percent of persons with disability in Bangladesh. People with disabilities are among the most ignored in any society and are more likely to live in poverty, experiencing higher rates of discrimination, neglect and exploitation in an occurrence of a virulent disease.

The United Nations Convention on the Rights of Persons with Disabilities (CRPD) was endorsed in 2006, soliciting considerable worldwide advancement aimed at eliminating the disparity and retrogression experienced by people with disabilities. The 2030 agenda and Sustainable Development Goals (SDGs) have renewed commitments to 'leave no one behind'.

Unfortunately, the health, social and economic crisis brought about by COVID-19 threatens to undo the progress made towards equal opportunity for people suffering from some or multiple disabilities. The greatest challenges of COVID-19 verily present itself to these persons who are heavily dependent upon caregivers for their existence. The threats lie in the fact that awareness of asymptomatic increase is hardly known among these persons with disabilities. Although highly contagious, knowledge about this disease and related consciousness has increased somewhat due to its life-threatening nature, but many have succumbed. The painful truth remains in the fact that adherence to social distancing remains a concern for persons suffering from disability, who in reality survive on physical support and dependence.

The world was ill-prepared for COVID-19. Bangladesh too was also caught unaware and vacuous. Corona infected patients suffer, and for many, it is severe and debilitating, while high treatment costs ensue for patients with complications. Compared to persons without any form of disability those with limitations have greater hardships. Men, women and children with disabilities often operate under a shadow of social stigma and experience financial and social dependency, and require caregivers, sighted guides and interpreters. Even during this pandemic, physical distancing is not possible. Moreover, travelling and manoeuvring patients with wheelchairs require more resources, manpower and structural designing, not to mention empathy, especially in nursing and care. Unfortunately, this is scarce.

Lack of appropriate vehicle services, preponderance of tertiary health care in primate cities, absence of training and awareness among nurses on specific needs of these vulnerable patients; physically impaired, neo developmental children, all add up to creating challenges. The primary objective of this study is to understand the severity of constraints, and inequality in access to healthcare of persons with disability, who coped with COVID-19 during this pandemic. In this study, the situation of the hospitals is reviewed and nurses who are at the forefront of this calamitous situation and persons with disability are interviewed to gauge nursing skills, preparedness, reaction and experience of patients, through 50 interviews of persons with disability and 15 stakeholders' interviews. Unbundling the issues could inform more sensitive policy formulation in favour of men, women and children with disability, who are inadvertently left out in the battleground of COVID-19.

Background

Disability is found among a large number of persons in Bangladesh. Some leading experts consider the official estimate to be too conservative. At approximately 9.2% (Kibria et al., 2020), the figure would be one crore 47 lacs and 20 thousand, estimated with a total population of around 16 crores. However, a figure closer to one crore 60 lacs, is far more plausible, organization heads assert. The reason being 11 types of disabilities exist and many are not in the official statistics. There is also a confusion regarding persons who are, in fact, autistic, having low intellectual capacity of 10–12 years old but physically competent, in the majority of the cases of autistic persons. Old people, individuals with chronic diseases, etc. are also persons who require care. Those who have become aged, often lose their faculty of eyesight. Moreover, they are often physically frail and require constant care. With COVID-19, most of these people have become unobserved as they are bereft of caregivers, distanced from family and friends, social workers, volunteers, so much so that such organizations are finding it difficult to trace the number of deaths.

Scope of the Study

Bangladesh has an extensive health infrastructure in the public and private sectors but is not equipped with adequate human and other resources such as drugs, instruments and supplies. There is a critical shortage of trained health providers and an inappropriate skill mix. Thus, the country remains at a ratio of doctors to nurses much lower than the WHO recommended ratio of 1:3:5. Due to various gaps in physical infrastructure and human resources, people's perception of the services provided at public sector health facilities is poor and as such, they mostly resort to unqualified informal providers (Cockcroft et al., 2007). According to the providers, lack of supplies and inadequate infrastructure is one of the major causes of inefficient services provided by these facilities (Cockcroft et al., 2011).

Bangladesh is suffering from a severe HRH crisis in terms of a shortage of qualified providers (when measured against the WHO estimate for achieving MDG and SDG targets), inappropriate skills-mix and inequity in distribution. This desperate situation demands immediate attention from policymakers. Reducing the 'income-erosion' effect of illness through a pro-poor health system is urgently needed in Bangladesh, a country besieged with large out-of-pocket payments for healthcare (Begum &

Mahmood, 2017). This augurs badly for patients suffering a disability as more often than not, they are hard up for cash.

Rationale

The objective of this study is to understand the severity of constraints, and inequality in access to healthcare of persons with disability, who coped with COVID-19 during this pandemic. Women's access to health service is also an important point which is addressed in this study. The unequal access of persons suffering from disability, in particular, inhibited and vulnerable women, is a reality in our cultural context where those with physical weakness and who are poor (lacking resources and voice/agency), are more often than not, discriminated against.

In Bangladesh there is uneven distribution of wealth, which is a product of policies, laws, institutions, social-cultural norms and practices, governance deficits and the unequal distribution of riches and control. The most plausible explanation for income inequality's apparent effect on health and social problems is 'status anxiety'. Income inequality varies by social factors such as sexual identity, gender identity, age and race or ethnicity, leading to a wider gap between the upper and working class. There is further categorization within the working class, gender groups namely those persons who suffer from disability. Limitations sometimes are so debilitating that joining the workforce becomes impossible. Rather, the onus is on family and friends to tend to them. It causes a depressing outlook that may be further deepened by their socio-economic status. Income inequality is harmful because it places people in a hierarchy that increases status competition and causes stress, which leads to poor health and other negative outcomes.

The predicament of persons with disability is two-fold. The labour market is almost inaccessible for them. Moreover, there is a categorization of sharp barriers to accessing basic essential services for the ones suffering with disability. They have innate helplessness to connect to remunerated employment and income, suffer from inability to access education and information and face routine restrictions in their access to assistance and aid support.

Methodology

To understand the severity of constraints, and inequality in access to healthcare of persons with disability, who coped with COVID-19 and those who accessed medical help for various problems during this pandemic relevant data was gathered. It is noteworthy that no vaccine was available from December 2020 through March 2021, during this empirical data collection. Due to the contagion, it is impossible to conduct face-to-face interviews. A list of persons with disability was made from collated information: those who had suffered corona belonging to an organization. A list of persons with disability who had suffered corona was made from the collated information taken from their organization. Also, personal contact with nurses and doctors was done. Their information has been solicited by this researcher through phone calls, which were mostly direct. In a few cases, family members spoke on their behalf as the member with disability is suffering from corona or cerebral palsy, Down's Syndrome, etc.

In this study, the approach of hospitals is reviewed and care of nurses who are at the vanguard of this hostile circumstance and persons with disability are interviewed to gauge nursing skills, preparedness, reaction and experience through 50 respondents who are suffering from disability, and 15 who gave services. Interviewee's names are pseudonyms and not their real names, in order to safeguard their identity. Exposing the state of persons with disability could incorporate into the picture and can lead to better and more robust policy formulation in support of men, women and children with disability, who have been involuntarily missing or camouflaged due to vulnerability, which bodes greater hardships during a crisis like the Corona Pandemic. During this crisis, there was a general concern, among public and private agencies, to safeguard the spread of this deadly disease. It was mandated that people would remain indoors, through a public announcement of 'lockdown' whereby only essential services would remain in operation but offices and shopping areas would be closed to minimize transmission. Hence, research investigators and persons with disability had to utilize telephones or computers to communicate.

Literature Review

Attempts have been made here, to situate the challenging issue of rights and responsibilities of persons with disability in a context that is realistic. Until now, this issue of persons with disability was viewed as individual limitations infused by cultural stigma and not, also in large part, a product of structural barriers that could exacerbate coping mechanisms and usurp individual rights. Many protagonists up-holding the role of structural functionalist approach (Gerold-Scheepers & Wim van Binsbergen, 1978; Mabogunje, 1970; Begum, 1999) have reasserted those individual actions may be thwarted by wider socio-economic and environmental structure. The wider socio-economic and structural milieu may commandeer individual action and impinge upon the predetermined individual perception and transcend individual awareness. It can mould the pattern of social and economic relationships: which affects to the degree that it can pre-determine individual actions.

Structural barriers are present in the everyday routine of persons who suffer from disability. This aspect is often not considered while cultural and attitudinal stigmas are highlighted in the analysis projecting the problems faced by persons with disability. Mehrotra and Solditac (2021) have underscored that literature dealing with Disability Studies (DS) in the Global South charted notable involvement through focussing on the implications of structural barriers in the lives of persons with disability in the past 20 years or so. They contextualized the limitations within a structural set-up and broadened the milieu that impinges upon such a population onto a wider canvas, away from contracted representational and cultural point of view.

They further underscore that the structural milieu of unfairness and repression, prevailing not in favour of persons with disabilities including policies simultaneously existing, at national and international levels, that augment social justice in diverse multi-cultural contexts and landscapes is needed.

In an integrated global world, the intermingling of the flow of resources, knowledge and comprehension render it unreasonable to narrowly conceive this problem in terms of secluded social and political perspective and practices. Disability rights, societal justice and disabled bias represent a process of hybridization of neighbouring, regional and global progression, vocabularies and sites of political deed. Effective discourse on disability within the Global South must therefore recognize the multifaceted layering and intertwining of thoughts, discussions, institutional performance and activist sensitization and mobilization.

Shajahan (2021) documents that the last four decades of war, ethnic clash, aggression, bloodshed and pecuniary state have made Afghanistan a country, which is home to many vulnerable people. At least a fifth of the population now lives with a serious physical, sensory, intellectual or psychosocial disability. Women suffering from disabilities in Afghanistan are looked down upon and said to be 'doubly stigmatized' due to gender disparity and physical incompetence viewed as a stigma and are often hidden from the social and political part of life. Even though in the post-Taliban era, expansion interventions supported by international aid have been designed to include women with disabilities, their impacts on cross-cutting income levels, traditions, constituency, different types of disability and other restrictions have not been explored to address different requirements, obstruction and inequalities across various regions. In this context, the COVID-19 crisis has made the lives of Afghan women with disabilities harder due to gender prejudice, shame and dishonour, unemployment, lack of mobility, lack of responsiveness and inadequate institutional grip and built environment coupled with widespread feelings of insecurity resulting from clash arising due to radical, fanatical assault.

The discussion above delineates women's coping mechanisms to the structural problems that have plagued the further development that was needed to move them to operate as effective citizens.

Some countries were able to keep schools open and safe even in difficult pandemic situations. Social distancing (a strategy which is not possible for children with a disability) and hygiene practices proved to be the most widely used measures to prevent the spread of the Coronavirus. They imposed significant capacity constraints on schools and required education systems to make difficult choices when it came to the allocation of educational opportunity. This opportunity was hardly explored in the case of students with disability (OECD, 2021a, b).

The organization, Women with Disabilities Development Foundation (WDDF), produced a booklet on the *Rights and Protection Act in Bangladesh for Persons with Disabilities*, in 2013 (SADF, 2013). It lays down the definition of Rights, the type of protection that they are entitled to, the types of disability that prevail in Bangladesh, the manner of mobilization through establishment of committee(s), the responsibilities of government officials and their routes to redress grievances within a legal arrangement.

Nayar et al. (2021) documents the challenges faced by young people with disabilities. This deadly disease has upset lives globally and among the persons suffering from disability. It has personified gender, social location, ethnicity and their individual bodies. For these persons with disability, public health amenities, ease of access to urban infrastructure, conservancy services and educational convenience in cities preceding the infectious disease were contingent upon the manner in which these people with disability are able to adapt to the current situation. It probes the challenges of young people living with visual impairments who reside in an urban low-income community in India and their unique confrontation such as the further reduction in accessibility to health and educational facilities that they are facing and the manner in which their carefully ordered everyday lives have changed. Young peoples' voices and needs in a COVID lockdown and the resultant vulnerability that solicit immense coping strategies are narrated in this paper, so that their real needs may be understood to structure more feasible policy support.

The calamitous nature of COVID-19, has brought about much discussion on the various impacts and coping mechanisms of different vulnerable groups especially persons with disability. Although epidemics and deadly diseases have historically disrupted the structured lives of most communities, such epidemics have had life-changing impacts upon those who are suffering from disability and are counted among the most vulnerable. To give some examples, Bano S. cites the Russian flu of 1889, the Spanish flu of 1918, the polio pandemic of 1949, H2N2 virus, 1956, HIV/AIDS 1981, Swine flu 2001, SARS 2002, etc. that have been the cause of uncountable deaths in modern-day documented narration. The paper points out that in the absence of any authoritative policy for persons with disabilities during COVID-19, there has been a universal lack of knowledge and ennui regarding persons with disabilities, which must be corrected.

Kandasamy et al. (2021) states that when a public health disaster is juxtaposed with a constitutional crisis, as in Sri Lanka, the logical consequence could be a 'doubling of the chaos'. This is especially true for the most downtrodden and victimized and marginalized communities, who are also highly vulnerable to the worst outcomes of COVID-19, particularly persons with handicaps and those living with chronic health conditions and illnesses. A survey of persons suffering from disabilities in Sri Lanka exposed the broad impacts of Sri Lanka's political disorder during COVID-19. The situation reveals categorization of sharp barriers to accessing basic essential services for the ones suffering with disability. They have innate helplessness to connect to remunerated employment and income, suffer from inability to access education and information and face routine restrictions in their access to assistance and aid support.

Bezbaruah (2018), in her paper, has documented a telephone conversation where the poignant, heavily depressed voice of an 83-year-old conveys fears of a silent death: 'For the first time I feel very alone …. (pauses) …. what if I die in my sleep …? Do you think they … will they? (a confused pause) just let me decompose (with an additional emphasis)? Will my children be able to even see me for the last time?

In that case, who performs my last rites?' It allows the 'manifold layers of meanings, attached to the very words as well as the sentiments behind it' to be interpreted.

When we explore the literature on persons with disability in the case of Bangladesh, we find that some measures to rectify the gross inequality is in place. The implementation of these measures would be beneficial for the community that has for decades been marginalized, in terms of rights and in the context of state responsibilities. Unfortunately gains could be compromised as evidence from surveys reveal that there is an increase over time in the number of girls who reported child marriage in their communities during COVID-19 (Population Council, 2020).

Mizan (2021) has explored the legal framework for the rights of persons with disabilities in Bangladesh and has brought forth positive developments in the arena of redress for persons with disability. The Constitution of the People's Republic of Bangladesh guarantees fairness for all citizens and confirmatory actions for the systemically down-graded and distinguished as marginalized sections of the community (Art. 27, 28(4), 29(3). The State vows to uphold its accountability to progressively ensure social security arising out of disablement (Art. 15). The initial State plan to acknowledge the rights of persons with disabilities was introduced in 1993. It began by setting up the National Coordination Committee on Disability under the auspices of the Ministry of Social Welfare, followed by the National Policy on Disability 1995, the Action Plan on Disability 1996 and the 2000 National Foundation for the Development of Disabled Persons (NFDD). The Disability Welfare Act 2001 was the original legal instrument for addressing the issue. Unfortunately, the 2001 Act was abortive in effect. It could not delineate the myriad needs of persons with disabilities and ineffectively articulated the redress mechanisms in Section 22.

Therefore in 2005–2006, the Department of Social Service launched the disability allowance, provided for the Disability Detection Survey and also employment for persons with disabilities (Hussain, 2020, 15). Following the country's ratification and being a party to the UN Convention on the Rights of Persons with Disabilities (CRPD) in 2007, Bangladesh (a dualist state) installed and enacted the domestic legislations. In 2013, Parliament endorsed the Rights and Protection of the Persons with Disabilities Act 2013 (RPPD Act), replacing the 2001 Act and the Neuro-Development Disability Protection Trust Act, 2013 to attend to the protection of the persons with neuro-developmental disabilities, i.e. autism, cerebral palsy, down syndrome, intellectual handicaps, etc. The RPPD Act (supplemented by the Rights and Protection of the Persons with Disabilities Rules, 2015) is the key instrument in ensuring disability rights in Bangladesh.

Overall, the opinion of persons with disabilities was not taken into consideration. The universal complaint was that their specific needs were never taken into cognizance, as none from the government sector approached them. Although 80% got information from television, the manner in which it was imbued left much to be desired. Persons with disability require important information on safety and precaution to be given to them in a way that they can understand and absorb easily. Surveys that have been conducted (i2i Innovation to Inclusion, 2021) in Bangladesh and Kenya have delineated the plight of such people. In the formal sector service, persons with disability were retrenched and their jobs were cut ahead of others. They needed to use their hands for support and the probability of contamination was considered to be higher in their case.

Analysis of Primary Data

The following section draws heavily on information, mainly qualitative views, from key individuals who facilitate people with disability. The answers were sought from persons with disability, who had corona as well as those who did not suffer from corona but had to seek medical care during the COVID-19 period. They had tried to avail health care services during the COVID-19 period, with some having suffered from the infection. All questions could not be equally answered by the respondents as many of the members were interviewed over the telephone and could not use a computer. Many respondents were quite poor and living in remote areas of Bagerhat, Barguna and Sathkhira of Bangladesh. Views of hospital heads and Senior Staff Nurses were taken from leading hospitals in Dhaka, Chittagong and Rajshahi.

Caregivers' opinions were also solicited. The persons interviewed were holding key positions such as Assistant Director, Coordinators, Assistant Coordinator, four Associate Coordinators, Union Facilitator, three Disability Inclusion Facilitators, two Computer Operators and an Inclusion Officer. Women who suffer from disability were mainly considered for their insights. The aim of this paper was to understand the milieu within which women operated in a culturally inhibited environment where women were often disregarded and their mobility, voice and decision-making prohibited. The extent to which these conscriptions prevailed while they sought medical care during COVID-19, was an important point to understand, given a situation of high contagion in reality. All respondents were unanimous in agreeing that health expenses presented a big problem for them during this disaster. Almost 35 of the respondents felt that expenditure on health was prohibitive for them, as they are often resource-poor.

Some of these women are from Bagerhat district, and to name a few, Beli, Champa, Sita and Bilkis who are suffering from blindness, lame in leg, visually impaired and a student with Down's syndrome, respectively. The costs they incur mainly arise from diagnostic tests, travel to health centre accompanied by one or two companions, cost of medicine, movement from one place to another and bed and breakfast for one or two days. These costs prove to be quite high for their families. There is little social security for them although one of them is registered for an allowance which is about Taka 600 per month (approximately $7 to $8 USD). This allowance is available to only one or two persons and it is not regular. They work as maids for households or remain within their homes as home-maker for husbands engaged as day labourers and cart-vendors.

From Barguna district, Manu Islam aged 21 years, Khan aged 28 years, Bashir aged 26 years and Hossain aged 45 are physically disabled. They did not suffer from coronavirus. They also said that they had very little information about this disease and known cases were few in the nearby district hospital. They had to seek medical care for their physical problems, and they could not access it during the lockdown. Costs of private service were quite high and often inaccessible for them as they did not know how to set an appointment. Their sources of income dwindled and food became scarce. They had to be resigned to lower rations in their homes as the able-bodied needed food to keep their energy and seek a livelihood, despite the disaster wrought by the disease.

One woman from Mymensingh district named Morjina, aged about 45, whose husband earns intermittently from vending seasonal vegetables or cereals during the dry months, started to become blind from the age of 25. By then she had two daughters. The third daughter was born while she could see through a hazy vision. Her elder daughter took her to the district hospital where the doctor on duty threw her out after cursorily examining her eyes. He shouted at her that she is destined to become blind. The thoughtless comment left her mentally depressed and she never managed to overcome it. Morjina recounted how:

> When I went to the hospital in Dhaka, I was partially blind. My elder daughter accompanied me. We waited in Islamia Eye Hospital in Farmgate, Dhaka. Then, after a long time, the nurse took us to the doctor. After the eye specialist checked me, he became very rough in his behaviour, sternly called the nurse on duty and told her to send me away as I would become blind eventually, so treatment was useless. Even the nurses became confused at his rage and muttered among themselves. We women have always bowed to men in this society. If my husband had been with me, maybe I would not face such rude behaviour. We are also poor and so we are deprived of rights and voice. I want my daughters to learn, earn and be independent. Not one woman or man protested on my behalf. Till this day, I am suffering from his callous remarks. Being poor is a curse and being a woman, more so. I will not go for treatment for my corona. My husband got some medicine for himself from the pharmacy. We may die.

Her whole family suffered from corona despite the fact that they are residing in the suburbs of Mymensingh district, which is quite near Dhaka. Due to financial constraints, they did not seek medical care from any hospital or clinic, preferring to pray and drink hot tea with herbs like ginger and lemon. During the first wave of COVID-19, and also the two festivals, huge influx of garment workers, manufacturing industry workers and small business in service industries travelled back to rural origins following lockdown in Dhaka. As there was little planning in containment, the inevitable spread of coronavirus was rampant.

They were exposed to countless people as their home is located near the district hospital. Their lack of money was the primary barrier to seeking healthcare. Morjina's blindness has made her resigned to being part of the family with the least power of decision-making. Her daughters try to support her with the household chores. Beyond this, seeking treatment for her eye presents an insurmountable hurdle for them. Her blindness is something which Morjina has accepted as inevitable. She rather seeks to get her daughters educated to a secondary level and then married them off without much ado.

While they suffered from coronavirus, there was silent enduring patience among the family members. The women's un-articulated and resigned behaviour was readily accepted by the head of the family. His mobility remained unhampered and he recovered quickly. They did not experience severe breathing problems. The positive part of their home is that it is made of temporary material and although very hot in the morning, it afforded them plenty of sunshine throughout the day. They usually take alms from acquaintances during the month of fasting (an obligatory money which Muslims pay to needy people, known as 'Zakat'). This financial support from charity is their only means of security in the instance of lean months when income is not possible from vending.

The level of physical suffering that they experienced as a result of their illness and disability, gauged on a three-level scale would show the greatest difficulty. Out of all respondents, no one said that they did not suffer, on account of their physical limitations. Only about a fifth of the respondents said that their suffering was bearable on account of support from well-off family members. However, about one-third reported that they experienced severe difficulties in accessing healthcare during COVID-19. Their problems arose mainly due to the attitude of doctors and nurses towards persons with disability. For example:

> I have Cerebral Palsy. I often require physical therapy; speech therapy; muscle exercises. I also face physical disability, having problems in walking. I often experience pain in my legs for which I need medical care. My parents have to accompany me all the time. (Jubaida Akhi, 13-year-old girl from Barguna)
>
> I face lot of problems: Hospital Doctor and staff misbehave; they talk so rudely. Staff sometimes take bribe from us; Cost of travel and waiting for service provider; Negligence of doctor; No proper treatment; Doctor are not available in the duty hour. Difficult for me to move everywhere. (Mr. Sujan, 20 years old from Barguna)

It emerges that the majority of those who had family or friend's support during this period, felt that their difficulty was much less on account of their support. During COVID-19, physical distancing was an imperative for general people but for those suffering from some form of disability especially lack of eyesight, lame in both legs, or dumb and/or with weak physique (due to old age or health complications), physical distancing was not possible and costly. For example:

> I had to take a private vehicle to go to the hospital, which proved to be quite costly. I had to take my parents with me to help me. Corona infection makes it difficult to breathe with mask on and enclosed in a 'tempo' (local transport). We were treated reluctantly after much waiting, at the hospital. And we had to remain in isolation and it was very difficult to manage the cost. (Ms. Maya, 16-year-old girl with speech disability)
>
> I had to be accompanied and taken in an ambulance. Cost was very high. I suffer from Cerebral Palsy. I often require physical therapy; speech therapy muscle exercises. (Mr. Farid, 10-year-old with Cerebral Palsy)

Further queries on whether they think that persons with disability who were patients with Corona, faced more challenges (compared to general patients), when accessing healthcare, during this COVID-19 period showed that the majority, 45 out of 50 respondents, felt that COVID-19 period was a real test for them, in accessing healthcare. Transportation, caregiver, resources, etc. were scarce. Out of 50 responses, one person did not find it too onerous, while four could not give an answer to this question.

Out of 50 responses 46 confirmed that lack of education and income (not being rich), make patients with disability more vulnerable. An overwhelming majority reported that lack of education and not being rich does make persons with disability more vulnerable. All the remaining persons, i.e. four respondents opined that maybe, it could adversely affect them.

> I need a chaperon all the time, sometimes both parents have to accompany me to the health centre. Our financial condition is bad, so getting treated from specialist is not possible. (Ankan, 15-year-old girl with physical disability)
>
> Need help from another person to travel to healthcare centre. No one pays attention as doctors are rude. I am scared to express my problem, also I cannot understand how to get service that is less costly. (Mrs. Sheuli Begum, 60-year-old with visual disability)

One pertinent point that requires attention of policymakers is the training of doctors and nurses with reference to handling patients with disability. This was not found among the nurses and doctors including heads of hospitals, who were interviewed. This was a vital question as none of the hospitals have specifically trained doctors and nurses who are adept at handling patients with disability. There were some patients with disabilities among these 50 respondents who did not know whether their caregivers were trained or not. This could be true for those who said that they received assistance from trained doctors and nurses, as nurses themselves claim that they do not get this training but their motto is basically to provide care for patients. Reports from the field, especially heads of well-known organizations for the disabled, opined that there were no doctors and nurses who are trained specifically to handle the patients with disability.

Fifty respondents answered the question on the quality of health care service that persons with disability, as Corona patients received, in the health centre that they visited. The responses were elicited, on the three scales, namely, basis of excellent service, passable service and very bad service. A sizable number, 45, reported their service to be very bad, followed by four respondents who found their service to be passable. The person who found her service to be excellent was one 48-year-old married lady, named Shebika Das, who also receives a disability allowance.

Respondent's response on whether the health care centre had enabling structures (Entrance, Toilets) for patients with disability, was sought. While explaining the question, it became obvious to the interviewer that patients were uninformed about their rights to permitted enabling structures in the hospitals. Many respondents, especially those who are blind, are dependent on their travel companion, and therefore are not able to give an account of the surrounding built environment of the hospitals they made trips to. About a fifth, ten persons among the respondents confirmed that facilitating arrangement in the building existed, while 14 respondents said that there was an absence of any easy entry to the hospitals/health care centres. About half of the interviewees, 26 respondents, said maybe, but they were not sure as most of them were blind or suffering and inattentive.

Responses from 50 respondents were sought on the query of whether they thought that patients/persons with disability were satisfied with the service they got during COVID-19. They were asked to rank their understanding on a scale of excellent, passable and very bad service.

The majority of them were dissatisfied with the service they received during COVID-19 with only three patients recording their moderate satisfaction with the service they received during COVID-19. Respondents were asked whether corona infection aggravated the problems of patients with disability, more than the able patients. Majority (48) affirmed this fact, while answering this question. They reported that it did aggravate such patient's problems, while two persons said 'maybe', it did, as they were not sure because they did not suffer from coronavirus. For example:

> I depend on my daughter to support me while walking. I am lame and cannot afford crutches. In this state I sought health service for my pain. I was turned away because only patients with cold and fever get treatment. I am mostly bed-ridden and cannot afford any private health provider now. (Mrs. Fazilatunnessa an 80-year-old female respondent with physical disability, Charfasson)
>
> Just like any other person, people with hearing impairment need health service from time to time. Getting sick with corona is a big problem due to lack of communication. I cannot understand what doctors tell me. I am blind too. Sadly, I unaware about how to protect myself, which makes me more vulnerable to infectious diseases like COVID-19. (Mrs. Mridula, Deaf and Blind 93-year-old female, Dacope)

While ranking the level of problems faced by persons with disability, almost all 50 respondents reported that they faced maximum problems, while one person opined that he faced obstacles while travelling to access service, but it was not too bad. The respondent was Mr. Chowdhury, a 33-year-old male suffering from speech disability, living in Dacope. He was supported by his nephew when he went for speech therapy. Hence, it was not too difficult as his nephew is an acquaintance of the person who runs the centre.

Respondents were asked about after-effects of coronavirus. Their responses ranged from high to low adverse effects. Even mental illness was reported to have occurred among one in five. Responses on whether they agreed that effects were highly detrimental, were recorded. Most of them were unaware about the effects of coronavirus. About 28 persons agreed strongly while the rest chose to remain neutral. Five respondents strongly disagreed with the suggestion. Seven were doubtful about the adverse effects of coronavirus. Their opinion was also sought on whether a female with a disability suffered much more hardship than a male with a disability, on the scale ranging from extreme suffering, passable suffering to little suffering. Maximum hardship was true for 41 who opined those women suffered more than men with disability. Second level was accepted by eight persons. One person claimed that little suffering existed between men and women's hardship, in case of corona infection.

Responses were sought on the level of healthcare in Bangladesh and its effect upon women with a disability. Opinion on quality of health service to females with disability, was ranked on the basis of excellent, satisfactory, passable and very bad. It appears that women do not get good health care service and this is evident from the responses of women themselves. About 25 of the respondents ranked their health care service as being very bad.

My son has Down Syndrome; hearing Loss, low vision, low intellectual capacity, bad memory, cannot communicate properly. He needs doctor's checkup. Due to corona, I could not take him for treatment as all transport service was disrupted. (Siraj a 12-year old's mother explained his problem, Charfasson)

I suffer from multiple disabilities. I have pain in my hips. Recently I was infected with Corona and needed treatment. Having physical disability (Spinal cord injury), every month I have to check my health for enabling sensory function, otherwise I cannot sustain my health. I could not get good treatment for my sickness. (Happy, 15-year-old girl from Charfasson)

This is followed by 15 respondents who chose level 2, i.e. passable. Ten respondents said that it was satisfactory. None said that their service was excellent. Education has been seriously disrupted for some

I have a son and a daughter. Unfortunately, my daughter suffers from autism. I am a working single-mother. It has been a hard struggle to sustain my family but my divorce has caused much distress. My daughter needs the support of her peers in school. After a lot of cooperation from teachers and students alike, she could overcome some of the inhibitions and confusions that occurred on account of her illness and a broken family. In 2019, she was becoming quite adept at understanding simple chores by observing her class mates. I find it difficult to explain to her the bodily changes that a 11-year-old girl is bound to experience. Since COVID-19, schools have closed. I kept a supportive young therapist to sit with her as she was losing all that she had learnt and becoming listless. Once again, in 2021, the lock down has disrupted the weekly sessions as the therapist cannot come. My daughter is suffering quietly and internally. This corona has undone all the gains she had acquired academically, physically and mentally. (Single Mother of an autistic girl in Dhaka)

Discussions with Key Stakeholders

This analysis comprises information that has been collected from qualitative interviews administered to 15 key informants who are at the key controls of management in hospitals and health care units. They are Managers of private hospitals in Dhaka, physicians of a district hospital, Health Manager of a large hospital, Nurse-in-Charge of a private hospital in Dhaka, Senior Staff Nurses, Nursing Superintendent and Staff Nurses. The Key Stakeholders were asked whether persons with disability come to access their services. As some of the well-known hospitals were included in this survey, many were not aware about persons with disabilities coming to their hospitals. Some answered that in all probability, persons with disability do access their service, but mostly the costs are exorbitant and hence present an invisible obstruction to their access.

Ten responses, to the question on persons with disability accessing healthcare in their hospital, were almost unanimous. Majority affirmed that those with disability do not access their health services, while two persons answered 'maybe'. The question on the percentage of total patients per month, who were disabled persons and had utilized their service, was almost universally not accepted by any of the respondents. They acknowledged that persons with disabilities require medical care. However, there is a dearth of nurses and doctors capable of managing such people so they are often given primary health care and sent for better treatment. The majority of hospitals refer them to other hospitals like Shishu Hospital or Dhaka Medical.

> Often such patients are not admitted in our hospitals because they require different management and their helpers keep away from using our service because of the costs involved. If they come, we refer them to other hospitals like Shishu Hospital. (Senior Staff Nurses)
>
> On account of the government's drive, most of the entrances are enabling but toilets are the same. Sometimes there is provision of commode. (Supervisor of Nurses)

In Chittagong Medical College, which is the largest hospital in the Chittagong region, such persons are given care. The problems arise on account of not having caregivers who can handle persons with disability even in district hospitals. Answers were sought to the question of whether they thought that disabled persons faced more challenges (compared to physically and mentally able people), when accessing healthcare, during this COVID-19 period. Majority answered in the affirmative with one person who said 'maybe'.

> I suffer from Cerebral Palsy. I often require physical therapy; speech therapy; muscle exercises. These out-patient services were not available during corona pandemic. (Mr. Munayem, 24-year-old from Dhaka)
>
> I got infected with Corona and the treatment was so expensive; I could not do tests as the doctor recommend their lab for test. Hospitals and doctors are not disabled friendly. (Mrs. Sabitri, housewife, Dhaka)
>
> I am always confused in hospital on account of their information, which is not disable friendly. Their test cost is more than I can afford. (Ajanta, female student from Charfasson)

The interviewees answered in practically the same manner, when they were questioned in presence of doctors and nurses in their hospitals who were capable of handling persons with disability. Majority of the respondents answered negatively, while 13 respondents said 'don't know'.

> Almost all with disability are referred to other hospitals. In the event of critical patients with disability, who are suffering from brain problems, they decide to keep them here for further brain treatment. It could be through surgery. (Senior Staff Nurse of Neuro Science Hospital, Agargaon)

In-depth questions on the level of healthcare that disabled Corona patients received, in hospitals during the pandemic, were posed to the interviewees. Answers were solicited on the level of care. Most preferred to say that care was satisfactory. None ventured to say that it was excellent or very bad. All respondents preferred to remain with average performance of their hospital caregivers. A point to note is that at the outset, all acknowledged that they did not possess the capability to handle persons with disability. Most, however, did not own up to referring them to other hospitals.

A clear majority have confirmed that Corona infection aggravated the problems of disabled persons, more than the able-bodied. Here, 45 respondents have confirmed the question while the rest have answered 'maybe'. There was no negative response to this question. For example:

> I have one prosthetic eye and the other has low vision, Often the prosthetic eye keeps on aching. I am in great difficulty, trying to get health service for my eye ache. No service is possible during Corona and lock-down. (Female NGO worker in Dhaka)

Questions were posed to rank the level of problems faced by disabled female persons, on a scale of four levels. Rejoinder was solicited on persons' experiences: first was 'No problems or excellent service' being least problematic, followed by 'Problems were present which had to be faced', then 'Problems were hard', lastly 'Extreme problems or great hardships experienced'. Levels 3 and 4, which denoted great hardships, were chosen by 45 of the respondents. Rest of the respondents chose level 2 which denoted the presence of problems which had to be tackled. None chose level 1 which would indicate that there were no problems.

> Most common and severe problem we invariably face while accessing health service is that unfortunately, doctors are not polite. They are very unprofessional. In this case, government health service providers are much more unprincipled and treat us badly. (Several female respondents, preferring anonymity, opined sadly)

Respondents answered the question on their satisfaction with services, graded on four levels, with one being excellent and four denoting 'very bad'. The excellent scores denoted by a very high level of service remained untouched. Very low-quality service represented by level 4 was chosen by 30 of the respondents, who were convinced that hospitals do not possess the skills for handling disabled persons and often refer them to other, more dedicated institutions. Level 1 was not chosen by any of the respondents. Level 2 was chosen by two respondents and level 3 by 18 respondents, that is, a sizable number of respondents.

Nearly all hospital proprietors and senior workers, despite their own deficiency of disability-specific training, opted for the higher performance levels with reference to their individual service. This gives emphasis to the universal breach in consideration of such a person's needs. Compulsory training of the hospital staff of those hospitals and clinics, in becoming disable friendly, is now imperative.

With the first onset of the virulence of corona in Dhaka in March 2020, large hospitals in Dhaka took a decision to refuse corona infected patients. They were uneasy about losing general patients. This continued for nearly two months and a lot of persuasion was required to convince private hospitals to set up separate corona units. After about two months of postponement, the largest and well-known private hospitals set up Corona units with around 25 beds devoted to patients with corona. These apex hospitals were yet to get hold of doctors and nurses trained in handling persons with disability. Thus, it emerged that patients with disability were further neglected and invisible even in times of this life-threatening corona pandemic. This fact was substantiated by some of the heads of organizations.

Nurses accepted that their syllabus and training was not designed for supervising patients with disability. They agreed that the prospectus of the nursing curriculum must incorporate requirements with special focus on four wide learning skills. They are emergency management, infectious disease management and treatment, chronic systemic disease treatment and geriatric care. Thus, the extra importance is accorded to those patients who have the need of the maximum skill and care. It follows that the position of patients with limited ability to manage independently now merit attention, as they are reliant upon caregivers.

COVID-19 and the Problem of Women in Accessing Healthcare

In this country, women have traditionally been accorded less importance in a culturally secluded environment. Women's position is subservient to men (Begum, 2015), as they are financially dependent, and especially if they lack education. If they are suffering from some disability or lack intellectual competence, a stigma exists with regard to such persons with disability, and where women are considered economically and socially weak, they are significantly vulnerable. In this situation, the infection has intensified the challenges to their survival as they cannot sustain without help.

Women have traditionally been the main actors who provide for water which is used in the household. However, their rights are not known as they are not considered to be capable of understanding with physical or mental limitations. It could be made available to them and they can learn about their right to use the healthcare and water and sanitation advantages available to the general public. They need awareness about public health facts and services they would require, especially in the instance of widespread COVID-19 eruption. Women, especially those suffering from disability are rarely inducted into decision-making at the community level.

Therapists and specialized caregivers are more often than not, trained on therapeutic workout, actions on a daily basis for active lives and use of assistive devices. These women are unable to perform therapeutic exercises, functions of daily living and use assistive devices in the absence of caregivers, which are a vital part of their regular healthcare.

This is of critical importance as those with special limitations have their own set of unique problems. As they are habitually reliant upon caregivers and personal assistants, who are physically assisting them in performing the tasks, their health situation deteriorated in times of corona. The true trial begins when the therapists are absent. Persons suffering from disability could face sensitive and obvious tests due to COVID-19. Basically, necessary cleanliness procedures may create impediments in execution, such as repeated washing of their hands may not be feasible due to a range of factors. If the persons with disability make use of wheelchairs, using a hand-basin which could be on an elevated level, might prove onerous; or alternately, tubs and buckets, hosepipes or other water sources may be in point of fact, difficult to get to; or a person with disability could be incapable of scrubbing both hands simultaneously and maintain cleanliness. Such persons with disabilities could find it impossible to maintain social distance as they are physically dependent. They experience problems in maintaining social space on account of helplessness, inability to be self-sufficient physically and they might require aid. Women, on account of their reproductive functions have to take special personal care but in situations when caregivers are absent, the chores become insurmountable. If they are part of an institution, conditions might exist where social (physical) division might not be practicable. Moreover, those who have impaired eyesight or cannot see at all will often understand the surroundings by touching objects to obtain information from the environs or for physical support.

Moreover, safeguards are an additional vital consideration for persons with disability. Contingent upon their overall health status and innate weakness or co-morbidity, persons with disability may be exposed to higher levels of severity if they contract this virus. There are chances of extra risks from incidence of COVID-19, to these persons as they are often unable to articulate their suffering or seek care independently, in case of infection.

Conclusion

Persons suffering limitations such as a disability often function under a gloom of societal dishonour and often face incidence of financial and social dependency, and require caregivers, sighted guides, interpreters. Still, under threat of a life seizing pandemic, physical or social distancing is not feasible. Furthermore, travelling and manoeuvring patients with wheelchairs necessitate additional funds, human resources, construction with specific designing, not to mention compassion, especially in tending and concern. Regrettably, these are scarce.

The most important purpose of this chapter is to comprehend the harshness of constriction, inequality in access to healthcare of persons with disability, who managed with COVID-19 during this pandemic. Evidence points to the fact that persons with disabilities such as cerebral palsy and down's syndrome are completely dependent upon caregivers and have found it difficult to maintain COVID-19 precautions such as maintenance of social distance. Girls suffering from autism have lost more than a year of educational gains they had developed with the help of assistance and peers. Moreover, persons in wheelchairs are unable to reach basins to wash their hands; often deaf persons are unable to lip-read due to the donning of masks. We also know that persons with disabilities are referred to specific hospitals only, as most hospitals do not have trained doctors and nurses. It is imperative to increase efforts to address their specific needs through targeted allocation of resources, such as training more doctors and nurses for treatment of disabled patients, or setting up especially designed washbasins for those in wheelchairs. While these options might not be immediately implementable, there should be plans of providing free masks and sanitizers to these marginalized people, or setting up subsidized medical schemes for them. Special training should be given to nurses and doctors and easing of the access to service for persons with disability, should be prioritized.

In Bangladesh, nursing has been disparaged due to culture, religion and other socio-economic factors; persons afflicted with disability often face the discouraging consequence of low standard service within this system. Women in particular are the foremost victims of this system.

Women's exposure to cultural conscriptions worsens prevailing low access to healthcare, employment and income, quality education and also deepen existing disparity in society. The severity of low access to healthcare for women has now forced an in-depth analysis to proffer inclusive and sustainable solutions to entrenched inequalities in society. Women with disabilities are among the most ignored in any society and are more likely to live in poverty, experiencing higher rates of discrimination, neglect and exploitation in an occurrence of a virulent disease. Unfortunately, the health, social and economic crisis brought about by COVID-19 threatens to undo the progress made towards equal opportunity for people suffering from some or multiple disabilities. The greatest challenges of COVID-19 inimically present itself to these persons who are heavily dependent upon caregivers for their existence. The threats lie in the fact that awareness of asymptomatic increase is hardly known among these persons with disabilities. Although highly contagious, knowledge about this disease and related consciousness has increased somewhat due to its life-threatening nature, but many have succumbed. The painful truth remains in the fact that adherence to social distancing, in this case, it is physical isolation, remains a concern for persons suffering from disability, who in reality survive on physical support and dependence.

References

Bangladesh Bureau of Statistics. (2001). *Census of Bangladesh 2001*. Ministry of Planning, Government of Bangladesh.

Bangladesh Bureau of Statistics. (2011). *Census of Bangladesh 2011*. Ministry of Planning, Government of Bangladesh.

Begum, A. (1999). *Destination Dhaka—Urban migration: Expectations and reality*. University Press Limited.

Begum, A. (2015). Gender in education: Policy discourse and challenges. *Journal of Development in Practice, 25*(5), 754–768.

Begum, A., & Mahmood. (2017). Chapter 9, on "Labour market and skill gap analyses: Health care (nursing and health technician)". In *Bids study report: Labour market and skill gap in Bangladesh (macro and micro level study)*, May 2017; published by Skills for Employment Investment Program (SEIP), Finance Division, Ministry of Finance, Government of the People's Republic of Bangladesh.

Bezbaruah, V. (2018). Uncertain personhood: Notes on ageing and disability in Guwahati during COVID 19. *Disability and the Global South, 2021, 8*(1), 1982–1992 (OPEN ACCESS). ISSN 2050-7364. www.dgsjournal.org © The Authors. This work is licensed under a Creative Commons Attribution 3.0 License 1982.

Cockcroft, A., et al. (2007). *What did the Public think of health services reform in Bangladesh? Three national community-based surveys 1999–2003*. Published by Springer.

Cockcroft, M., et al. (2011). *Health services reforms in Bangladesh*. Published by Springer.

Gerold-Scheepers, T. J. F. A., & van Binsbergen Wim, M. J. (1978). Marxist and Non-Marxist approaches to migration in Tropical Africa. In M. J. van Binsbergen Wim & A. Meilink Henk (Eds.), *Migration and the transformation of modern African Society*. Afrika-Studiecentrum.

Hussain, M. S., Ferdous, S., & Siddiqee, M. (2020). Mass panic during COVID-19 outbreak–A perspective from Bangladesh as a high-risk country. *Journal of Biomedical Analytics, 3*(2), 1–3.

i2i Innovation to Inclusion. (2021). Insights and stories from Bangladesh and Kenya, published by Leonard Cheshire, European Disability Forum and UK AID.

Kandasamy, N., Perera, B., & Soldatic, K. (2021). COVID-19 from the margins: Gendered-disability experiences in Sri Lanka. *Disability and the Global South, 2021, 8*(1), 1873–1879 (OPEN ACCESS). ISSN 2050-7364. www.dgsjournal.org

Kibria, et al. (2020). *Barriers to healthcare services for persons with disabilities in Bangladesh amid the COVID-19 pandemic.* Elsevier. www.journals.elsevier.com/public-health-in-practice

Mabogunje, A. L. (1970). Systems approach to a theory of rural-urban migration. *Geographical Analysis, 2,* 1–18, Ohio State University Press, USA.

Nayar, M., Juvva, S., & Lakshman, C. (2021). Psychosocial consequences of COVID-19 on persons with visual impairments. *Disability and the Global South, 2021, 8*(1), 1958–1971 (OPEN ACCESS). ISSN 2050-7364. www.dgsjournal.org © The Authors. This work is licensed under a Creative Commons Attribution 3.0 License 1958.

Mehrotra, N., & Soldatic, K. (2021). COVID-19 in South Asia: State practices, responses and the experiences of persons with disability within the region. *Disability and the Global South, 2021, 8*(1), 1873–1879 (OPEN ACCESS). ISSN 2050-7364. www.dgsjournal.org © The Authors. This work is licensed under a Creative Commons Attribution 3.0 License 1873.

Mizan, A. S. (2021). Invisible to the law: COVID-19 and the legal consciousness of persons with disabilities in Bangladesh. *Disability and the Global South, 2021, 8*(1), 1873–1879 (OPEN ACCESS). ISSN 2050-7364. www.dgsjournal.org © The Authors.

OECD. (2021a). *Rights and protection of the persons with disabilities rules of 2015.*

OECD. (2021b). *The state of school education: One year into the Covid pandemic* (p. 50). OECD.

Population Council. (2020). Bangladesh: Covid-19 Knowledge, (2020), Attitudes, Practices & Needs Responses from Three Rounds of Data Collection Among Adolescent Girls in Districts with High Rates of Child Marriage; UNICEF and Population Council, Knowledge Commons.

Rights and Protection Act in Bangladesh for Persons with Disabilities in 2013 (User Friendly). Booklet: WDDF, the Asia-Pacific Development Center on Disability APDC, and South-Asian Development Forum (SADF).

Rights and Protection of the Persons with Disabilities Act 2013 (RPPD Act), replacing the 2001 Act, and the Neuro-Development Disability Protection Trust Act, 2013.

Shajahan, S. (2021). Life becomes harder: Intersectional feminist lens to dis/abled experience of women in Afghanistan during Covid 19 pandemic and post Covid development context. *Disability and the Global South, 2021, 8*(1), 1873–1879 (OPEN ACCESS). ISSN 2050–7364. www.dgsjournal.org ©The Authors. This work is licensed under a Creative Commons Attribution 3.0 License 1873.

United Nations Convention on the Rights of Persons with Disabilities (CRPD) in 2007.

Chapter 11
How Do Pandemics Affect Frontline Health Interventions? Insights from the National Tuberculosis Elimination Programme in Bengaluru, India

Sobin George, Aditi Paranjpe, and Prajwal Nagesh

Abstract Available literature shows that lockdowns and reassignment of health infrastructure carried out in response to the COVID-19 pandemic adversely affected several national health programmes in India. The National Tuberculosis Elimination Programme (NTEP) is one such important health programme that faced serious setbacks due to the pandemic since TB interventions require constant follow up of patients by frontline workers. We endeavoured to understand how TB frontline activities are affected by the ongoing COVID-19 pandemic interventions. The chapter draws on qualitative in-depth interviews with TB health visitors (TBHV) and patients, which were conducted before and after the outbreak of the pandemic. Our findings show that the pandemic situation has weakened the critical frontline interventions of NTEP since the frontline activities of DOTS, including active case finding, follow up of sputum examination, distribution of medicine, monitoring of patients with side effects and patient support measures, were either slowed down or temporarily suspended in several instances. Also, the existing vicious cycle of TB and poverty got exacerbated with the pandemic for female patients due to job loss, lack of supporting systems and improper adherence to treatment regimen. Most importantly, the pandemic has exposed the weaknesses of Indian health delivery system that fell short of health personnel and physical infrastructure, especially doctors, nursing staff, hospital beds, medical supplies and equipment. Hence, there is a need for restructuring of the health system in India with equitable distribution of infrastructure and development of a dedicated public health cadre to respond effectively to the crisis such as the present one so that other equally prioritised public health interventions are not hampered.

S. George (✉) · A. Paranjpe
Institute for Social and Economic Change, Bengaluru 560072, India

P. Nagesh
Department of Human Geography and Spatial Planning, Utrecht University, Utrecht, Netherlands
e-mail: p.nagesh1@uu.nl

Keywords COVID-19 pandemic · TB frontline interventions · TB Health Visitors · Health delivery systems · India · COVID-19 · Tuberculosis interventions · Health visitors · Health delivery systems · India

Introduction

The COVID-19 pandemic has been a litmus test on the preparedness of the health care delivery system of India and available studies show that the pandemic has exposed the systemic weaknesses, rigidities and flaws of the health and health service delivery systems of India (Bhatia & Abraham, 2020; Chetterje, 2020; Kumar & Reddy, 2020). There is already evidence that health care delivery in India is constrained by lack of sufficient infrastructure and diagnostic facilities, non-availability of qualified medical personnel, corruption, poor health management system, absenteeism of staff and apathy of service providers (Acharya, 2010; George, 2019; Hazarika, 2013; Jaysawal, 2015; Motkuri et al., 2017; Saikia, 2018). Potnuru (2017) estimated that India has only 4.8 practising doctors per 10,000 population against the standard ratio of 7 per 10,000. As per the rural health data provided by the Government of India, there is a shortfall of 19,644 doctors in rural and 1,812 in urban India as of December 2018. Further, data from rural health statistics showed that there was a shortage of 7,092 pharmacists (in PHCs and CHCs), 13,194 nursing staff (in PHCs and CHCs), 18,347 specialists (in CHCs), 10,112 female health workers (PHCs and SCs) and 99,572 male health workers (in SCs) as of December 2017. There was a shortfall of 627 doctors and 3,369 specialist doctors in tribal areas as of 2017 (Saalim, 2020).

Shortage of physical infrastructure is also a major problem that India faces. For instance, availability of hospital beds in public sector is as low as 0.55 beds per 1000 population and it is much lower than the national average in states including Bihar, Jharkhand, Gujarat, Uttar Pradesh, Andhra Pradesh, Chhattisgarh, Madhya Pradesh, Haryana, Maharashtra, Odisha, Assam and Manipur (Singh et al., 2020). George (2016) showed that tribal areas have the worst infrastructure shortage problem in India and highlighted that several states have shortage of PHCs and CHCs in tribal areas and the deficit also increased considerably in some states, including Gujarat, Madhya Pradesh and Bihar between 2006 and 2014. Further, micro-level studies have pointed out that tribal India suffers from severe shortage of health care infrastructure, such as sub-centres, PHCs and nutritional service infrastructure like Anganwadis (Das et al., 2010). Studies have also linked the problems with health care delivery to poor health outcomes, especially in rural India with special focus on women, children and marginalised groups (Borooah et al. 2012).

It is in this context that one needs to understand and assess the pandemic response that the Indian states have undertaken. As highlighted by the media reports, the pandemic significantly stressed the already overburdened health care workforce both in public and private sectors and even states such as Kerala, which has relatively better health responsiveness, faced considerable challenges to manage the situation.[1] Media reports have shown that public and private hospitals in several states could not recruit additional health workers to meet the requirement of COVID care due to problems with availability of staff, low pay, short term contract and poor safety facilities available. There is also evidence that lockdowns and reassignment of health infrastructure as part of COVID-19 responses adversely affected several national programmes to control and eliminate infectious and non-communicable diseases (Behera, 2021; Glaziou, 2020). The National Tuberculosis Elimination Programme (NTEP) is one such important health programme that faced considerable challenges due to the pandemic since TB treatment regimen requires constant follow up of patients with the help of frontline workers. Glaziou (2020) predicted that weekly counts of reported cases of TB in India dropped by 75% in the initial three weeks of lockdown, possibly due to factors such as 'delays in entering the data onto the real-time national online TB surveillance system, reduced attendance to health services, reassignment of health personnel and a reduction in TB testing and detection'. Similarly, Behera (2021) noted that redeployment of health care workers, diversion of TB diagnostic facilities for COVID-19 work, conversion of hospitals exclusively for COVID-19 care and diversion of budgets adversely affected the NTEP programme in India. This chapter tries to understand how TB frontline activities which include active case detection, Directly Observed Treatment, Short-Course (DOTS) regimen and disease prevention are affected by the pandemic. It also aims to reflect on the structural, systemic, cultural and institutional barriers for the successful adherence to treatment for female patients working in informal arrangements.

Methods

This chapter is based on a qualitative study conducted among TB patients and TB Health Visitors (TBHVs) in the city of Bengaluru, Karnataka, India. Data were collected through in-depth interviews conducted in two phases. The first phase, which was conducted from January to August 2019, collected data from eighty working women TB patients who were undergoing DOTS treatment and eight TBHVs from eighteen DOTS centres across four regions of Bengaluru city. An interview guide was developed for in-depth interviews, which were conducted in the first phase. The questions asked in the interviews with TB patients in the first phase included treatment pathways, work-life balance, construction of employability through various channels, experience of working while affected with TB, employability of women TB patients in various intimate work spheres, work-induced health-seeking behaviour, follow up of TB regimen while in the workforce, etc. Questions asked in the interviews with TBHVs in the first phase included those related to compliance of working

---

[1] scroll.in/article/969107/indias-health-centres-are-facing-staff-crunch-even-as-coronavirus-cases-continue-to-rise.

patients with the new DOTS regimen, facilities given to working patients and suggestions for better compliance to treatment by TB afflicted women in the workforce. We conducted telephonic follow up interviews with ten previously interviewed TB patients who continued treatment and seven TBHVs in the months of April 2020 (during the period of the nationwide lockdown) and August 2020 (during the phasing out period of lockdown). Same questions of the first phase of the interview, however in the context of the pandemic, were asked to patient respondents and TBHVs in the follow-up interviews.

We used the grounded theory method for analysing the data. All interviews were conducted in the local language of *Kannada*. Interviews were recorded and the verbatim was transcribed and translated to English by bilingual experts. Sufficient care was taken to reproduce the information in respondents' own words, phrases and expressions. The data was analysed using qualitative software *Atlas-ti 7*. The transcribed data was anonymised in order to conceal the identity of the patients and TBHVs who participated in the study. Further, we developed three core themes from the sub themes identified from the transcripts (Table 11.1).

Limitations

The fieldwork in the first phase of the study was very intensive; however, data in the second phase (follow-up) was collected through telephonic interviews due to lockdown and other pandemic related restrictions. The first phase of the study focused only on women patients working in the informal sector. Hence, the follow-up interviews among patients were limited to the same group of respondents, although it is evident that the pandemic adversely affected all TB patients. Further, the sample size was small in the follow-up interviews since only a small number of patients who participated in the first phase were continuing DOTS regimen when the follow-up interviews were conducted.

Findings

We have analysed the responses of patients and TBHVs to the questions asked in the interviews on treatment-seeking, DOTS administration and monitoring, active case detection, TB prevention activities and problems faced by TBHVs and patients during pre- and post-pandemic situations. Major findings are presented below.

Table 11.1 Core themes and sub themes emerged

Core themes	Sub themes
Exacerbation of the vicious cycle of TB and poverty with the pandemic	Job loss
	Lack of social security
	Falling back to poverty
	No access to short term remedial measures by the state
	Impoverishment and increased vulnerabilities to TB
Intersections of gender, informality and exigencies of the pandemic leading to unmet needs of working female patients	Continuing gender expectations in the family
	Avoidance of family members
	Apathy of family members
	Increased violence faced in the family
	Informality at work and fear of loss of job
	Clash of timings of work and DOTS
	Coping to work and violation of treatment protocol
Disruptions, delay and suspension of TB frontline interventions	Flexibilisation of DOTS regimen
	Slow down/suspension of ACF and follow up investigations
	Failure of follow up with patients
	Lack of patient support measures
	Redeployment of NTEP resources
	Lack of information on compliance of migrant patients
	Job insecurity and apprehensions of frontline health workers

Source Developed by authors from interview transcripts

Balancing Treatment, Work and Family: DOTS Regimens for Female Patients

All participants from the group of patients were women working in informal arrangements and hence, balancing of life, work and treatment was a dominant theme in the initial interviews as also the follow-up interviews. We attempted to understand how disease conditions and treatment of working female TB patients interacted with their life worlds. It emerged from the interviews that there still exist families that inflict stigma and practice avoidance once a female member is diagnosed with tuberculosis. It emerged from the interviews that there still exist families that inflict stigma and start avoiding the female member who is diagnosed with tuberculosis. Such families often asked the patient to leave her home and find some other location until she gets well. Often, if allowed by the religion, the man marries again, citing her disease as the reason for second marriage. The female from such a family can never return to her married family as the disease becomes a permanent blight on her. One of our patient respondents noted:

> The day my husband knew I had TB, I knew my days in the home were over. I myself just said that I will go to the village and stay there.

Patients also experienced apathy from family members. They noted that the family members did not consider her problems and treatment regimen seriously, whether she consumes tablets properly, or takes regular medications. It is found that patients in such families cannot stay away from their gender roles as well. The work at home must get done. The female patient, especially in the low socio-economic group, has to fight on several fronts at the same time. On the one hand, there are debilitating symptoms of disease and coping with the hardship and drudgery of household work. On the other hand, there are concerns of losing employment if the disease is disclosed to the employer and also the concern of secrecy imposed on oneself with regard to neighbours, relatives and friends so that the TB status is not disclosed to them. An even greater concern is that often, in reality, she is the sole breadwinner of the family. There may be a spouse who is earning, but in a majority of the low socio-economic cases, the husband is often an alcoholic or simply unavailable and hence, his earnings do not find their way into the household spending. This leads to the occurrence of large debts upon the female, which sends the entire household into a poverty spiral. Moreover, once the tenacious hold on a decent life is lost, it is difficult for the whole family to climb out of the poverty spiral. Often the basic requirements such as the school fees and house rents do not get paid and the family is forced to move out of a *pucca* house into a smaller tenement. Also, the nutrition of the family gets affected. In a few cases, the family members of some patients were aware of the difficulty of working with TB women patients; however, they were unable to do anything to help the situation. Most of these families were headed by women patients themselves and they were the main earners/or significant contributor to the income of the family. Quitting employment, while trying to recover from TB, is not an option for such female patients as it would push them into poverty and hence, they are often forced to work. The following narrative from a patient reflects the situation:

> Where do we have the luxury of being concerned about the disease? We know that unless we both earn, we cannot survive.

Further, their narratives reflected the conflicts between work-related issues and DOTS regimen that had implications for treatment-seeking by the patients. They noted that DOTS and work timings always clashed for them. Although the DOTS programme introduced flexible timings as part of the guidelines of patient support programmes, it was not followed in several of the locations where we conducted interviews in the first phase. Respondents also noted that employers did not allow them to make DOTS visits on working days. They explained how work and DOTS centre timings clashed:

> There is a problem to manage both [work and DOTS visits] properly. The work timings clash with the treatment timings and hence, I struggle to obtain my medicines properly. Since the

employers do not give time off repeatedly, it is difficult to reach the DOTS centre on time. Commuting to and from the workplace to DOTS centre is also tiring and difficult to manage.

Another major factor that interfered with balancing work and treatment was the conveyance required for travelling to work and treatment centre. Long distance between the place of work and the DOTS centre was a barrier for some patients. Although they initially tried to manage the DOTS centre visits during work hours by hiring a taxi (mainly auto-rickshaws), they could not continue it due to the high cost. Patients found that the travel to DOTS centres along with the usual travel to work and back home increased their fatigue and clashed with the timings of work and DOTS. Some patients also noted that DOTS visits on working days had been a major stress factor for them since they were constantly worried about meeting the timings at both locations. They also had to change their daily routine of sleep and preparation for the working day. Patients who visited the DOTS centres in the morning noted that they had reduced sleep hours since they needed to wake up earlier than usual. Further, some of the patients shed light on the problem of transport services. The DOTS Centres or their residences often did not have access to public transport services, which increased their burden in an effort to access DOTS services. Respondents explained how commuting to work and reaching the DOTS Centres increased their burden of TB treatment:

> I am always worried about commuting between my workplace, the DOTS Centre and going back to work and again and then back home. I get too tired. Earlier I used to sleep till 6 am, now I have to get up by 4 so that I can finish the work at home and reach the DOTS Centre and then the workplace, all on time.

For patients, the constant travel between DOTS centres, workplace and home not only increased the fatigue but also added to the financial burden. They noted that either the workplace or the DOT centre was far from home and in order to reach both the locations on time, they were left with the sole option of hiring a taxi or a three-wheeler. A few patients opted to go to the DOTS centre during lunch break in order to avoid the conflict of work and DOTS Centre timings, as otherwise, it would have increased their spending since they had to hire a vehicle.

> I have too many problems with commuting. My home is a far distance away from the main road. So, I must walk 15 minutes every time to catch a bus. There is no good bus route connection either. The DOTS Centre is far from work. It is expensive to travel between the two. If I do not take an auto-rickshaw, I would never reach my workplace on time, and this would lead to loss of pay for the day. But then, hiring a three-wheeler is too expensive.

Follow up interviews conducted during the lockdown period showed that conflicts in work, life and treatment have aggravated during the COVID-19 pandemic period. Lack of adequate family support was an important issue that the patient respondents considered as an unmet need while balancing work, family and treatment. The patients experienced lack of empathy and care from family members. Most of them noted that they expected more care, consideration, assistance in household work [rest] and emotional support from family members. They also pointed out that the family members, especially the significant others, can play a major role in the timely intake of medicine and food of the patients. Patients shared their unmet needs from family members:

> The TB patient must be treated with care and love by family members. They should be provided good food & rest to recover soon.
>
> They [family members] should help us in check-ups and taking nutritious food. They should let us take enough rest.
>
> The patient should be given all support by family members, by accompanying her to hospital and providing her emotional support.

For married patients, spouse violence was a major issue during the COVID-19 period. They noted that spouses should be considerate about their physical and mental health and avoid picking up fights. Similarly, some of the patient respondents experienced negligence and isolation within the family, which was found to have further stressed them. They noted that providing emotional support is one of the major needs of female patients who are struggling to balance home, work and treatment. They elaborated:

> He [husband] should not fight. He should provide a good atmosphere for living a peaceful life, good food and help in every way.
>
> The family should be very loving and not speak rudely to them [to the patient].

While hostile conditions of work were the problems during pre-COVID-19 period, loss of work and earning were the major problems for patients during the COVID-19 period. Decline in earnings led patients to borrow money and sell assets [mostly ornaments], especially those who were the principal earners of the family and did not have other support mechanisms. Patient respondents reported that they could not find money for regular household expenditures such as house rents and school fees. It was also noted by the patients that they fell back into the poverty spiral, which further increased their vulnerability associated with TB due to lack of nutritional supplementation and poor compliance to treatment regimen. One of the patients who worked in a private school as a 'cleaner' explained how the COVID-19 pandemic and loss of work affected her TB treatment, nutritional status and financial conditions of the family:

> I enquired [for a job] everywhere, I did not get [an opportunity] anywhere. Currently, I am at home and not going anywhere... I tried in some 3–4 places [for a job] [...] in hospitals and in offices, but it did not happen anywhere... They say that they will call back, but no one called back.... He [husband] also lost job and started enquiring in different places. [...] We have not paid rent since April [2020]. [...] We somehow managed till now. Now going forward with it will be very difficult. All four of us [including two children] are sitting at home, no work, no rent, not enough food. It is becoming difficult now. Now even the loan people [money lenders] do not understand the situation. One woman came in the evening and made a scene [asking for recovery of loan]. Knowing the situation also, they are asking for money. Don't know what to do.

Patient respondents who continued to work during the pandemic noted that support from health care providers is paramount in balancing work, life and treatment. DOTS timings, stringent treatment regimen, side effects and follow up medical investigations tended to affect the work hours of the patients. Most importantly, patients felt that the providers need to be aware and sensitive to this conflict and working patients need to be prioritised at DOTS centres. Some of them also noted that flexible timing at DOT centres could be an option so that the patients could consult and collect medicines whenever they are free. Patients also preferred DOTS visits in the evenings rather than mornings and felt that medicines supply should be provided to suffice for longer periods at one time so as to avoid frequent visits. Similarly, they opined that it would be convenient if the patients can be provided medicines at their location itself so that they can avoid regular DOTS visits.

> They (Doctors, Nurses, DOTS service providers) must be concerned about the waiting time as we leave our work and get late but still sometimes, we have been asked to wait, which is very troublesome.
>
> The DOTS centre timings are not convenient [for me]. I cannot go when I am free, after 5pm, since they are not available then. I feel that there must be flexible timings at DOTS Centres.

Challenges of Frontline TB Interventions for Health Workers

It emerged from the interviews with TBHVs that poverty, non-adherence to treatment, stigma associated with TB [for women], lack of support in family and at workplace, difficulties in following up with substance users/alcoholic and poor and migrant patients have been the common barriers for the successful completion of DOTS regimen. They explained these barriers:

> Some patients try to bargain in this [intake of medicine] also. They say, sir, it is for six months. Can I take it only for two months or three months? Some take the medicines for two months. After this, in the follow- up test, it will be negative. Since it is negative, they feel that they do not have TB and decide that they can discontinue the medicines.

The pandemic situation, on the one hand, aggravated some of these problems and opened up fresh challenges on the other. Lockdown and restrictions were imposed hurriedly in India without much planning or preparation. Restrictions on travel that were imposed were reported to have affected the DOTS visits during lockdown. Further, TBHVs noted that they did not get adequate time to come up with a better alternative plan for DOTS regimen since the lockdowns were imposed hurriedly. Most importantly, the deployment of NTEP staff for COVID-19 response was reported to have affected the routine DOTS programme. They noted:

> Since the lockdown was declared without much warning, it became difficult for patients to come to the DOTS centre. Due to lockdown, even if they were close to the DOT Centre, they often had to take an exceedingly long route to reach us.
>
> The police would stop them each time they tried to come to us. Then we spoke to the policeman every time to endorse that the TB medicine was important and they should be allowed to come to us.
>
> We are asked to do COVID-19 work also. We are going to the houses of second line contact of COVID-19 patients and inform them about quarantine. There is absolutely no ACF [Active Case Finding] going on at all. We will try to start after 17 May [2020] when the lockdown may be lifted. Actually, we don't know.

Subsequent to the imposition of lockdown and related restrictions on travel and work, several changes have been made in the administration of DOTS programme. Most importantly, the frequency of DOTS centre visits was reduced (which ranged from once in a month during lockdown to once a week after lockdown). Medicines were given for a period of one month for migrant patients as well as for those patients who could not make regular visits. Physical follow up visits were replaced by virtual follow up through mobile phones. However, it should be highlighted that there were situations wherein the staff could not distribute drugs to patients due to lockdown even with the introduction of these flexibilities. One of the TBHVs noted:

> We have a two-month stock of medicines ready with us. But we could not distribute due to lockdown. All these patients are now defaulters for sure.

Similarly, TBHVs noted that diluting of DOTS regimen by allowing unsupervised DOTS administration and virtual follow up led the vulnerable patient groups to defaulting on medicines or improper intake of medicines. This group comprised primarily migrant workers, substance users/alcoholics, patients who had side effects and patients who did not have family support. TBHVs, during lockdown, could follow up only the patients who stayed in close proximity to the DOTS centres. The reverse migration of patients who were under treatment was another major problem. It was reported by TBHVs that although the migrant patients could continue the treatment in their native places since all information of the patients was available through their unique Nikshay identification number; the coordination with patients and local DOTS centres was difficult. In some cases, patients who returned to remote areas could not access DOTS centres since the service was not available near their locality. It was also reported by TBHVs that patients hesitated to go to local DOTS centres for the fear that they would be quarantined since they returned from cities where COVID-19 spread was high. They explained the difficulties of DOTS administration and follow up among vulnerable patients during the pandemic period as follows:

> We are able to track only those patients who live near the DOTS centres. If they are now outside Bangalore, we can contact the local DOTS centre and ask them to provide the medicines. But it requires a fair amount of coordination.
>
> Many patients from the families of migrant workers already left the city and went to their villages. We are concerned about them since they are not reachable. Some of them have switched off their mobiles for the fear of quarantine since they come from a zone which is categorised as red zone [place where infection is high]. We don't know whether they will be able to buy medicines locally so that they can continue treatment.

There were also efforts to follow-up patients through mobile phones during the pandemic period. While this was found useful among those patients who continued to stay in the city, mobile phone-based follow-up of migrant patients was not successful due to issues such as deactivation of phone numbers, switching off mobile phones by the patients and technical problems associated with mobile phone networks. TBHVs noted that lack of follow-up would lead to defaulting, especially by new patients who cannot manage the side effects of TB medicines, which are common in the initial days of medication. As noted by TBHVs, it is important that patients with severe side effects (such as extreme fatigue, vomiting and skin eruptions) should immediately be attended and taken to hospitals. However, such follow-up activities did not happen during COVID-19 period, which would lead to defaulting. TBHVs explained their experiences of phone-based follow up and its possible consequences:

> Mobile phone networks in many interior places are still bad and it is difficult to continue conversation. Some patients were under the V-DOTS scheme where they can send us an immediate message upon consuming the medication. Not all patients are under the V DOTS scheme which is initiated by a private entity.
>
> My previous experience shows that although many patients say that they take medicine over the phone, they might be irregular. Most of the patients who started treatment recently are reluctant to take medicines regularly due to side effects. Patients with severe side effects of drugs are in problem since they don't get treatment now [COVID-19 period].

Their narratives also reflected the problems faced by patients with comorbidity, reduction in the number of active case findings, delay of TB diagnosis due to shortage of laboratory facilities, unavailability of outpatient facilities for TB patients due to COVID-19 care and lack of proper patient support mechanism, which are integral to the tuberculosis elimination programme during the pandemic. There were instances that TB patients could not avail treatment for comorbidity since most of the public hospitals were either partially functioning or reserved exclusively for COVID-19 care. One of the TBHVs narrated the difficulties that a TB patient, who also had HIV, faced while accessing treatment for both diseases from two different health centres.

> I can narrate to you the big challenge I am facing with a patient who has both TB and HIV. He must collect TB medicines from me and the HIV medicines from the ART centre located elsewhere. He came to me saying [that] he had severe blurring of vision. I was concerned but could not help him at our OPD since there was nobody to check him up. Since it was an eye issue, I referred him to Minto hospital [public hospital in Bengaluru]. He went there. However, due to COVID-19, that hospital was not functional. Then I referred him to Victoria hospital [public hospital in Bengaluru]. He was told there that all beds were kept for COVID-19 patients.

Our interviews with TBHVs further showed that deployment of NTEP staff, including TBHVs, to COVID-19 care and management considerably hampered their routine work, especially the active case finding (ACF). As it is discussed earlier in the chapter, TBHVs were given additional work as part of COVID-19 response interventions. It was reported by TBHVs that they were deployed for survey and awareness generation on COVID-19 and contact tracing of COVID-19 patients. As per their estimation, ACF was reduced considerably during the lockdown period. They noted:

> There is absolutely no ACF going on at all. We will try to start after 17 May [2020] when the lockdown may be lifted. Actually, we don't know
>
> I was asked to go for a house-to-house COVID-19 survey and awareness mostly. Some were also sent for tracing the contacts of COVID-19 patients. Our Active case finding is at least 50 % less right now. The [TB] cases could spike after lifting the lockdown.

Similarly, TBHVs noted that closing down of outpatient departments (OPDs) in public hospitals due to the pandemic delayed TB diagnosis. Another major issue was the unavailability of laboratory facilities for TB diagnosis due to COVID-19 care. All DOTS centres are not adequately equipped with laboratory facilities and follow up examinations are usually undertaken in other public laboratories. As a result, the number of sputum and other follow up investigations came down during lockdown, which can have implications for early detection and confirmation of TB cure rates. Other issues such as unavailability of Personal Protective Equipment (PPE) kits for lab technicians in government labs and reluctance of symptomatic patients to get tested due to fear of COVID-19 diagnosis and possible isolation and stigmatisation, since most of the symptoms of TB and COVID-19 are similar, were also identified as barriers of ACF and diagnosis by TBHVs.

> We can't do the sputum exam as PHCs won't do the sputum test. The patients cannot go to hospitals since they don't entertain these TB patients since they are committed right now to COVID-19 care. No inpatient services are available now in government hospitals. It is a matter of great concern that some patients who may be in the initial stages of TB will not get properly diagnosed until lockdown is lifted. At the moment, we have 50% less cases due to the lockdown.
>
> The lab technicians have no PPE and therefore, [they] are refusing to take any risks.
>
> Patients now do not go to hospital if they have persistent cough for the fear of being diagnosed for COVID-19 and the attached stigma of isolation and quarantine of family members.

Finally, the pandemic has exposed the precarious conditions of work associated with the frontline health interventions in India which are performed by health workers/visitors/volunteers. The national tuberculosis elimination programme depends heavily on TBHVs for delivering the crucial frontline activities that include initial home visits, active case detection, defaulter visits, health education, documentation and reporting. Our discussions with TBHVs showed that other than these responsibilities, they also distribute medicines, follow up with the patients, conduct chemical prophylaxis, undertake patient counselling, ensure the reach of patient support services (such as nutritional allowance) and facilitate follow up investigations. However, TBHVs who lead the frontline interventions are temporary workers on fixed-term job contracts without social security entitlements. They are also at high risk of disease infection. One of the respondents explained the vulnerable position of TBHVs:

> We are all working on a contractual basis. Our job is not secure. We have no PF [provident fund], insurance, sick leave and other allowances. We also do not have a risk allowance. Daily, we see a minimum 50 cases, out of which there will be minimum 10–20 pulmonary cases. While interacting with such patients, they might cough and we might get an infection. The staff has no special facilities in the eventuality that they get infected. In our department itself, many are infected with MDR TB and have died. Some of our colleagues have died due to accidents while doing [TB] fieldwork.

There was a general feeling of apathy and de-motivation among TBHVs who were deployed for COVID-19 response—primarily due to the informalities associated with their work, overwork, non-recognition of their contribution, poor payment and risk of infection. TBHVs who were assigned the pandemic related work also had to undertake their routine TB work and achieve the stipulated targets of DOTS. This had increased their work burden and disturbed the TB programme at the ground level.

One of the TBHVs explained how the pandemic exacerbated their already precarious conditions of work:

> I have worked non-stop since COVID-19 lockdown was declared, even on all weekends and holidays. We are doing so much work in COVID-19 times. But there is no credit [recognition] given for that work at all. If we develop any health concern due to COVID-19, there is no provision for any medical facility to take care of us at all. Now I am sure I will get a notice concerning why I have no new diagnosed cases. No one has asked us what our problems on the ground are. They just want statistics and that is all. My salary after 18 years of work is only 21,000/. How is it possible to survive? I have two grown up daughters too.

Discussion

Our results shed light on the barriers that could come in the way of realising the goal of elimination of tuberculosis in India by 2025 due to the continuing structural problems of poverty and poor conditions of employment for vulnerable group of people, as well as the challenges that frontline TB interventions face during health emergencies such as the present pandemic. These are discussed below.

Pandemic Exacerbation of Tuberculous and Poverty Cycles

The findings presented in the previous section clearly show that the COVID-19 pandemic situation exacerbated the already existing vicious cycle of TB, employability and poverty. The vicious cycle of TB and poverty is already well illustrated in India (Grange & Zumla, 1999; Killewo, 2002). Further, studies in the context of the COVID-19 pandemic have predicted that loss of jobs and decline in food consumption can lead to worsening of the problem of under-nutrition, which, in turn, can increase TB incidents. Bhargava and Shewade (2020) estimated that COVID-19 would heighten the problem of under-nutrition among the poor in India and could result in an additional 185 610 cases of TB. The double burden of TB infection and COVID-19 pandemic led to the loss of job and earnings for working patients, especially the vulnerable population who include women and migrants. The interconnectedness of TB and poverty has been a matter of concern in the NTEP programme in India, realizing the huge share of the population below poverty and the possibility that TB could push families further into poverty and increase the vulnerability to other diseases. For instance, under the programme a patient is given Rs. 500/- per month as nutritional allowance. However, such remedial measures were found to be inadequate in the event of pandemics such as COVID-19, which led to a loss of employment and earnings for workers engaged in informal arrangements. We note that the economic implications of TB on patient and family are long-lasting and should be approached more comprehensively, especially for more vulnerable families wherein the patient is a woman and sole earner.

Unmet Needs of Patients at Multiple Intersections

It is already brought out by studies that several structural, systemic, social, economic and cultural reasons, including lack of knowledge of the patients, constraints related to family life, constraints as part of work status and religious practices, were found to have interacted with the compliance of DOTS regimen (Bagchi et al., 2010; Deshmukh et al., 2018; Talukdar et al., 2015). We found several unmet needs pertaining to balancing of work, life and treatment related to women TB patients who work in informal arrangements. Married female patients reported unmet needs related to managing household works and balancing or retaining relationships subsequent to TB diagnosis and treatment. There were families which inflicted stigma on the patients and subsequently sent the patient out to natal families; families that behaved indifferently with the patient; families which were sympathetic but helpless and a very few families which were concerned and helpful to the patients. Except for the last category, TB infection did not change family's expectation of women patients performing gender roles such as cooking, cleaning, preparing children for schools, care of elderly and small children and special care for husbands in addition to the financial contribution that they make to the family by working. Patients in such families continued these routine household works that they had been doing irrespective of their fatigue, exhaustion and increased physical burden due to wage work, disease and intake of drugs. In some cases, patients also skipped food due to workload and lack of time, although they were required to follow special dietary practices as part of the treatment regimen.

Further, we found that except a few, most of the significant others were neither responsive nor sensitive to the physical exhaustion that the patients faced during the symptomatic and treatment phase. For instance, several significant others of patients believed that working while undergoing TB treatment may not add to the fatigue of the patients. Like other studies have pointed out (Mukhopadhyay and Roy this volume) the married patients faced more violence from spouses and in-laws during the lockdown period. It should also be noted that while some of the family members acknowledged the increased fatigue of the patients, they were left with no option other than forcing/letting the patient work as the said patients were the major wage earners.

Another significant sphere of conflict was the workplace, especially the informal work environments.

The common response that emerged from our interactions with the patients was that the employment and working conditions were hostile and not encouraging for TB patients in several ways. The first issue is related to the unfavourable physical conditions of work in the informal work arrangements. The other major concern is the precariousness associated with informal work, especially pertaining to intensification of work. While such unfavourable conditions at the workplace can adversely affect the health of even the healthy worker, it increases the exhaustion of TB patients. Finally, there was no medical assistant or support provided to TB patients in informal work arrangements. Patients felt that there should be a more conducive environment at the workplace so that they can work and follow their treatment without fear. They felt that they may be given flexible working hours, paid leave, work breaks and time for rest and most importantly, they should not be stigmatized.

Modalities of the DOTS regimen also created conflicts for working female patients in their ability to balance work, life and treatment. Timings of DOT centres, regimen, side effects and requirement of follow up investigations tended to conflict with the work timings of patients. Such conflicts ultimately led to non-supervised treatment or violation of DOTS protocol with irregular DOTS visits, lack of follow up examinations and improper intake of medication. Working women patients felt that the health providers should be considerate about their conflicts and provide support in managing the spheres of work, life and treatment. They suggested flexible timings, especially the availability of health personnel and medicine during lunch breaks and evenings after work hours and supply of medicine for a longer duration.

Slowing Down of Frontline TB Interventions

There is already evidence that under-detection during COVID-19 lockdown increased TB mortality in India. Bhargava and Shewade (2020) estimated that TB mortality, attributable to under-detection, could be as high as 87,711 in 2020. Our findings showed that lockdown and subsequent restrictions, as well as the additional burden on the already stressed health service delivery system at the ground level due to COVID-19 response, disrupted the frontline activities of the TB elimination programme. It should be viewed in the context that there are already several factors that contribute to delay in TB diagnosis among the poor socio-economic sections of the population in India. For instance, the perception of the patient regarding symptoms, as being normal or not as serious, was one of the major socio-cultural reasons for the delay that these studies identified (Mistry et al., 2017). Late diagnosis, which is attributed to both patients and providers, was another reason for the delay in initiation of treatment (Mistry et al., 2017). While a set of studies identified that lack of proper knowledge and awareness led to delayed diagnosis of TB of people from poor socio-economic background (Chakravarty et al., 2019; Purohit et al., 2019), studies in other settings noted that TB knowledge did not correlate with treatment delays (Ness et al., 2017). Studies also illustrated the gender related reasons for delay in TB diagnosis that included lower intra-household spending for women's health, social stigma, fear of labelling and family responsibilities which led poor women in India to prioritize their health and they tended to resort to home remedies and non-formal healers (Das et al., 2018; Jayakumar et al., 2019).

Our interviews with working female patients showed that structural and systemic issues pertaining to family, work and access to health services delay TB diagnosis and adversely affect the adherence to treatment regimen, which are discussed earlier in the chapter. The COVID-19 pandemic situation has particularly exacerbated the systemic issues of health care delivery with the deployment of frontline TB health

workers for COVID-19 management, restricting the access to OPD, IPD and laboratory facilities for non-COVID-19 patients and return of migrant patients who were
untraceable for follow up medication. The short-term remedial measures such as
minimizing DOTS visits and issuance of drugs for longer duration tended to back-
lash, especially among new patients and vulnerable sections. Virtual follow up of the
patients through mobile phones was also not successful, especially among migrant
patients. All these factors resulted in lowering of ACF, reduced follow up of sputum
examination, reduced initiation of chemical prophylaxis, higher odds of defaulting,
irregular intake of drugs and reduced counselling of TB patients with comorbidities.
Another systemic weakness was related to the organization of frontline TB interventions. TBHVs and the Accredited Social Health Activists (ASHA), who are at the
war front of the programme, are temporary staff without any social security entitlements. Additional tasks assigned to them as part of the COVID-19 management
interventions are reported to have increased their work significantly, worsened their
conditions of work and most importantly hampered the regular DOTS programme.
It is, hence, important to ensure that the nature of work is formalised, conditions of
work are decent and tasks are limited and defined for the TB frontline interventions.

Conclusion

The COVID-19 pandemic brought about several operational barriers to NTEP in
realising its goal of elimination of tuberculosis in India by 2025. Although the TB
elimination programme in the country is strong, several challenges continue to exist.
These are related to early detection, completion of treatment regimen, managing of
multi drug resistant (MDR) and extremely drug resistant (XDR) TB, supporting of
vulnerable population and management of comorbidity. Inadequate attention to these
issues can hold up the goal of elimination of TB. Our study shows that pandemics
such as the present one has the potential to adversely affect active case finding,
early diagnosis and adherence to treatment regimen and follow up of vulnerable
groups including poor, migrants and women due to the systemic problems related
to the organization of the health programmes at the ground level and the structural
problems of the society and economy. We found that almost all frontline interventions
of NTEP got halted during lockdown. Similarly, patients and their family members
from vulnerable groups of population fell back into the spiral of poverty and under-
nutrition since they lost work and earnings. This could increase the risk of poor
treatment outcomes, recurrence of the disease and drug resistance for the patients
on the one hand and increase in disease incidence on the other. Although the NTEP
programme flexibilized the DOTS regimen in order to cope with the present crisis,
the outcomes are yet unknown. Since follow up of patients is done largely through
phone calls, TBHVs were unable to confirm regular medication of patients. Side
effects of medication for new patients and follow up of MDR/XDR patients and TB
patients with HIV are other major constraints that the health workers are facing at

the ground level. Most importantly, the deployment of NTEP staff to COVID-19 response can significantly weaken the programme.

To sum up, the COVID-19 pandemic has exposed the weaknesses of Indian health delivery system that fell short of health personnel and physical infrastructure, especially doctors, nursing staff, hospital beds, medical supplies and equipment. Hence, there is a need for a major restructuring of the system with equitable distribution of public health infrastructure and a dedicated public health cadre to respond effectively to the crisis such as the present one without hampering other equally prioritized public health interventions. It is also equally important to prevent the falling back of vulnerable groups of patients into poverty during such eventualities by appropriate social assistance programmes.

Acknowledgements Part of the data used in this chapter was extracted from a study titled 'Tuberculosis and the Social Construction of Women's Employability: A Study of Women with History/Symptoms of Tuberculosis in Bangalore City', funded by the Indian Council of Medical Research (ICMR), New Delhi. Usual disclaimers apply.

References

Acharya, S. S. (2010). Caste and patterns of discrimination in rural public health care services. In S. K. Thorat & K. Newman (Eds.), *Blocked by caste: economic discrimination in Modern India* (pp. 208–229). Oxford University Press.

Bagchi, S., Ambe, G., & Sathiakumar, N. (2010). Determinants of poor adherence to anti-tuberculosis treatment in Mumbai, India. *International Journal of Preventive Medicine, 1*(4), 223–232.

Behera, D. (2021). TB control in India in the COVID-19 era. *The Indian Journal of Tuberculosis, 68*(1), 128–133. https://doi.org/10.1016/j.ijtb.2020.08.019

Bhargava, A., & Shewade, H. D. (2020). The potential impact of the COVID-19 response related lockdown on TB incidence and mortality in India. *Indian Journal of Tuberculosis, 67*(4), 139–146. https://doi.org/10.1016/j.ijtb.2020.07.004

Bhatia, R., & Abraham, P. (2020). Lessons learnt during the first 100 days of COVID-19 pandemic in India. *Indian Journal of Medical Research, 151*(5), 387–391.

Borooah, V. K., Sabharwal, N.S., & Thorat, S. K. (2012). *Gender and caste based inequality in health outcomes in India*, Working Paper Series. 6(3), Indian Institute of Dalit Studies

Chakravarty, A., Rangan, S., Dholakia, Y., Rai, S., Kamble, S., Raste, T., Mistry, N. (2019). Such a long journey: What health seeking pathways of patients with drug resistant tuberculosis in Mumbai tell us. *PLOS One, 14*(1), 1–25.

Chetterje, P. (2020). Gaps in India's preparedness for COVID-19 control. *The Lancet Infectious Diseases, 20*(5), 544. https://doi.org/10.1016/S1473-3099(20)30300-5

Das, B. M., Kapoor, S., & Nikitin, D. (2010). *A closer look at child mortality among ain India, policy research*, Working Paper No 5231, The World Bank South Asia Region. https://doi.org/10.1596/1813-9450-5231.

Das, M., Angeli, F., Krumeich, A., & van Schayck, O. (2018). The gendered experience with respect to health-seeking behaviour in an urban slum of Kolkata, India. *International Journal for Equity in Health, 17*(1), 24. https://doi.org/10.1186/s12939-018-0738-8

Deshmukh, R. D., Dhande, D. J., Sachdeva, K. S., Sreenivas, A. N., Kumar, A. M., & Parmar, M. (2018). Social support a key factor for adherence to multidrug-resistant tuberculosis treatment. *Indian Journal of Tuberculosis, 65*(1), 41–47. https://doi.org/10.1016/j.ijtb.2017.05.003

George, S. (2019). Reconciliations of caste and medical power in rural public health services. *Economic and Political Weekly, 54*(40), 43–50.

George, S. (2016). Health for not All: Mapping the discriminated and detached terrains of health services in rural India. *Journal of Health System, 1*(1), 20–27.

Glaziou, P. (2020). Predicted impact of the COVID-19–19 pandemic on global tuberculosis deaths in 2020. *MedRxiv.* Retrieved September 17, 2020, from https://www.medrxiv.org/content/10.1101/2020.04.28.20079582v1.full.pdf.

Grange, J., & Zumla, A. (1999). Tuberculosis and the poverty-disease cycle. *Journal of the Royal Society of Medicine, 92*(3), 105–107. https://doi.org/10.1177/014107689909200301

Hazarika, I. (2013). Health workforce in India: Assessment of availability, production and distribution. *WHO South-East Asia Journal of Public Health, 2*(2), 106–112. https://doi.org/10.4103/2224-3151.122944

Jayakumar, B., Murthy, N., Misra, K., Burza, S. (2019) "It's just a fever": Gender based barriers to care-seeking for visceral leishmaniasis in highly endemic districts of India: A qualitative study. *PLOS Neglected Tropical Diseases, 13*(6). https://doi.org/10.1371/journal.pntd.0007457.

Jaysawal, N. (2015). Rural health system in India: A review. *International Journal of Social Work and Human Services Practice, 3*(1), 29–37.

Killewo, J. (2002). Poverty, TB, and HIV Infection: A vicious cycle. *Journal of Health Population and Nutrition, 20*(4), 281–284.

Kumar, S., & Reddy, D. C. S. (2020). Response to COVID-19 pandemic in India: How can we strengthen our response? *Indian Journal of Community Medicine, 45*(3), 251–255.

Mistry, N., Lobo, E., Shah, S., Rangan, S., & Dholakia, Y. (2017). Pulmonary tuberculosis in Patna, India: Durations, delays, and health care seeking behaviour among patients identified through household surveys. *Journal of Epidemiology and Global Health, 7*(4), 241–248. https://doi.org/10.1016/j.jegh.2017.08.001

Motkuri, V., Vardhan, T. S., & Ahmad, S. (2017). Quantity and quality of human resources in health care: Shortage of health workers in India. Retrieved August 15, 2020, from https://mpra.ub.uni-muenchen.de/84332/1/MPRA_paper_84332.pdf.

Ness, S., Chandra, A., Sarkar, S., Pleskunas, J., Ellner, J. J., Roy, G., & Hochberg, N. S. (2017). Predictors of delayed care seeking for tuberculosis in Southern India: An observational study. *BMC Infectious Diseases, 17*(1), 567. https://doi.org/10.1186/s12879-017-2629-9.

Potnuru, B. (2017). Aggregate availability of doctors in India: 2014–2030. *Indian Journal of Public Health, 61*(3), 182–187.

Purohit, R. M., Purohit, R., & Mustafa, T. (2019). Patient health seeking and diagnostic delay in extrapulmonary tuberculosis: A hospital based study from Central India. *Tuberculosis Research and Treatment, 2019,* 1–8. https://doi.org/10.1155/2019/4840561

Saalim, M.P.K. (2020). *Public healthcare infrastructure in tribal India: A critical review*, ISEC Working Paper No. 477, Institute for Social and Economic Change.

Saikia, D. (2018). Nursing shortages in the rural public health sector of India. *Journal of Population and Social Studies, 26*(2), 101–118.

Singh, P., Ravi, S., & Chakraborty, S (2020). COVID-19: Is India's health infrastructure equipped to handle an epidemic? Retrieved November 7, 2020, from https://www.brookings.edu/blog/up-front/2020/03/24/is-indias-health-infrastructure-equipped-to-handle-an-epidemic/.

Talukdar, N., Basu, A., & Punekar, R. M. (2015). An ethnographic study on the factors affecting adherence to directly observed treatment short-course in typical Indian settings. *Journal of Tuberculosis Research, 3*(01), 19–25. https://doi.org/10.4236/jtr.2015.31003

Chapter 12
Lone Warriors in the COVID-19 Lockdown: Impediments and Resilience of Women in Allahabad District, India

Firdaus Fatima Rizvi

Abstract The 'New Economic Theory of Migration' incorporates the social dimension in the decision to migrate. The decision is often taken collectively, especially within households. Migration of selected family members is used to mitigate risks by providing remittance to support their families at home. However, due to sudden lockdown in the pandemics, the household's economies came to standstill and the remittance that was once sent to households stopped. Workers in the informal sector lost their jobs, whether self-employed or regular salaried. During the lockdown (in the absence of male members), women are additionally burdened with managing rations for their family, looking after children's education and dealing with other social issues. Many households faced sudden cessation of children's schooling, family's survival depended upon the public distribution system, they had no rents to pay, borrowed goods from general shops/vegetable/meat/milk vendors and thus had huge debt. The financial crisis of households worsened with the increase in lockdown period; while the migrant workers still left at bay with no monetary support. This paper takes up issues and challenges faced by women; specifically, in a woman-headed household struggling to mitigate the COVID19 predicaments. Finally, it provides policy implications for the social inclusion of women in development planning.

Keywords Migration · Lockdown · Remittances · Children · Education

Introduction

In early December 2019, the news flashed on national television showing coronavirus spread in China. It was just casual news for the people staying in other parts of the world. None would have imagined that this endemic would turn into an epidemic. Shortly, the disease spread across the globe and the media started referring to this

F. F. Rizvi (✉)
Department of Development Studies, School of Social Sciences and Policy, Central University of South Bihar, Gaya, India

© The Author(s), under exclusive license to Springer Nature Singapore Pte Ltd. 2022   233
S. S. Acharya and S. Christopher (eds.), *Caste, COVID-19, and Inequalities of Care*,
People, Cultures and Societies: Exploring and Documenting Diversities,
https://doi.org/10.1007/978-981-16-6917-0_12

disease as a 'global pandemic'. The term was new to this generation, however, people adapted to this new vocabulary later.

A Pandemic is the worldwide spread of a new disease. An influenza pandemic occurs when a new influenza virus emerges and spreads around the world, and most people do not have immunity. The viruses that have caused past pandemics typically originated from animal influenza viruses (WHO).

The first case of COVID-19 was reported in India by the end of January 2020. As the cases increased gradually and the fear grew, the Prime Minister of India addressed the nation and asked people to follow social distancing and avoid going out of the house to check the spread of coronavirus. One day voluntary *Janta (Public) Curfew* was announced for 22nd March 2020 from 7 am to 9 pm, cautioning people against any complacency in dealing with COVID-19. He said, it is a curfew for the people and imposed by the people themselves. This was the beginning of a long battle.

Soon after this, the Government of India announced the first phase of nationwide lockdown from 25 March 2020 to 14th April 2020 without analysing the consequences of lockdown on society. It was an abrupt and blunt call. By the end of the first phase of lockdown, the government extended the lockdown period with a recommendation from state governments and the advisory committees. The second phase of lockdown started from 15th April to 3rd May 2020 and the third phase from 4th May to 17th May 2020. Further to tackle the COVID-19 disease more efficiently, the government demarcated affected areas into three containment zones i.e. Green, Red and Orange based on the severity of the disease. Later when the number of corona cases reduced, services were resumed all over India in a phased manner in the name of Unlock-1 to Unlock-6 starting from 8th June onwards.

Due to a sudden lockdown announcement on 24th March 2020, the migrant workers got trapped in host cities with no work or food. The remittance that was once reaching their families at home was unexpectedly stopped. The Indian Economy was on halt and this directly led to cessation of many households' economic activities. The social distancing norms during the pandemic acted as a catalyst in increasing the inequalities among the households. The support from the distanced relatives also was not possible during these days.

Railways, air flights, road-ways, educational institutions, markets and even many health institutions were closed during the lockdown. The unexpected decision by the government for a lockdown had many repercussions on women-headed households where male members have migrated or where no male member was present in the households.

Roadmap

This study provides a brief literature through some newspapers, reports and websites publishing articles on pandemic issues. The study looks into some theoretical framework fitting with the current economic and social issues faced by the community followed by research methodology. The study supports its findings with the help of case studies in detail, followed by analysis and discussion. The study concludes with policy interventions required by the state and other supporting agencies.

Literature Review

The Centre for Monitoring Indian Economy (CMIE) conducted a survey of Indian households during April 18–30, 2020 and revealed that the economic impact of the lockdown was not equally distributed across people and places. Significantly, 14% of the sample were already out of economic resources and would be in severe deprivation if they are not able to borrow or receive additional benefits. According to a survey conducted in June 2020 across India, 34% of households confessed that they will not be able to survive for more than one week without additional assistance. About 84 per cent of Indian households have seen a decrease in income since the lockdown began. The economic distress in India caused by the lockdown is dire. (Wharton UoP, 2020). Direct and immediate transfer of food and cash is of high priority. The study found that the fall in income affected people mostly in the lower and middle segments of the income distribution.

According to a study conducted by the National Council of Applied Economic Research, Delhi and Nossal Institute for Global Health, University of Melbourne in Uttar Pradesh and Odisha during June 2020, 79% households reported a fall in income and 29% were left with no source of income. The households are dwindling between incomes and emerging supply shortages. They adopted different strategies to meet expenditure on essential items. About 53% confessed to receiving government assistance and 41% borrowed money. In addition to this, 20% households even reduced consumption expenditure on household essentials (Ghosh, & Kumar, 2020).

The Census Bureau's Household Pulse Survey conducted in America, launched in April 2020, provided real-time weekly data on how the unprecedented health and economic crisis is affecting the nation. It provided data on the overall number of adults struggling to cover usual household expenses such as food, rent or mortgage, car payments, medical expenses or student loans. Around 35% of all adults reported it was somewhat challenging for their households to cover usual expenses. Data from this and other sources, such as unemployment data from the Census' Current Population Survey and the Department of Labour, show that tens of millions of people are out of work and struggling to afford adequate food and pay the rent in America.

Data from several sources show a dramatic increase in the number of households struggling to put sufficient food on the table. According to Household Pulse Survey data collected on March 17–29, 2021, some 18 million adults (9% of all adults) in the country reported that their household sometimes or often did not have sufficient food in the last seven days. This was far above the pre-pandemic rate that was 3.4% of adults reporting that their household had 'not enough to eat' at some point over the last 12 months of 2019 (Jansen et al, 2020). When asked about the reason, they said that they could not afford to buy more food, besides some non-financial factors like lack of transportation or safety concerns due to the pandemics. Black, Latino and other non-American adults were more than twice as likely as white adults to report that their households did not have sufficient food (Centre on Budget and Policy Priorities, 2021). About 20% of renters were unable to pay rents during the pandemics, with renters of colour facing greatest hardship. Children in renters' households also face high rates of food hardship.

In developing Asia, around three-fourths of the countries had negative growth in the year 2020. India reported an economic downturn of nine per cent in the same year (Rooks, 2020). Global remittance has also fallen. There was a sharp decrease in expenses and outflows during April and May 2020 following the lockdown. The World Bank also predicted further decline of remittance because of high global unemployment among migrants and the economic catastrophe (Prange, 2020).

According to *India Covid-19 Survey* conducted by 'Save the Children' foundation, 84% of urban households lack livelihood opportunities compared to 64% of households in rural areas. About 50% of households lack sufficient food supplies, a quarter of households reported having no family income whatsoever and little less than half of the households resorted to credit/loans to meet daily expenses. Eight in ten households are struggling to meet their daily expenses. Worst happened, 40% of the household children did not receive support from school to study at home.

Furthermore, there has been an exponential increase in unpaid care work with the closing of schools and additional care needs of family members at home. In a study by CARE, women were almost three times as likely as men to suffer from anxiety, worry and emotional fatigue from the coronavirus pandemic. When schools were closed and children were left with an online mode of learning, the burden was disproportionately on women to keep them focused and check their assignments. Women were also more subjected to economic stresses (Kluger, 2020).

Because pandemics rarely happen, there is less literature available on the current social and economic problems. This study tries to explore some of the economic and social issues that a single woman faced during the lockdown in the pandemics. This knowledge can also help policymakers to develop much-needed interventions at community, household and individual level.

Theoretical Perspective

For the vast majority of the world's poor whose labour is their primary asset, migration offers one of the best opportunities to escape unemployment and poverty. For the many poor whose labour is their only asset, migration to a richer country offers an opportunity to escape poverty. The poorest of the poor, however, tend to migrate internally, as they are unable to afford the costs associated with moving abroad (Borjas, 1987). Migration can reduce unemployment and underemployment and facilitate access to more-productive and higher-paying jobs. Large-scale emigration can raise employment and wages in origin countries (Dustmann et al., 2015). But sudden cessation of employment may reduce/eliminate parent's wages that will have immediate effects on food intake and health outcomes of children (Ravindranath, & Daniel, 2020; Yadav, 2020).

The new economic theory of migration incorporates the societal dimension in the decision to migrate. The migration decision is often taken collectively, especially within households. Migration of selected family members mitigates risks by providing remittance to support their families at home. However, a common pattern seen in men migrating in developing countries is that they leave their wives and children at home while they migrate in search of work (Kanaiaupuni, 2000). A study suggests that the migration of men typically involves increasing responsibilities of their wives and attaining more skills in household tasks not usually undertaken by women (Hondagneu-Sotelo, 1992). Women not staying with extended families have to face more responsibilities and greater autonomy when male members migrate. While women who live with extended household members do not have to experience high responsibilities or autonomy (Desai & Banerji, 2008). When an economically active family member migrates, it puts a heavier burden on those who stay behind and have to spend more time on household chores. Families which get disturbed by migrations, face poor diets and increased psychological problems (Démurger, 2015).

The lockdown rules of physical and social distancing have larger implications on women in their lives. With the high rise in unemployment and limited accessibility to social protections, they are unable to absorb the economic shocks and are at greater risk of falling into poverty. Hence, this study will analyse how women (in the absence of male members) were physically and mentally stressed during the lockdown and the impediments and resilience they faced in the COVID-19 Pandemics.

Research Methodology

The study is a descriptive research. It is a cross-sectional study conducted during the lockdown in the month of June–July 2020 in India. The study was conducted in Allahabad district of Uttar Pradesh. Only those households were selected where only women members were taking care of their families during the pandemics. Primary data was collected from the female respondents through a structured interview. Findings and analysis are qualitative in nature. This paper reflects on the impediments and resilience confronted by women with the help of case studies at household level, the analysis of which will be discussed later under different subheadings. Indicators of study include vulnerability of households in terms of income and earnings, indebtedness, food insecurity, children's education, house rent, availability of public health services, emotional and mental stress faced by women, loss of social cohesion, etc.

Findings

The research undertaken led to some interesting findings which are discussed through the following case studies. The names mentioned in the case studies are pseudonyms.

Case Study-1

SAMINA KHAN

Age: 32 years.

Occupation: Housewife.

Place: Allahabad (U.P).

Samina is a 32-year-old housewife. She was born and brought up in Jabalpur (M.P) and soon after her father's demise, her mother shifted to Delhi where her maternal uncle stayed. She got her schooling till standard VIII and at the tender age of fourteen she got married to Mohammad. Her husband is from the Fatehpur district (U.P) who migrated to Delhi in search of employment. He works with an employer in North-East Delhi who is in the retail business of school uniforms and bags. Basically, Mohammad is a tailor by job. They had three children, Fiza (daughter) aged 17, Arif (son) aged 15 and Ginnu (daughter) aged 5.

About five years ago, Mohammad sent his family to Allahabad (nearest to his native place) and he himself stayed back at Delhi for livelihood generation. Hence, Samina shifted to Allahabad with her new born daughter and her two elder children in a rented house. Since then, the whole household responsibility was laid on her from managing rations, children's schooling, family health, etc.

Samina's husband was the only earning member of the household who got stuck at Delhi during the lockdown phase. As the schools in Delhi closed, the uniform business was indirectly affected. Hence his employer's business was also closed down. There was no job for him. Mohammad was locked in a house for four months. There was nothing for him to cook and eat. Even the local hotels in the vicinity were also closed on which he was totally dependent. Knowing the circumstances of her husband, Samina felt mentally sick. Spouses were providing strength to each other via phone calls all through the day.

During this period of economic crisis, Samina was over burdened with household responsibilities; with no money left to survive in a complete lockdown situation. The family depended upon the Public Distribution System (PDS) for food grains, a programme supported by Government of India (GoI) for the people below poverty line (BPL). Under the Antyodaya Anna Yojana (AAY) scheme, she used to get 30 kg of grains including rice and wheat per month at a subsidised rate (rice for Rs. 3 per kg and wheat for Rs. 2 per kg). She also benefited through free distribution of rations run by GoI for all poor (irrespective of BPL cards) during the COVID-19 lockdown each month. Nonetheless, availability of food grains is not the only thing for a family to survive. As to maintain the day-to-day requirements, she used to exchange the surplus PDS rice in lieu of money from a local General Merchant. However, she took vegetables, milk, meat and other groceries on credit from General Stores and local vendors in the lockdown period and thus had huge debt on her till date.

She felt helpless whenever cash was immediately required for buying cooking gas and other important necessities that was not possible through burrowing. Owner of the house and her family were a little generous towards her during the critical phase. They were helping her at times of such urgencies. As the auspicious month of Ramadan (according to Islamic calendar) fell during the initial phase of lockdown, many people came forward to help by providing food and other items during the fasting season (Begum, this volume).

Samina's daughter passed class VIII and her son passed class VII in March 2020. Managing school fees was really tough for her as in the new academic session (that begins in April), the fees are comparatively high against the rest of the year. The messages from school kept pouring in on her mobile to submit Rs. 10,000 and Rs. 8000 as tuition fees of her daughter and son, respectively. However, the online class started before the school fees were submitted. The class teachers continuously called parents over the phone to pay the school fees and they warned that if the fees were not paid by April end, they would drop the name of the student from the school register. Samina tried to convince the teachers that she herself is not in a position to afford food for her family, then how come she will be able to pay the school fees. The requests made to the class teachers were ineffective. The teachers were compelled by the school administrators to force students to pay fees without which their monthly salary is not possible. Samina went twice or thrice to meet the school principal but in vain. The office staff always made some or the other excuses and she had to return back without justifying her needfulness. She never had an opportunity to meet the school principal.

Being unable to pay the fees, Fiza's name was dropped from online classes by April end while Arif studies continued. Both the class teachers of Fiza and Arif behaved differently. The family was also burdened with an extra expenditure on recharging internet data for two different mobile phones that cost around Rs. 800 per month for children to continue their online classes.

The health issues also added fuel to the fire in the economic crisis. Samina had stones in kidney and was suffering for a long time. The problem aggravated more during the COVID-19 lockdown. Visiting the doctor was also riskier during the period as there were high chances of contacting corona. In between this phase, her children also suffered mild fever and other minor diseases.

When there was slight relaxation during the lockdown period in June, her husband managed to reach Allahabad with the help of some distant relatives. It provided some mental strength to the family in the catastrophe. By the month of July 2020, the family was unable to pay five months' rent to the owner of the house. The unpaid rent increased to Rs. 22,000. Besides this, they were indebted to many vendors and shopkeepers. The worst happened when the schools asked for another set of fees for the month of July to September including the previous dues. Unable to pay the school fees and thinking that debt will increase while staying here, the family decided to return to their native place Fatehpur; with a promise to pay back the money they owe to the owner of the house in future. No way out to escape poverty, the family left Allahabad in July 2020 and hence it was a case of reverse migration for a family of five.

Case Study-2

FARHA QASIM

Age- 43.

Occupation- Housewife.

Place- Allahabad (U.P).

Farha is a 43-year-old housewife. She was born and brought up in Allahabad city. She is a Bachelor in Arts. Seventeen years back, she got married to Ishaq who belonged to a rural village of the same district. During the initial years of marriage, her husband worked in Mumbai and later he migrated to Jordan for work. He works in a retail tailoring business as a 'Cutter'. They have two sons Sunny and Sonu aged 14 and 9.

Ishaq has a story that goes back before the corona pandemics. Ishaq last visited India in 2017 for two months. It is the condition of his job that he will be allowed to visit his home every two years and the travel cost is to be borne by his employer. However, after more than three years of his stay in Jordan, his employer did not allow him to visit India. He even kept his passport with him. After being far away from his family for so long, Ishaq resigned from his job in February 2020. His employer cancelled his visa and delayed booking his tickets. Amid this, the COVID-19 pandemic happened. International flights were closed and economies were shut. Ishaq was locked at home in Jordan.

Ishaq received his last salary in the month of February just before the lockdown. This salary got exhausted by spending on the younger son's admission. Ishaq got his remaining dues of Rs. 30,000 by his employer in April 2020. This was the total monetary reserves that Farha had during the initial COVID-19 lockdown, of which one-third was spent on her elder son's school fees and the remaining was given to the house owner for already pending two months (April and May) house rents.

Now it was a complete financial crunch for Farha. She was incapable of managing food and other household items for the family. Being from a middle-class family, she does not hold BPL card; hence she didn't benefit from government food programmes and she also shy away from receiving any help from other local charities. Knowing the helplessness, Farha's sister stood by her and provided food and other household requirements. However, when the financial crisis continued, her mother (who stays nearby) called her and her children to stay with her.

Her husband is still in Jordan. His ex-employer only provides food once in the day time and for the rest of the day he has to manage his food himself. Till date, his employer has not booked his return ticket to India nor allows him to work elsewhere (till the time of interview).

Farha's mother also helped her in providing two months (June–July) pending house rent. Farha is back to her rented house in October 2020, with not much change in her situation. As of now, four months' rent is still pending on Farha. Her younger brother who works in Oman is helping her these days. She has not paid the tuition fees of her children for the last three months (July to September) and her economic crisis continued.

Case Study-3

NORAH KHAN

Age: 30.

Occupation: School Teacher.

Place: Allahabad (U.P).

Norah is a 30-year-old single woman. She is a native of Allahabad. She lost her mother ten years back and her father almost two years back. No properties were left by her parents except a small house in which she lives. Being a senior, she has to take care of her younger sister aged 25. Norah is a Bachelor in Computer Applications (B.CA) and has an education degree as well. She works in a private school situated about 45 kms away from the city. Her salary is Rs. 12,000 per month, but during her father's illness, she borrowed a huge amount of money from her school administration, hence she was getting around Rs. 6000 in hand after all the deductions. Her sister Sarah is also a primary school teacher in the nearby private school and was earning a meagre amount of Rs. 3000 per month. Her sister somehow manages additional earnings by giving tuition at home.

During the COVID-19 lockdown, schools were shut and tuition was closed. Both the sisters were taking classes in online mode during this period. Classes continued irrespective of parent's inability to pay fees of their wards. Parents themselves were helpless to pay school fees (very much clear from the above-mentioned case studies). As schools were not generating income, they were unable to pay salaries to their employees as money did not float from one sector to another in the economy.

It was good that Norah stored ration and other basic necessities for the approaching two months just before the commencement of the lockdown. Norah's employer did not provide salary for the first three months of the lockdown. After teachers compelled parents to submit their ward's fees, little income was generated by the schools after two months. Hence, in the month of June, Norah received one-third of her April's salary. However, her younger sister did not receive any wages instead of work performed. Therefore, it was a hand-to-mouth situation for the family when her food reserves finished.

During the Corona pandemics, Norah's younger sister's health also deteriorated with liver infection increasing the burden on her. Public health facilities were not available during that period so she had to consult a doctor running his own private clinic (Begum, this volume). Every fortnight, she had to spend Rs. 2000–3000 on medical expenses. According to the doctor, her sister's health requires medication for the next six months. Managing this was arduous for her. She had to borrow money from her distant relatives for the same. Till now, Norah is getting only one-third of her salary each month and her sister earned nothing hence the economic crisis continues. There was no support from the running government programmes as the family didn't own any BPL card and they even shy off from availing food and other charities sponsored by the community because of their self-esteem and dignity in society.

Case Analysis and Discussion

Analysing the three case studies, we derive to certain impediments and resilient faced by the women during the pandemic lockdown under the following points.

Burden of All Responsibilities of Household and Non-Household Chores

As the economic theory of migration says that it is the joint decision of a family for a male to migrate for employment purposes and earn livelihood, henceforth in these cases women have to face all the responsibilities of household and non-household chores. Here, the first two cases augment the theory that women were the sole sufferers of COVID-19 lockdown when the males left for job. In all the three cases, women had to face huge impediments for managing their families alone (George et al., this volume).

Loss of Purchasing Power Parity and Difficulty Getting Enough Food

The cases clearly show that women face a significant financial crunch during the pandemic. They lost the purchasing power parity to buy things that range from food to non-food items. In the cases referred above, only in the first case, the family was supported by an existing public food programme during the food crisis and the other two families were out of food soon after two months of lockdown. Only households under BPL were somewhat food secured either by the PDS programme or through community charity. However, food insecurity (inequality) rose among the households who were above the BPL category. They had no government supported food programme nor they received charity from local community and other organizations because of self-esteem.

Inability to Afford Children's Fees and Online Education

Previous literature suggested that the fall in income severely affects people who are in the lower and middle class hence these households dwindle over income and emerging supplies. In the first two cases mentioned, the women were struggling to cover usual household expenses such as food, medical expenses and children's school fees. During the online classes, families were loaded with extra expenses for recharging data for mobile phones for each school going children. Worst of all, neither children received any sort of fee concessions from schools nor any support from the government to study at home. Even the school Administration/Principal denied meeting parents regarding fee issues. Rather, there was continuous harassment by the class teachers to pay ward's fees and hence children's names were deleted from school registers for not paying the fees.

Inability to Pay Rent and High Indebtedness

India Covid-19 Survey and many other reports suggested that people were out of work and were struggling to afford adequate food thus many households resorted to credit/loans to meet their daily expenses. They were struggling with daily expenses therefore paying the house rents was probably an impossible thing. Similar conditions were found true in the first two cases mentioned above. As already overburdened, women were unable to pay the house rents. Even now, around five to six months of house rents are still pending.

Failed Public Health System

During the COVID-19 lockdown, all public hospitals were closed in Allahabad excluding Swaroop Rani Hospital that was admitting only level three (L3) and level four (L4) degree of corona patients. A few camps were formed in the outskirts of the city where level one (L1) and level two (L2) degree coronavirus patients were admitted. Even in Swaroop Rani Hospital, the Outpatient Department (OPD) was closed during the lockdown. Besides this, private hospitals and clinics were also closed except few. The burden of health was totally laid on the poor people in the absence of a public health system (George et al., this volume). In above cases also, women confronted health issues of their family members including self in the absence of public health facilities when they had no earnings but had to pay for the treatment in private hospitals.

Loss of Social Cohesions

Neighbours and relatives are the real support system for individuals or families during any exigencies; perhaps when one is going through an economic, health and other crisis. The physical and social distancing norms in the lockdown broke this system as well. In the first case referred above, many distant relatives of the woman were present in town but were unable to help; forget about financial support, they were not even there for emotional and mental support. Whereas in the second case study, the women got economic and social support from her family members that stayed nearby. In the third case, the women were isolated with no help from the government or from distant relatives.

Conclusion

The decision of members to migrate for livelihood purposes is taken collectively within households according to the new economic theory of migration. But this theory does not take into account the consequences of sudden cessation of employment of these migrant workers leading to immediate impact on food intake and health outcomes on their families (Ravindranath, & Daniel, 2020; Yadav, 2020). During the lockdown, women are facing great difficulties as they bear the burden of household responsibilities. Single parents or female headed households face difficulty in supporting themselves and their families (Mathews, 2020). All the responsibility of household and non-household chores, taking care of economic, social (health and education) and other issues has made the single women most vulnerable during the lockdown.

Policy Implications

Many public funded programmes are specifically implemented for the people below poverty line (BPL); nonetheless no programmes are there for the families who are above poverty line (APL) and have higher chances of slipping down under poverty at times of calamities and economic depressions. It is clear from the case studies that most of the provisions of food were made for the BPL card holders during the lockdown period, however, no provisions were made for households who were devoid of earnings for the same period. The government should come up with certain programmes for the families who are insecure during exigencies such as pandemics/natural disaster/economic depression, etc.irrespective of their class category.

Apart from the food security programmes, some programmes need to be implemented for households who lose jobs during exigencies. The government should provide some sort of remuneration to these families as 'Unemployment Allowances' for the restricted period during catastrophes. The programme should have a 'women specific component' into it as they are the flag bearers of a household. Some norms have to be implemented for private schools to stop the harassment of students during the economic depression. Hence private schools and private clinics should also come into purview of the State at least to some extent.

Not only the role of the Indian state, but interventions by communities, NGOs and individuals are equally important to tackle issues and help families who are in dire need of economic, social and mental support. As major responsibilities are placed on women to sustain their families, households and communities during difficult times, they need to be included and represented in economic planning and policy decision-making and also during emergency response planning (Mathews, 2020). The Government needs to prevent food insecurity, malnutrition and other related issues by in-kind or cash transfer programmes. By reaching the demands of the people and promoting health, the country will recover soon from economic slowdown when reopening. Not all the public hospitals and OPDs are supposed to be closed down during the health emergencies.

References

Borjas, G. J. (1987). Self-selection and the earnings of immigrants. NBER working paper 2248. National Bureau of Economic Research.

Centre for Budget and Policy Priorities. (2021). *Tracking the covid-19 recession's effect on food, employment and employment hardship.* Retrieved March 10, 2021, from https://www.cbpp.org/research/poverty-and-inequality/tracking-the-covid-19-recessions-effects-on-food-housing-and.

Démurger, S. (2015). Migration and families left behind. *IZA World of Labour.* Retrieved December 15, 2020, from https://wol.iza.org/uploads/articles/144/pdfs/migration-and-families-left-behind.pdf?v=1.

Desai, S. & Banerji, M. (2008). Negotiated identities: Male migration and left behind wives in India. *NIH Public Access.* Retrieved December 17, 2020, from https://www.ncbi.nlm.nih.gov/pmc/articles/PMC2916725/.

Dustmann, C., T. Frattini, & A. Rosso. (2015). The effect of emigration from Poland on Polish Wages. *Scandinavian Journal of Economics, 117*(2), 522–64. Retrieved December 11, 2020, from https://onlinelibrary.wiley.com/doi/abs/10.1111/sjoe.12102.

Ghosh, P. K, & Kumar, S. (2020). Covid-19 and the resilience of our household economy. *Financial Express.* Retrieved December 15, 2020, from https://www.financialexpress.com/opinion/covid-19-and-the-resilience-of-our-household-economy/2060144/.

Hondagneu-Sotelo, P. (1992). Overcoming patriarchal constraints: The reconstruction of gender relations among Mexican immigrant women and men. *Gender and Society, 6*(3), 393–415. Retrieved May 27, 2021, from https://www.jstor.org/stable/189994?seq=1.

Jansen, A. C., Rabbit, M. P., Gregory, C. A., & Singh, A. (2020). Household food security in the United States. *USDA, economic research service.* US Department of Agriculture. ERR Number 275. September 2020.

Kanaiaupuni, S. M. (2000). Reframing the migration question: An analysis of men, women, and gender in Mexico. *Social Forces., 78*(4), 1311–1348.

Kluger, J. (2020). The corona pandemic outsized effect on women's mental health around the world. Retrieved December 27, 2020, from https://time.com/5892297/women-coronavirus-mental-health/.

Mathews, R. (2020). Covid-19: Why are women more vulnerable to mental health issues?.

Prange, A. (2020). Global poor hit as covid-19 causes drop in remittances. Retrieved December 15, 2020, from https://www.dw.com/en/global-poor-hit-as-covid-19-causes-drop-in-remittances/a-55306293.

Ravindranath, D, & Daniel, U. (2020). The wire. *Understanding the implications of the covid-19 lockdown on migrant workers' children.* Retrieved November 30, 2020, from https://thewire.in/rights/covid-19-lockdown-migrant-workers-children-implications.

Rooks, T. (2020). *Asian economies to shrink for first time in 60 years.* Retrieved November 31, 2020, from https://international.thenewslens.com/article/140619.

India Covid-19 Survey. (2020). *Eight in ten households are struggling to meet their daily expenses, warns save the children.* Survey conducted by 'Save the Children' Organisation. Retrieved November 31, 2020, from https://www.savethechildren.net/news/india-covid-19-survey-eight-ten-households-are-struggling-meet-their-daily-expenses-warns-save.

Wharton, UoP. (2020). *How the covid-19 lockdown is affecting India's household.* Wharton, University of Pennsylvania.

Yadav, Renu. (2020). Impact of covid-19 on Indian migrant workers. *Critical Edges.* Retrieved November 23, 2020, from https://criticaledges.com/2020/07/12/covid-19-on-indian-migrant-workers.

Chapter 13
COVID-19 and Violence Against Women in India

Trisha Mukhopadhyay and Sumanta Roy

Abstract Women have long been facing oppression and violence. There are various forms of violence which include domestic violence, intimate partner violence, sexual harassment, sexual abuse and sexual exploitation. The violence against women is often associated with power and dominance. With the COVID-19 pandemic there has been a sudden increase of cases being reported of violence against women. It has been seen in various studies that whether it is a pandemic or natural disaster women face additional burden. As the number of COVID-19 cases increased, the Government of India took the step of lockdown to curb the spread but there were certain social discriminations which rose in the shadow of the pandemic. Men and women have been affected indifferently during the pandemic. The pandemic led to the loss of jobs of men and women. The men vented out their stress and frustration on the women. The women who lost their jobs became more dependent on abusive partners. The lockdown phase obstructed women seeking help when facing violence. The chapter focuses on complaints received by the authorities (National Commission for Women), the state-wise variation of crimes reported against women, cases of violence against women using newspaper articles, the impact on women and strategies to help women facing violence.

Keywords Domestic violence · COVID-19 · Cybercrime against women · Strategies of help · India

T. Mukhopadhyay (✉)
Research Scholar at Centre of Social Medicine and Community Health, Jawaharlal Nehru University, New Delhi, India

Indian Institute of Public Health, New Delhi, India

S. Roy
Centre of Social Medicine and Community Health, School of Social Sciences-II, Jawaharlal Nehru University, New Delhi, India

© The Author(s), under exclusive license to Springer Nature Singapore Pte Ltd. 2022   247
S. S. Acharya and S. Christopher (eds.), *Caste, COVID-19, and Inequalities of Care*,
People, Cultures and Societies: Exploring and Documenting Diversities,
https://doi.org/10.1007/978-981-16-6917-0_13

Conceptualizing Violence

Violence is associated with power. It is determined to feel a sense of power continue as a tool of oppression. Anyone facing the threat of oppression or being forced to act in a way by another individual or group is meant to be violence. Physical violence is prevalent against women, but it can also emerge in other forms to give rise to an atmosphere of threat or revenge (Krishnaraj, 2007). There are many forms of violence against women such as sexual, emotional, physical and economic. Globally, the most common forms of violence includes domestic and intimate partner violence, sexual harassment and emotional or psychological violence sexual violence (including rape), prostitution, domestic violence and pornography, sexual abuse, sexual exploitation. The forms of violence may vary between cultures and societies, but it is universal that male violence always exceeds female violence.

Other extensive forms of violence around the globe are sexual abuse, sexual crime, trafficking practices such as female genital mutilation, forcible wedlock and child marriages. In addition, there are other types of violence carried out against women which are crimes committed in the name of honour, femicide, prenatal sex selection, female infanticide, economic abuse, political violence, elder abuse, dowry-related violence and acid throwing (Ending violence towards women and girls: programming essentials, 2014).

Walby (1990) suggested that rape and wife beating considered as individual acts, are social facts and can be best understood with the already existing patriarchal social structures. She has described violence in three theoretical approaches and critiqued other authors:

Liberalism: It discusses the violence in terms of psychological disorder of a small number of men. They focus on psychological derangement rather than the social contexts. The liberal response to state and male violence is to say that the state is little incapable and faces technological difficulties due to the nature of the crimes taking violent men to court. According to them violence against women is rather rare.

Class Analysis: It is in terms of the frustrations of men who are oppressed in a class society. As a result of the anger caused by their circumstances, men who are at the bottom of the class hierarchy are violent towards women. The violence is the result of the functioning of class cultures. There are two major models: general model where male violence against women is most prevalent in situations of economic stress, high unemployment, lack of housing, acute stress and a sub-cultural model where rape is only created as one more form of violence. Walby (1990) critiqued and argued class-based analysis of men's violence has one good point that it examines social not psychological processes but it is unable to deal with the gendered nature of this violence of why some might be more prone to violence than others.

Radical Feminism: They talk about male control in a patriarchal society. Radical feminist believes male violence is based on both its gender and its social character. They analyse social forces that cause this violence and its consequences for women's inequality. Under this approach, violence and sexuality both are believed to be socially formed.

In this scenario of forcing socially sanctioned values and practices, domestic violence is itself a part of it. A significant part of the norms is the male privilege in marriage of women's bodies. In many societies, the high incidence of violence against women within the private sphere of families being viewed normally in marriage and family life, which again represents dominance of men over women and the generally prevalent patriarchal structure. Rather than being extraordinary, in the sense of marriage and family, it is symptomatic of the sexuality of daily life as women live it. Husbands tried to control their wives by representing their social status, economic and familial power. They express masculinity in the context of marriage through sexual demands. Domestic violence is not about direct confrontation or direct assault, it can take the form of deprivation through a pattern of food distribution, wealth distribution, restricts mobility, obstructs the interests. Studies have found that, as in the case of rape, domestic violence stresses the victim with shame for her 'mistakes' in not performing her assigned duties to husband and in-laws appropriately. She has to sacrifice her own well-being to the demands of husbands and in-laws.

Early marriages are overburdened with roles and responsibilities for the young girls who get married and invite violence for not performing the responsibilities assigned to them. This can be anything from not being at home when the husband comes home, not finishing work assigned, refusing sex or quarrels with in-laws. The young girls in the marital family have the least power, least voice, no capacity to negotiate in decision-making including delaying pregnancy. Women have been the victims of patriarchal sexual practices through abuse of landlords during caste riots, in marital rape, in state reproductive policies, and of course, the battering of women (Krishnaraj, 2007).

Intersectional Determinants of Violence

In a patriarchal society like India, gender is a very important issue to be discussed. Functionalist perspective of gender is in terms of behaviour and tasks, gender division of labour is the focus. Social conflict perspective is, gender cannot be defined only in terms of behaviour and tasks, it sees in the lens of power. They say functionalists didn't see it as a power on inequality. Marxist understanding is that control of private property goes to men. Marxists track the rise of inequality between men and women. They look much more at structural factors, power and inequality. Symbolic interactionist see gender as the play out of the power in everyday lives. For example, in the Indian wedding, the widow's presence in the gathering is considered as polluted and she has not been treated equally, Nirbhaya like cases are coming in everyday life, people suffering from leprosy are treated unequally. Symbolic interactionists talk about stigma, they work on stigma extensively.

For us caste is an institution of inequality which has a role in women's lives. Different scholars gave several arguments of how caste plays an important role in

Indian society. Ghurye (1969) explained everything about the caste system: the upper castes and lower castes, he talks only about them (their lifestyle, structure of their society, forms of punishments if anyone violates the established principles). He didn't talk about the exploitative relations between them; he missed out the relation between dignity, exploitation and oppression in his explanation. On the other hand, Srinivas (1952) asked the lower caste to follow Sanskritization in order to achieve upward mobility in the society which is clearly a vague concept. As Singh (1994) critiqued by saying Sanskritization missed out cultural changes and non-Sanskritic traditions in the past and contemporary India. The researcher wants to reject both of these theories as it did not talk about the relationship between dignity, exploitation and oppression which Mencher talked about. Mencher (1974) talks about objectivity, she argued from top-down view for an upper caste the position of the lower castes is perfectly alright but caste in bottom-up approach where the structure has two striking characteristics, first as the perspective of people at the lowest end and the other is caste derives its viability from the drastic socio-economic disparities. She talks about the socio-economic and political exploitation of the lower caste and the privileges of each caste by his study on Untouchable labourers in Tamil Nadu but he missed to discuss the gender relations though.

Walby (1990) starts from the very point where Mencher didn't talk about. She has explained different concepts of feminism and power relations. Radical feminism which only talks about male domination over women (patriarchy, sexuality) as the sole reason for gender inequality which was critiqued for false universalism, Marxist feminism which says gender inequality is derived from capitalism and male domination over women is a byproduct of capital domination and power was also critiqued for reducing gender inequality to economic relations of capitalism. Liberalism which refers prejudice against women is responsible for gender inequality but the deep-rootedness of gender inequality and its interconnectedness between its various forms has not yet been acknowledged. Dual system theories which are a synthesis of both Marxist and Radical feminism which was critiqued by many as it is an impossible task to synthesize both of them. However, the researcher thinks that all the forms of feminism is responsible for not the domestic violence, as a women may be oppressed in the form of patriarchy and sexuality, where they may also be oppressed by the capital domination and power relation in their household and the place where they work, prejudice against women is always there in Indian society or it may be both.

Velaskar (2012) rightly pointed out how the notions of caste, class and patriarchy shape the health and well-being of a woman, how they are being discriminated against in accessing the basic facilities, how the patriarchy exploits labour, sexuality and fertility of women and oppresses them. She has also described how a lower caste woman always becomes a victim of patriarchy from her husband and from upper caste men. First, they were abused by their husbands in the households for not doing well/making them happy in household duties and then the upper caste men also exploited them sexually and tortured them if they did not perform well in the assigned work. Velaskar talked about these multiple layers of oppression where intersections of caste class and gender plays crucial roles. For example, a women sanitation worker face multiple forms of discrimination, first for her position as a woman in society, second as a Dalit woman which is at the lower strata in the society, third as a Dalit sanitation worker because of her considered as polluted job in the society.

As Yadav (2009) discussed, Khap is an old social administration followed predominantly in Haryana, Rajasthan and Uttar Pradesh and other north-western states. These are extra-constitutional bodies, not to be mistaken for elected gram panchayats, that began in the tribal era as clan organizations but have literally turned into kangaroo courts. The influence of the Khap Panchayats is that the women of their society have always been targeted without exception. Khap or caste Panchayats have far more jurisdiction than the present Panchayats and they take punitive action against women if Khap rule is violated. Khap Panchayat's key critique is that women's rights are not respected, the outdated notions of equality and docility of women are somewhat exclusively imposed on men on the basis of patriarchal society. They enforce society's age-old patriarchal concepts and threaten those who tried to break them. Women are oppressed and their problems are never dealt with. This is how they have normalized violence as a practice to control women.

Pandemic Forms of Exclusion and Impediments Towards Inclusion

The meaning and concept of pandemic has gone through evolutions since the initiation of the word. The word epidemic and pandemic were often used interchangeably in the seventeenth and eighteenth century in both the medical and social field. The word pandemic was first supposed to be used in 1666 which meant, '*a Pandemic, or Endemic, or rather a Vernacular Disease (a disease always reigning in a country)*'. In the nineteenth century the word epidemic was mostly used. But as the societies developed there were changes in the disease patterns as well as the scientific understanding on the spread of diseases. The global spread of cholera in the year 1831–1832 gave shape to the usage of pandemic. Therefore, when the influenza pandemic occurred in 1889, the concept of pandemic had found its existence (Morens et al., 2009).

Many definitions came up to explain the term pandemic, 'extensively epidemic', 'an epidemic over a very wide area and usually affecting a large proportion of the population', 'distributed or occurring widely throughout a region, country, continent or globally'. Still confusion remained as to the identification of occurrence of pandemics. This confusion was aggravated at the time of H1N1 influenza virus in the year 2009 (Morens et al., 2009). The World Health Organization (WHO) came up with a definition to explain the word pandemic. According to WHO, 'A pandemic is the worldwide spread of a new disease'.[1]

The occurrence of a pandemic not only causes health issues but brings with it various forms of exclusion, some to be mentioned are—discrimination towards the

---

[1] https://www.who.int/csr/disease/swineflu/frequently_asked_questions/pandemic/en/.

Table 13.1 Crime against women in India from January to October, 2020

Month	Jan	Feb	Mar	Apr	May	Jun	Jul	Aug	Sep	Oct
Total crime against women	1462	1424	1347	800	1500	2043	2914	2128	2318	1294

Source National Commission for Women, 2020

person affected with the virus, social exclusion (education, person with disability, health disparities), gender inequality. To understand the exclusions associated with pandemic we need to first understand the concept of exclusion. Exclusion consists of dynamic, multidimensional processes driven by unequal power relationships inter-acting across four dimensions—economic, political, social and cultural—and at different levels including individual, household, group, community, country and global levels. It results in a continuum of inclusion/exclusion characterized by unequal access to resources, capabilities and rights which leads to health inequali-ties", (Popay et al., 2008). Social exclusion refers to the concept where people are not able to participate fully in the spheres of economic, political, social and cultural.

Pandemic also hinders the process of inclusion. For example, the lockdown in India during COVID 19 to reduce the spread of the virus, was decided all of sudden without taking into consideration the need of migrant workers, the elderly population, persons with disability and violence against women. The COVID-19 pandemic has caused an increase in the unemployment rates, income loss and gender inequality. The current pandemic has also affected the homeless and the refugees who have been affected disproportionately. Women have been affected during the pandemic as violence against women has increased; they were unable to reach out to authorities. The immediate need was to curb the spread of the virus and neglect of other important issues. Hence another example of how the pandemic has hindered in the process of inclusive measures (Tables 13.1, 13.2, 13.3, 13.4, 13.5 and 13.6).

COVID-19 and Gender Violence

As the number of COVID-19 cases was increasing in India and the Government took the step of lockdown, there were also some social issues which were increasing in the shadow of the pandemic. To be mentioned it was the violence against women or the gender-based violence (GVB).

> Without a doubt, the most grievous violation of women's rights during COVID-19 is the rise of gender-based violence (GVB) (Guidorzi 2020).[2]

Due to the pandemic the lives of women and men have been affected differently. According to a report by UN Women, the pandemic has led to increased gender

---

[2] GBV is any harmful act that is perpetrated against someone's will and based on socially ascribed gender differences and can include acts of physical, sexual or mental harm, and threats or acts of coercion in public or private (Inter Agency Standing Committee, 2015: 5).

Table 13.2 Percentage of reported cases of crime against women in India, (Jan–Oct, 2020)

Crimes against women	Percentage of cases reported
Acid attack	0.040626814
Bigamy/polygamy	0.603598375
Cyber crime against women	3.360417876
Denial of maternity benefit	0.452698781
Dowry death	1.468369124
Free legal aid for women	0.237957052
Gender discrimination including equal right to education & work	0.052234475
Harassment of married women/dowry harassment	15.02611724
Indecent representation of women	0.150899594
Not categorized yet	1.630876378
Outraging modesty of women/molestation	7.968659315
Police apathy against women	5.3801509
Protection of women against domestic violence	23.02959954
Rape/attempt to rape	5.089959373
Right to exercise choice in marriage/honour crimes	1.816598955
Right to live with dignity	29.94776553
Sex selective abortion/female foeticide/amniocentesis	0.011607661
Sexual assault	0.481717934
Sexual harassment	1.42774231
Sexual harassment of women at workplace	0.87637841
Stalking/voyeurism	0.725478816
Traditional practices derogatory to women rights i.e. sati pratha, devdasi pratha, witch hunting	0.005803831
Trafficking/prostitution of women	0.168311085
Women's right of custody of children in the event of divorce	0.046430644

Source National Commission for Women, 2020

Table 13.3 Crimes against the right to live with dignity

Crime	Jan	Feb	Mar	April	May	Jun	Jul	Aug	Sep	Oct
Right to live with dignity	374	436	388	239	474	611	778	612	889	359

Source National Commission for Women, 2020

Table 13.4 Reported cases of domestic violence against women

	Jan	Feb	Mar	April	May	Jun	Jul	Aug	Sep	Oct
Protection of women against domestic violence	271	302	298	315	393	461	660	539	492	237

Source National Commission for Women, 2020

Table 13.5 Reported cases of cyber crime against women in India

Crime	Jan	Feb	Mar	April	May	Jun	Jul	Aug	Sep	Oct
Cyber crime against women	32	21	37	55	73	103	110	68	59	21

Source National Commission for Women, 2020

inequality and gender discrimination globally and it has disproportionately impacted the women and girls (UN Women, 2020). There was an increase in the calls in police stations and helpline numbers during the lockdown period. Some incidences of rape and sexual assault against women in the quarantine centres were also reported (Deccan Chronicle Staff, 2020; The Wire Staff, 2020; Nightmare, 2020). Due to the lockdown which was a measure to curb the spread of the virus, women were confined to stay at home all the time with the abusive partners. COVID-19 led to the loss of job, overcrowded family environment, financial dependency due to job loss, role expectations of women from abusive partners, all these contributed to the triggering of violence on women (Vranda & Febna, 2020). The mentioned reasons led to development of stress and a sense of loss of power which in turn increased the severity and frequency of the abusive behaviour of the offenders (Vaeza, 2020). There has been a rise in Intimate Partner Violence (IPV) as well during the COVID-19 situation. According to the WHO, IPV is 'a physical, sexual, or psychological coercive act by a current or former partner or spouse to a woman' (WHO, LSHTM, SAMRC, 2013).

Amidst the lockdown phase beginning from March 23 which extended till May 25 saw a rise in the crime against women in India. This is not the case only in India but globally as well there has been an increase in the number of cases reported. According to the National Commission for Women, the total cases reported till October 2020 has been 17,230. Of the ten months July alone has the highest number of cases reported of violence against women which accounted to 2914 cases (Fig. 13.1).

During the lockdown phase the number of cases being reported has been low. As it can be seen from the graph that the reporting of crime against women has been the lowest during the month of April i.e. 800. This month was part of the lockdown phase in India. From May the lockdown was being gradually lifted in certain parts of the countries with the number of the cases being reported were also increasing. From the month of May the reporting increased, reaching a peak in the month of July i.e. 2914 cases.

The lockdown further added to the barrier for women to access the lifesaving services, seek counselling, legal advice, justice resources, lack of social support, medical assistance, sexual health and refuge provision. These led to negative health impacts and increase in the risk of extreme violence. Women including older women, teenage girls, disabled women/girls, LGBTQ/trans women, migrant women, refugee women, indigenous women, rural women face higher obstacles in accessing the essential services (Vaeza, 2020).

Table 13.6 State-wise reported cases of crime against women in the lockdown period (March–May, 2020) and post lockdown (June–July, 2020)

FID	ST_NAME	LP	LP_P	Post_LP	Post_LP_P
0	ANDAMAN AND NICOBAR ISLANDS	1	0.027419	0	0
1	Andhra Pradesh	82	2.248423	78	1.57353237
2	Arunachal Pradesh	0	0	1	0.02017349
3	Assam	23	0.630655	12	0.24208190
4	Bihar	184	5.045242	244	4.92233205
5	CHANDIGARH	9	0.246778	13	0.26225539
6	Chhattisgarh	29	0.795174	31	0.62537825
7	DADRA AND NAGER HAVELI	3	0.082259	1	0.02017349
8	DAMAN AND DIU	1	0.027419	3	0.06052047
9	Goa	6	0.164518	1	0.02017349
10	Gujarat	45	1.233890	51	1.02884809
11	Haryana	189	5.182341	284	5.72927173
12	Himachal Pradesh	20	0.548395	20	0.40346984
13	Jammu and Kashmir	13	0.356457	23	0.46399031
14	Jharkhand	43	1.179051	73	1.47266491
15	Karnataka	117	3.208116	98	1.97700221
16	Kerala	39	1.069372	25	0.50433730
17	LAKSHADWEEP	0	0	1	0.02017349
18	Madhya Pradesh	141	3.866191	174	3.51018761
19	Maharashtra	265	7.266246	283	5.70909824
20	Manipur	3	0.082259	2	0.04034698
21	Meghalaya	2	0.054839	3	0.06052047
22	Mizoram	0	0	0	0
23	Nagaland	NA	NA	NA	NA
24	Nct of Delhi	499	13.68247	578	11.6602783
25	Orissa	27	0.740334	26	0.52451079
26	Pondicherry	0	0	5	0.10086746
27	Punjab	89	2.440361	93	1.87613475
28	Rajasthan	170	4.661365	200	4.03469840
29	Sikkim	NA	NA	NA	NA
30	Tamil Nadu	105	2.879078	111	2.23925761
31	Tripura	0	0	0	0
32	Uttar Pradesh	1388	38.05867	2337	47.1454508
33	Uttarakhand	47	1.288730	88	1.77526729
34	West Bengal	107	2.933918	98	1.97700221

(continued)

Table 13.6 (continued)

FID	ST_NAME	LP	LP_P	Post_LP	Post_LP_P
	Total	3647		4957	

Source National Commission for Women, 2020

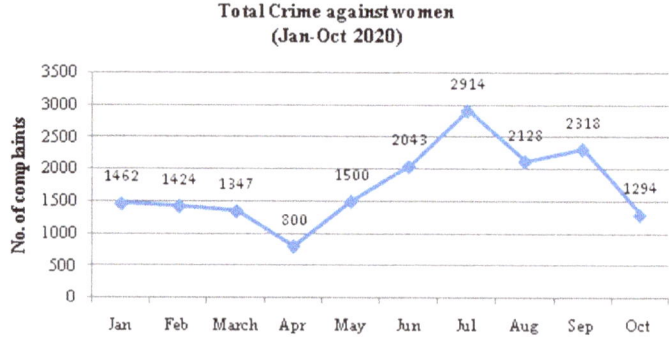

Fig. 13.1 Total crime against women in India (Jan–Oct 2020). *Source* Report of the Complaints by NCW in 2020

Complaints

Of the total number of cases reported of crime against women to National Commission for Women (NCW) till October (17,230), the highest percentage of complaints has been in the category of Right to live with dignity i.e. 29.94% and the second highest category has been Protection of Women against Domestic Violence with a percentage of 23.02. Cybercrime against women was reported to be 3.36%. In the category of outraging modesty of women/Molestation percentage of cases reported were 7.9%. Rape/attempt to rape reported 5.08% of cases. 1.4% of cases were reported in the category of dowry death. Cases were also reported of police apathy against women which was approximately 5.38%. The percentage of cases reported for acid attack on women was 0.04% (According to Fig. 13.2—Nature wise Report of the Complaints by NCW in the Year: 2020).

Right to Live with Dignity

This is the category which reported the highest number of complaints among the crimes against women. Number of cases being reported in the pre-lockdown months was high with a decrease beginning from March dipping in the month of April, the month during the lockdown phase. The number of complaints increased from the

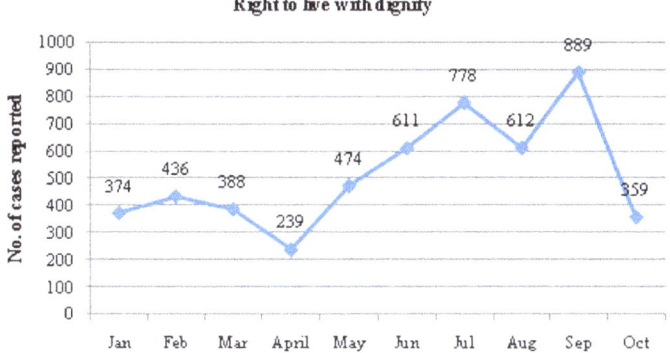

Fig. 13.2 Right to live with dignity. *Source* Report of the Complaints by NCW in 2020

month of May with a slight peak in the month of July i.e. 778 complaints. Of the ten months, September has shown the greatest peak with 889 complaints (Fig. 13.3).

Domestic Violence

Domestic violence is the second category with the highest complaints. The peak is in the month of July with 660 complaints. Complaints analyzed by NCW have revealed that there was an increase in domestic violence complaints and cybercrime complaints in May 2020 in the Indian districts under the red zones having strictest lockdown measures in comparison to the green zones.[3]

A study by the researchers from the University of California, Los Angeles noted that during the lockdown period there has been a fall in the rape and sexual complaints. This fall has been due to the decreased mobility in public spaces, public transport and workplaces. Though in India many cases are unreported and marital rape is not considered as a crime which may have been increasing in the lockdown period. Marital rape in India if reported gets reported under the domestic violence category (Bhattacharya, 2020).

The highest number of domestic violence complaints has been from Uttar Pradesh followed by Delhi i.e. 5470 and 1697 respectively in the COVID-19 induced lockdown (Jadhav, 2020).[4] According to a report compiled by the Himachal Pradesh Police, the crime against women fell down drastically with the initiation of lockdown but as the lockdown was gradually being lifted the number of complaints rose sharply (Fig. 13.4).

---

[3] https://qz.com/india/1882497/cases-of-domestic-violence-cybercrime-rose-in-indias-lockdown/.

[4] https://www.thehindubusinessline.com/data-stories/data-focus/abuse-of-women-at-home-rose-during-lockdown/article33060560.ece.

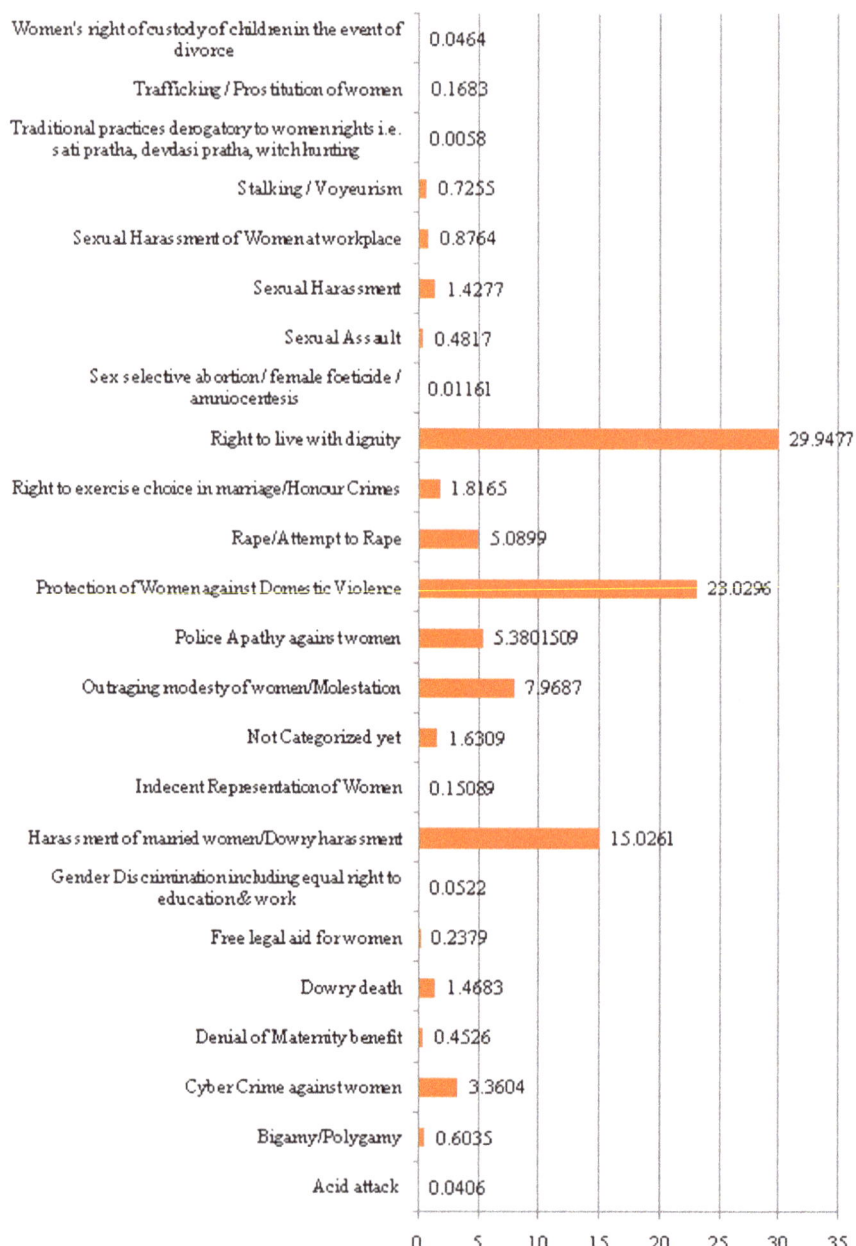

Category wise cases reported in % (Jan-Oct 2020)

Category	%
Women's right of custody of children in the event of divorce	0.0464
Trafficking / Prostitution of women	0.1683
Traditional practices derogatory to women rights i.e. sati pratha, devdasi pratha, witch hunting	0.0058
Stalking / Voyeurism	0.7255
Sexual Harassment of Women at workplace	0.8764
Sexual Harassment	1.4277
Sexual Assault	0.4817
Sex selective abortion / female foeticide / amniocentesis	0.01161
Right to live with dignity	29.9477
Right to exercise choice in marriage/Honour Crimes	1.8165
Rape/Attempt to Rape	5.0899
Protection of Women against Domestic Violence	23.0296
Police Apathy against women	5.3801509
Outraging modesty of women/Molestation	7.9687
Not Categorized yet	1.6309
Indecent Representation of Women	0.15089
Harassment of married women/Dowry harassment	15.0261
Gender Discrimination including equal right to education & work	0.0522
Free legal aid for women	0.2379
Dowry death	1.4683
Denial of Maternity benefit	0.4526
Cyber Crime against women	3.3604
Bigamy/Polygamy	0.6035
Acid attack	0.0406

Fig. 13.3 Category wise cases reported in % (Jan–Oct 2020). *Source* Report of the Complaints by NCW in 2020

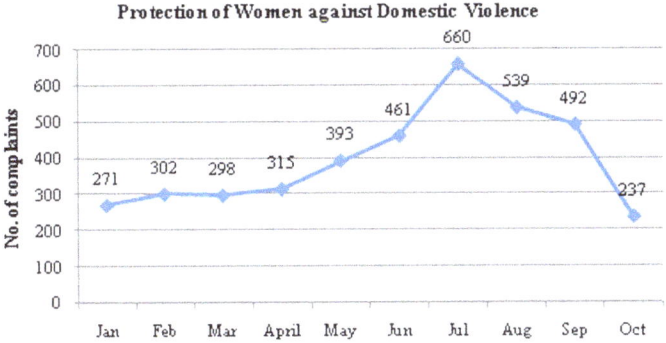

Fig. 13.4 Protection of women against domestic violence. *Source* Report of the Complaints by NCW in 2020

The reason for rise in domestic violence during the lockdown period was mainly the already existing gender inequalities, crisis created in the pandemic situation, stress, frustration and loss of job (Guidorzi, 2020).

Lockdown Gendered Violence

A study was based on articles published in three newspapers, *The Hindu*, *Times of India* and *Dainik Jagran* on domestic violence against women in India revealed that the total number of published articles on domestic violence increased during the lockdown period in the months of April, May and June. The articles published during this period on domestic violence were higher than all the articles ever published (Maji et al., 2021).

During the lockdown period there was an increase of 47.2% of domestic violence complaints in India (Pandit, 2020). The connection between alcohol abuse and domestic violence was reported in Uttar Pradesh. The study found that on 1st, 2nd and 2rd of May the complaints of domestic violence were 29, 34 and 34 respectively but with the opening of the alcohol shops the number of complaints increased to 92, 123 and 143 (Agnihotri, 2020; Chakravarty, 2020). In many parts of India women are not allowed to go anywhere except to the office or school. As a result, during the lockdown period men went out of the house for essential purposes, while the women were confined to the house which left them to the place of conflict facing the brutality of physical violence. In Ludhiana a woman was beaten by her husband, mother-in-law and father-in-law (Kumar, 2020a). An article reported that a woman was forced to commit suicide by her husband in Chandigarh and a case had been filed against the husband (Kumar, 2020b).

A case from Malda, West Bengal was reported where a 26-year-old woman was strangled to death by her husband. Another case of a man killing his wife was reported because she protested against the extra-marital affair of her husband (Nigam, 2020).

State's Women Commission of Kerala got a call from Chennai from a man who asked for help for her sister and her daughter. They were residents of Idukki district and they were hiding in a forest after both of them were ejected by her husband. The husband was taken into custody while investigating the case (Dhamini, 2020).

A 25-year-old woman living in a slum in Chennai was brutally beaten by her alcoholic husband on 25th March 2020 which was just at the beginning of the lockdown period. Earlier before the lockdown if any such incident would take place she would go out of the house and call the neighbours for help. But on this day, there were police barricades and she could not go out to seek help from the neighbours (Nigam, 2020).

In Vadodara, Gujarat, a man broke his wife's spine after she defeated him in an online ludo game. His ego was hurt as she defeated him consecutively in the game and she contributed to the family income by taking tuition classes (Pachchigar, 2020).

In Assam a woman in order to seek refuge from her abusive husband went to her parents' home with her five-month-old child after crossing two paddy fields during the lockdown period (Nagpal, 2020).

Bunty, a worker at the garment factory and her husband, collected garbage. Her husband was an alcoholic and physically abused her during the lockdown. Her husband used to get angry over little things, hit her and broke the TV (Rukmini, 2020).

In Delhi the calls received by DCP in lockdown period increased to 1000–1200 per day as compared to 900–1000 calls (India Today, 2020). The cases of violence were reported not only from rural areas but also from the cities (Nigam, 2020). From Delhi alone 2500 cases were reported during the lockdown period (Dhamini, 2020). The child helpline numbers also reported increased number of calls pertaining to physical and sexual abuse and also child marriage (Tyagi, 2020).

Cybercrime Against Women

During the lockdown period the usage of the internet went up and with it there was a surge in cybercrime against women.

> There has been a spurt in cybercrimes against women for years and the lockdown has made the stalkers much bolder, said speakers at a webinar on 'Cybercrime against women' organized by the APCID and Cyber Peace Foundation.—Cybercrimes against women on the rise- The Hindu.

The NCW had opened the online intake of complaints during the lockdown phase. According to the NCW data, last year in 2019 during April they received 37 complaints but in April 2020 it was 54. Indraveni K, the joint director of Centre for Development of Advanced Computing said there were 412 complaints of cyber abuse from March 25 till April 25, 2020, of which 396 were complaints of serious nature. The harassment done to women in social media is mainly done by messages,

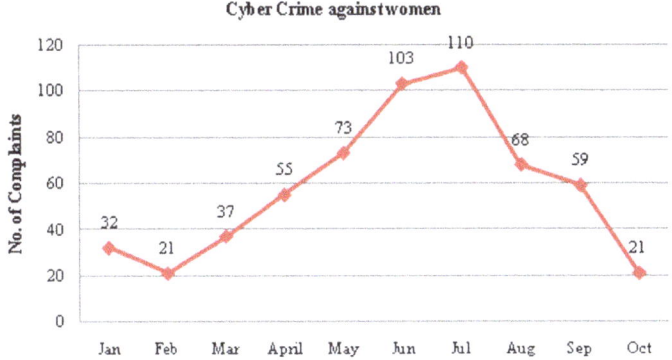

Fig. 13.5 Cyber crime against women. *Source* Report of the Complaints by NCW in 2020

calls, video, photo morphing, profile hacking, dating scams, link baiting, information theft, cyber bullying, etc. Complexity exists in cyberspace, for instance the 'Bois Locker Room' incident which took place a few months back. Cyberspace has been promoting sexual violence, toxic masculinity and rape culture upfront. In India where women's bodies are considered as a symbol of chastity and pride for the family, it makes them an easy target for the cyber criminals. Despite this pandemic situation, the cyber criminals have an easy spot on the women and girls who have been using the internet for work, talking to friends, watching movies, web series or study. As it can be seen from the graph that the peak of the complaints has been in the month of July i.e. 110 cases. From the month of March, the number of complaints has been increasing, when the various types of cybercrimes were surging (Fig. 13.5).

Sextortion was one of the rising crimes against the women in the lockdown phase. What is Sextortion? It is a virtual blackmail where the abuser threatens the woman or girl to publish real or morphed photographs or videos in the online platform if she refuses to perform sexual or financial favours towards them. It is sexual extortion. In this lockdown period, the couples not being able to meet each other, having long distance relationships have taken their relationship online, sharing intimate pictures which has given opportunity for increased threats. But as per many cyber experts this is just the tip of the iceberg. Many women do not know whom and where to approach for the complaint.

As mentioned earlier this is just tip of the iceberg as women do not want to make official complaints because it will impose a question on their dignity and the social stigma associated with it and want the NGO's or other organizations to handle such cases unofficially.[5]

Cybercrimes can be reduced through education, awareness on the usage of technology. Certain suggestions came from the cyber experts to create strong passwords, spreading awareness on phishing emails, fake videos and sharing confidential content

---

[5] https://cio.economictimes.indiatimes.com/news/digital-security/significant-increase-in-cybercrime-against-women-during-lockdown-experts/75500549.

securely, talking to friends or people around you can help in strengthening the security. There is a presence of cyber police in every district which people are not aware of, whom they can approach in case such a situation arises. Also, there is a need to train the police officials to handle such situations with delicacy and without any sort of stigma. It would be safe for women and girls not to share any personal images or details on social media. Although India has enacted the IT Act 2000, still the laws need to be more stringent to tackle such situations. The Government of India launched a programme in 2019, Cyber Crime against women and Children to introduce awareness on cybercrimes and cyber hygiene as a component of school curriculum at the early stages of education has been an important step.[6] Despite the efforts of the Government and Non- government organizations, there has been an upsurge in the cybercrimes against women.

Statewide Analysis

The map given below shows the state-wise percentage of crimes reported against women in India in the lockdown period i.e. March–May 2020. It can be seen that Uttar Pradesh and Delhi have had the highest percentage of reported cases. Uttar Pradesh reported approximately 38.05% of total cases and Delhi about 13.68% of total cases. During the lockdown period states like Arunachal Pradesh, Mizoram, Lakshadweep, Pondicherry and Tripura has not reported any cases of violence against women.

From Table 13.6, it can be seen that the total cases reported during the lockdown months was 3647, which increased to 4957 cases in the post lockdown months of June and July.

As the lockdown was lifted in a phased manner, women got a chance to go out of their houses and report the cases and thus an increase in reported cases was seen post the lockdown period. In the post lockdown period, again the state of Uttar Pradesh reported the highest percentage of reported cases to the total reported cases of about 47%. The absolute figure being 2337 cases in the post lockdown period as compared to 1388 cases in the lockdown period (Fig. 13.6).

Impact of Gender Violence

Violence against women has been and is still a public health issue, but during the lockdown the discrimination, inequalities, oppression and patriarchal violence has seen a surge. Earlier women facing violence would take refuge in their parental home but the lockdown has affected this accessibility. The women also fear that with their

---

[6] https://www.mha.gov.in/division_of_mha/cyber-and-information-security-cis-division/Details-about-CCPWCCybercrimePreventionagainst-Women-and-Children-Scheme.

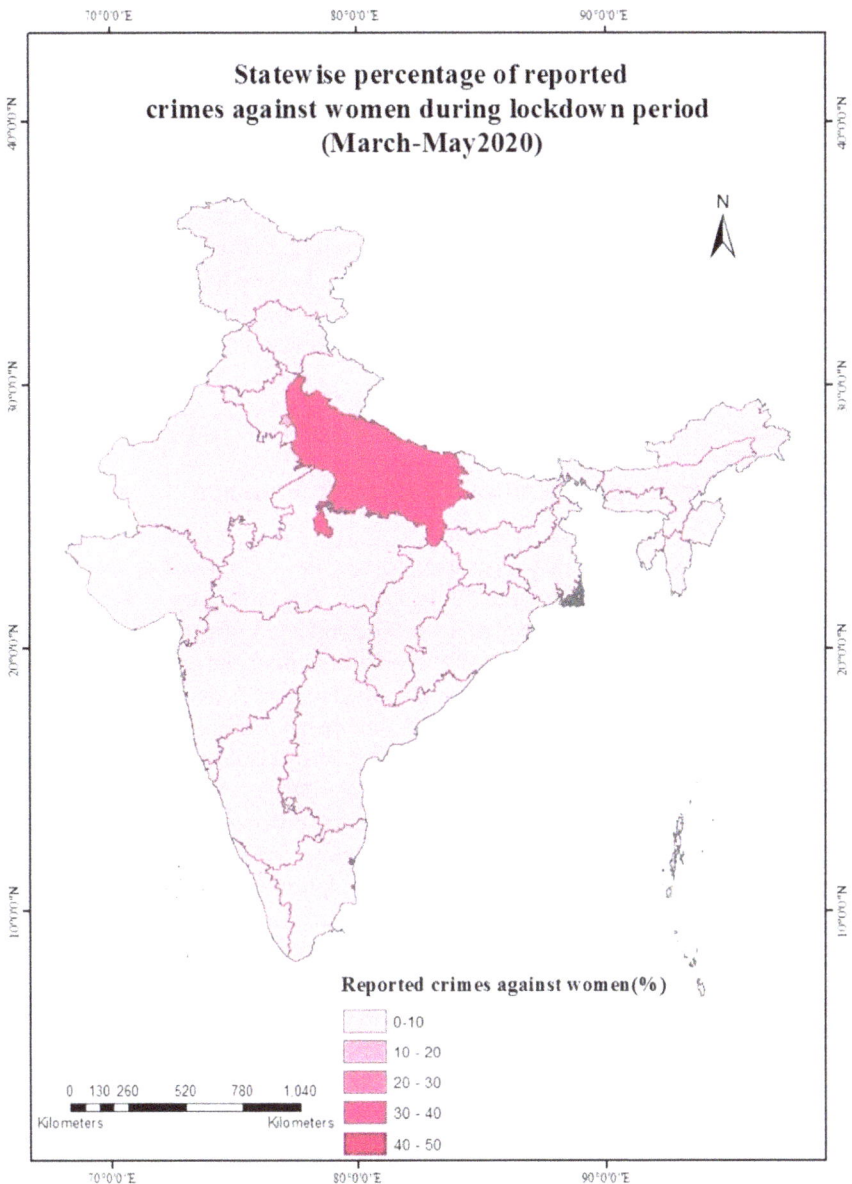

Fig. 13.6 State wise percentage of reported crimes against women during lock down period (March–May 2020). Uttar Pradesh has a disproportional number of crimes against women. *Data source* National Commission for Women, Report 2020

movement they might expose their elderly parents to the virus and thus acting as an obstruction to take refuge in the parental homes (Nigam, 2020).

It is mostly the women who take care at home; therefore, women are at a higher risk of contracting the virus. The work participation rate of women is low in India and the lockdown has further pushed the women out of work. Thus, the economic dependence on abusive partners have also increased adding to the vulnerability. Women are also being affected with sexual violence and being forced to take abortion drugs without supervision in the absence of medical help (Srivastava, 2020). Women and children are being harassed mentally, physically and this is leading to taking up of drastic steps of suicide. Women face a lot of risk due to domestic violence like isolation, mental health issues, high-risk pregnancy, Sexually Transmitted Disease (STD), HIV infection.

Strategies for Helping Victims of Gender Violence

Provisions of basic needs and measures to fight the COVID-19 is required but the violence against women cannot be neglected. The Protection of Women from Domestic Violence Act, 2005 needs to be implemented effectively at this hour. Media both print and broadcast can create awareness among the general public of the domestic violence issue, whom to reach, helpline numbers, shelter homes and legal assistance available for women. The ASHA workers and other health workers need to be educated and trained to identify signs of domestic violence while conducting door-to-door surveys about COVID-19 (Vora et al., 2020).

In France warning systems have been set up at the pharmacies to help the victims of gender and family violence and alert the respective authorities. Some code words can be used to alert staff (Guenfound, 2020). Helpline numbers can be posted in pharmacies to help the women. Similar steps can be taken up in India.

In India the National Commission for Women started a Whatsapp number during the lockdown period to provide assistance for the victims of domestic violence. Many authors have suggested the use of mobile health and telemedicine as a technique to discuss and counsel the victim by the usage of yes or no questions.[7]

Discussion

Violence against women as defined by United Nations as 'any act of gender-based violence that results in, or is likely to result in, physical, sexual or mental harm or suffering to women, including threats of such acts, coercion or arbitrary deprivation of liberty, whether occurring in public or in private life'.[8] About 30% of women around

---

[7] Emezue (2020).

[8] UN (1993): http://www.un-documents.net/a48r104.htm.

the world face violence at least once in their lifetimes (WHO, 2021). According to the National Crime Records Bureau, a crime is committed against women every three minutes. Due to violence women suffer from social isolation, unemployment, income loss, and lack of self-care, mental health issues and also failure of childcare. Violence by intimate partners and associated sexual violence leads to high risk of pregnancy, sexually transmitted diseases and HIV infection.[9]

With the increase in the COVID-19 case, violence against women has also been increasing in the shadow of the pandemic. When the entire country was going through lockdown, for safety from the virus, safety of women was decreasing. The National Commission for Women has been publishing monthly reports of Crime against Women in India. According to the National Commission for Women, the total cases reported till October 2020 has been 17,230. Of the ten months July alone has the highest number of cases reported of violence against women which accounted to 2914 cases. During the lockdown period the reporting of complaints decreased but as the lockdown was being lifted gradually, the reporting of cases increased simultaneously. Of the total number of cases reported of crime against women to NCW till October (17,230), the highest percentage of complaints has been in the category of Right to live with dignity i.e. 29.94% and the second highest category has been Protection of Women against Domestic Violence with a percentage of 23.02. Domestic violence against women increased in the lockdown period. This was mainly because of the crisis created in the pandemic situation, stress, tension, frustration and loss of job. Women face a lot of risk due to domestic violence like isolation, mental health issues, high-risk pregnancy, Sexually Transmitted Disease (STD), HIV infection.

During the lockdown period the usage of the internet went up and with it there was a surge in cybercrime against women. The harassment done to women in social media is mainly done by messages, calls, video, photo morphing, profile hacking, dating scams, link baiting, information theft, cyber bullying, etc. According to the NCW data, last year in 2019 during April they received 37 complaints but in April 2020 it was 54. Indraveni K, the joint director of Centre for Development of Advanced Computing said there were 412 complaints of cyber abuse from March 25 till April 25, 2020, of which 396 were complaints of serious nature. Sextortion was one of the rising crimes against the women in the lockdown phase. There are government schemes to make people aware of cybercrimes. Despite all the efforts of the government and NGOs the women are still at risk.

During the lockdown months the percentage of reported cases was less but as the lockdown was being lifted the percentage of cases reported began to increase. This was mainly because women got a chance to go out of their houses, contact various organizations and report the crime.

Women with disability in general face lower income, high levels of poverty, lower education, poor health conditions and the patriarchal values existing in the society. But COVID-19 further added to this distress and ongoing discrimination towards disabled women. Some women faced lack of information about the lockdown, lack of

---

[9] WHO   (2005):   www.who.int/reproductivehealth/publications/violence/9241593512/en/index.html.

access to relief resources like food and medicine and also lack of personal assistance for taking care of daily needs. Women with disabilities living in rural areas were affected more than those in the urban areas because of the presence of urban home deliveries. Other scholars note how the pandemic has magnified the distress of the differently abled (Nayar, Mehrotra, this volume).

Conclusion

Violence against women is a major health and human right issue. The Declaration on the Elimination of Violence Against Women, adopted by the United Nations General Assembly, in 1993, defines violence against women as 'any act of gender-based violence that result in, or is likely to result in, physical, sexual, or mental harm or suffering to women, including threats of such acts, coercion or arbitrary deprivation of liberty, whether occurring in public or in private life'.

The complaints received by the National Commission for Women are just tip of the iceberg, women who took the courage to complain. There are many cases which go under reported due to lack of awareness as to whom to approach, associated social stigma. There is a need to provide comprehensive care pro-actively. A multidimensional and multi-agency team is required to provide psychological support. There is a need to implement primary prevention programmes, gender sensitization, sex education in schools, colleges, to boys and girls for a sustainable solution.

Cybercrimes can be reduced through education, awareness on the usage of technology. Certain suggestions came from the cyber experts to create strong passwords, spreading awareness on phishing emails, fake videos and sharing confidential content securely, talking to friends or people around you can help in strengthening the security. The Government of India launched a programme in 2019, Cyber Crime against women and Children to introduce awareness on cybercrimes and cyber hygiene as a component of school curriculum at the early stages of education has been an important step. The laws need to be made more stringent. We have a long way to go in making this country a safe place for women and girls.

In the lockdown period women had lesser opportunity to go out of their houses, interact with people and thus lesser cases were reported. The lifting of lockdown gave women a chance to go out of their houses and report the crime inflicted towards them (Charkha Features and Youth ki Awaaz, 2020; Dang and Nguyen, 2021; Dixit and The Week, 2020; DNA Web Team, 2020; Emezue, 2020; Express News Service & Indian Express, 2020; Global is Asian Staff, 2020; Harbishettar and Suresh Bada Math, 2014; Kaur and Garg, 2008; Malik and Khansa, 2020; National Crime Record Bureau, 2017–2019; National Herald, 2020; NE NOW NEWS, 2020; PACS INDIA, 2021; Peterman and O'Donnell, 2020; Rakshit and The Swaddle, 2020; Suhasini and Vogue India, 2020; The Hindu, 2020; Thomas and Bangalore Mirror, 2020; UN Documents, 1993).

Acknowledgements   We dedicate this paper to the women, who have been the victim of patriarchy, the physical and mental violence throughout the lockdown and so. We would also like to thank several authors including student researchers who have researched thoroughly on this topic; their contribution helped us to write on this topic.

References

Agnihotri, S., & Dainik Jagran. (2020). *Domestic violence, murder and suicide increased after open wine shops.* Retrieved April 15, 2021, from https://www.jagran.com/uttar-pradesh/kanpur-city-domestic-violence-murder-and-suicide-increased-after-open-wine-shops-20253265.html.

Bhattacharya, A., & Quartz India. (2020). *Cases of domestic violence, cybercrime rose in India's lockdown.* Retrieved November 24, 2020, from https://qz.com/india/1882497/cases-of-domestic-violence-cybercrime-rose-in-indias-lockdown/.

Chakravarty, S., & Dainik Jagran. (2020). *Incidents of domestic violence escalated due to opening of liquor shops, phones rang on dial 112.* Retrieved April 15, 2021, from https://www.jagran.com/uttar-pradesh/varanasi-city-incidents-of-domestic-violence-escala ted-due-to-opening-of-liquor-shops-phones-rang-on-dial-112-pirv-20247052.html.

Charkha Features, & Youth ki Awaaz. (2020). Retrieved November 24, 2020, from https://www.youthkiawaaz.com/2020/06/increasing-cases-of-cyber-crimes-against-women/.

Dang, H. A. H., & Nguyen, C. V. (2021). Gender Inequality during COVID-19 pandemic: Income, expenditure, savings, and job loss. *World Development, 140,* 105296, 1–10.

Deccan Chronicle Staff. (2020). *Outrage in Kerala over sexual assault on COVID patients.* Retrieved April 21, 2021, from https://www.deccanchronicle.com/nation/crime/080920/outrage-in-kerala-over-sexual-assault-on-covid-patients. Not available currently.

Dixit, R., & The Week. (2020). Domestic violence against women on the rise amid nationwide lockdown. Retrieved November 24, 2020, from https://www.theweek.in/news/india/2020/04/02/domestic-violence-cases-against-women-on-the-rise-amid-nationwide-lockdown.html.

Dhamini, R., & The Hindustan Times. (2020). *Domestic violence during Covid-19 lockdown emerges as serious concern.* Retrieved April 15, 2021, from https://www.hindustantimes.com/india-news/domestic-violence-during-covid-19-lockdown-emerges-as-serious-concern/story-mMRq3NnnFvOehgLOOPpe8J.html.

DNA Web Team. DNA. (2020). *Cyber crime against women at its peak, close to 60 percent victims of online abuse.* Retrieved November 24, 2020, from https://www.dnaindia.com/india/report-dna-special-cybercrime-against-women-at-its-peak-close-to-60-percent-women-a-victim-of-onl ine-abuse-2847984. Not available online currently.

Emezue, C. J. (2020). Digital or digitally delivered responses to domestic and intimate partner violence during COVID-19. *JMIR Public Health Surveillance, 6,* e19831. https://doi.org/10.2196/19831

Express News Service, & Indian Express. (2020). As govt eased curbs, crimes against women shot up in Himachal. Retrieved November 24, 2020, from https://indianexpress.com/article/cities/cha ndigarh/as-govt-eased-curbs-crimes-against-women-shot-up-in-himachal-6543014/.

Ghurye, G. S. (1969). *Caste and race in India.* Popular Prakashan.

Global is Asian Staff. Global is Asian. (2020). *India's shadow pandemic and trends of violence against women.* Retrieved November 24, 2020, from https://lkyspp.nus.edu.sg/gia/article/india-s-shadow-pandemic-and-trends-of-violence-against-women.

Guenfound, I., & ABC News. (2020). French women use code words at pharma-cies to escape domestic violence during coronavirus lockdown. Retrieved April 15, 2021, https://abcnews.go.com/International/frenchwomen-code-words-pharmacies-escape-dom estic-violence/story?id=69954238

Guidorzi, B. (2020). "The Shadow Pandemic": Addressing gender-based violence (GVB) during Covid-19. In P. Carmody, G. McCann, C. Colleran, & C. O'Halloran (Eds.), *Covid-19 in the Global South* (pp. 117–126). Bristol University Press. https://doi.org/10.2307/j.ctv18gfz7c.18

Harbishettar, V., & Suresh Bada Math. (2014). Violence against women in India: Comprehensive care for survivors. *Indian Journal of Medical Research, 157–159.*

India Today. (2020). New Delhi. *Domestic violence spikes in lockdown, govt told to step in.* Retrieved April 15, 2021, from https://www.indiatoday.in/mail-today/story/domestic-violence-spikes-in-lockdown-govt-told-to-step-in-1671460-2020-04-27

Inter-Agency Standing Committee. (2015). *Guidelines for integrating gender-based violence interventions in humanitarian action: Reducing risk, promoting resilience and aiding recovery.* IASC

Jadhav, R., & The Hindu Business Line. (2020). Pune. *Abuse of women at home rose during lockdown.* Retrieved April 15, 2021, from https://www.thehindubusinessline.com/data-stories/data-focus/abuse-of-women-at-home-rose-during-lockdown/article33060560.ece

Kaur, R., & Garg, S. (2008). Addressing domestic violence against women: An unfinished agenda. *Indian Journal of Community Medicine, 33*, 73–76.

Krishnaraj, M. (2007). Understanding violence against women. *Economical and Political Weekly, 42*(44), 90–91.

Kumar, V., & Dainik Jagran. (2020a). Woman's arm broken due to beating. Retrieved April 15, 2021, from https://www.jagran.com/punjab/ludhiana-woman-arm-broken-due-to-beating-by-husband-mother-in-law-and-father-in-law-20378905.html

Kumar, V., & Dainik Jagran. (2020b). Case against husband for forcing wife to commit suicide, Chandigarh News. Retrieved April 15, 2021, from https://www.jagran.com/punjab/chandigarh-case-against-husband-for-forcing-wife-to-commit-suicide-20237288.html

Maji, S., Bansod, S., & Singh, T. (2021). Domestic violence during COVID-19 pandemic: The case study for Indian women. *Journal of Community & Applied Social Psychology*, 1–8.

Malik, S., & Naeem, K. (2020). *Impact of Covid-19 pandemic on women: Health, livelihoods and domestic violence.* Sustainable Development Policy Institute.

Mencher, P. J. (1974). The caste system upside down. In D. Gupta (Ed.), *Social stratification.* Oxford University Press.

Morens, D. M., Gregory, K. F., & Anthony, S. F. (2009). "What is a pandemic?" *The Journal of Infectious Diseases, 200*(7), 1018–1021.

Nagpal, A. (2020). Activists urge roping in ASHA workers and other novel approaches as domestic violence rises during lockdowns. *India Spend.* Retrieved April 15, 2021, from https://www.indiaspend.com/activists-urge-roping-in-asha-workers-and-other-novel-approaches-as-domestic-violence-rises-during-lockdowns/

National Commission for Women. (2020). Nature wise report of the complaints by NCW in the year: 2020.

National Crime Record Bureau. (2017–2019). *Crime against women (IPC+SLL).* Retrieved November 15, 2020, from https://ncrb.gov.in/sites/default/files/crime_in_india_table_additional_table_chapter_reports/Table%203A.1_2.pdf

National Herald. (2020). *NCW received 2043 complaints of crimes against women in June, highest in 8 months.* Retrieved November 24, 2020, from https://www.nationalheraldindia.com/national/ncw-receives-2043-complaints-of-crimes-against-women-in-june-highest-in-8-months

NE Now News. (2020). *Northeast Now. Assam Tripura among states registering maximum domestic violence case during lockdown.* Retrieved November 24, 2020, from https://nenow.in/north-east-news/assam/assam-tripura-among-states-registering-maximum-domestic-violence-case-during-lockdown-ncw.html

Nigam, S. (2020). COVID-19, lockdown and violence against women in homes. independent research. ORCID 0000-0002-9518-4804.

Pachchigar, J., & Times of India. (2020). Retrieved April 15, 2021, from https://timesofindia.indiatimes.com/city/vadodara/defeated-in-online-ludo-man-breaks-wifes-spine/articleshow/75394992.cms

PACS INDIA. *What is social exclusion?* Retrieved March 31, 2021, from www.pacsindia.org/about_pacs/what-is-social-exclusion.

Pandit, A., & Times of India. (2020). *Domestic violence accounts for over 47% complaints to NCW in lockdown.* Retrieved April 15, 2021, from https://timesofindia.indiatimes.com/india/domestic-violence-accounts-for-over-47-complaints-to-ncw-in-lockdown/articleshow/76161829.cms

Peterman, A., & O'Donnell, M. *Covid-19 and violence against women and children.* Center for Global Development.

Popay, J, Escorel, S., Hernandez, M., Johnston, H., Mathieson, J., & Rispel, L. (2008). *Understanding and tackling social exclusion. Final Report to the WHO Commission on Social Determinants of Health From the Social Exclusion Knowledge Network.* World Health Organization.

Rakshit, D., & The Swaddle. (2020). Retrieved November 24, 2020, https://theswaddle.com/cybercrime-cases-against-women-spike-under-covid19-lockdown/

Rukmini, S. A. (2020). Retrieved April 15, 2021, https://www.aljazeera.com/news/2020/04/locked-abusers-india-domestic-violence-surge-200415092014621.html

Singh, Y. (1994). *Modernization of Indian tradition: A systematic study of social change.* Rawat Publications.

Srinivas, M. N. (1952, March 1). Social anthropology and sociology. *SAGE Journals.*

Srivastava, R., & Reuters. (2020). Retrieved April 15, 2021, from https://www.reuters.com/article/us-health-coronavirus-india-abortion-trf/abortion-in-a-lockdown-india-says-yes-but-women-wonder-how-idUSKCN21Y2HO

Suhasini, L., & Vogue India. (2020). *Vogue warriors: Meet the social entrepreneur leading the fight against the rising rate of cyber crime during the lockdown.* Vogue India.

The Economic Times. (2020). *The Economic Times.* Retrieved November 24, 2020, from https://cio.economictimes.indiatimes.com/news/digital-security/significant-increase-in-cybercrime-against-women-during-lockdown-experts/75500549

The Hindu. (2020). *Cybercrimes against women on the rise.* Retrieved January 15, 2021, from https://www.thehindu.com/news/national/andhra-pradesh/cyber-crimes-against-women-on-the-rise/article32399536.ece

The Wire Staff. (2020). *Delhi: 14-year-old sexually assaulted at COVID care centre.* Retrieved April 15, 2021, from https://thewire.in/rights/delhi-14-year-old-sexually-assaulted-covid-care-centre

Thomas, B., & Bangalore Mirror. (2020). *Nightmare in HSR quarantine centre.* Retrieved April 15, 2021, from https://bangaloremirror.indiatimes.com/bangalore/cover-story/nightmare-in-hsr-quarantine-centre/articleshow/76473988.cms

Tyagi, T., & The Hindustan Times. (2020). Child helpline receives double the usual number of calls amid lockdown. Retrieved April 15, 2021, from https://www.hindustantimes.com/noida/child-helpline-receives-double-the-usual-number-of-calls-amid-lockdown/story-gzup46Dt2U66be8TvMkoRK.html

United Nations. (1993). *Declaration on the elimination of violence against women. Gathering a body of global agreements, A/RES/48/104.* Retrieved November 22, 2020, from http://www.un-documents.net/a48r104.htm

UN Women. (2020). *The first 100 days of the COVID-19 outbreak in Asia and the Pacific: A gender lens.* UN women regional office for Asia and the Pacific. Bangkok. Retrieved April 15, 2021, from https://asiapacific.unwomen.org/en/digitallibrary/publications/2020/04/the-first-100-days-of-he-covid-19-outbreak-in-asia-and-thethepacific

Vaeza, M. N. & UN Chronicle. (2020). *Addressing the impact of the COVID-19 pandemic on violence against women and girls.* Retrieved April 15, 2021, from https://www.un.org/en/addressing-impact-covid-19-pandemic-violence-against-women-and-girls

Velaskar, P. (2012). Structural subordination of Dalit women. In I. Qadeer (Ed.), *Glimmerings of an awakening—Dalit women's health and rights.* Yatra/Penguin (Hindi). Zubaan (English translation available)

Vora, M., Malathesh, B. C., Das, S., & Chatterjee, S. S. (2020). COVID-19 and domestic violence against women. *Asian Journal of Psychiatry,* 1–2.

Vranda, M. N., & Febna, M. (2020). Response to sexual and gender-based violence against women during COVID-19. *Indian Journal of Psychological Medicine, 42*(6), 582–584.

Walby, S. (1990). Theorizing patriarchy. In *Introduction* (pp. 1–25). Basil Blackwell Ltd.

WHO. (2005). *Multi-Country study on women's health and domestic violence against women.* Retrieved November 15, 2020, from www.who.int/reproductivehealth/publications/violence/924 1593512/en/index.html.

World Health Organization. (2010). WHO. Retrieved March 31, 2021, from https://www.who.int/csr/disease/swineflu/frequently_asked_questions/pandemic/en/.

World Health Organization. (2021, March 9). Violence against women. https://www.who.int/newsroom/factsheets/detail/violence-against-women. Accessed 31 Mar 2021.

WHO, LSHTM, SAMRC. (2013). *Global and regional estimates of violence against women: Prevalance and health effects of intimate partner violence and non-partner sexual violence.* WHO.

Yadav, B. (2009). Khap panchayats: Stealing poverty. *Economic and Political Weekly, 44*(52), 16–19.

Part III
Health Inequalities

The cumulation of historical deprivation among tribals, Dalits, rural non-literate peoples, the disabled, and religious minorities is correlated with disparities at multiple levels of analysis. The oft-proposed explanation, constantly backed up by new rounds of social science data, is that health inequalities cannot be explained away simply by differences in health care expenditures or by absolute levels of affluence (Singer and Ryff, 2001). Financial barriers alone are argued to be the key barrier to accessing health care services in South Asian countries, as Out-of-Pocket Expenditures (OOPE) constitutes a significant proportion of health care cost borne by users (McIntyre et al., 2006; Leive, 2008; Joglekar, 2012). These health care expenditures, sitting on top of pre-existing economic precarity, further drive the poor into poverty (Duggal, 2007, WHO, 2012). This explanation overlooks the correlation between poverty and SC/ST status and, therefore, minimizes intersectional social inequalities in favour of a monocausal economic explanation. To resist such trends, the chapters in this section all address social identity-induced health care disparities. Economic subordinations, while universally present, are placed in a wider social milieu.

The opening chapter by **Sanghmitra S Acharya** analyzes persistent inequalities and their impact on health. Through a quantitative consideration of parameters of inequality and commitments to reduce inequality, she reflects on the health gap—which is significantly larger in India than neighbouring South Asian countries. She analyzes health inequalities as being symptomatic of systemic social and economic discrimination (Kabeer, 2000; Thorat, 2002; Shah, et al. 2006). She argues that social disadvantages underpin economic inequalities, which in turn drive differential access to health care resources. These systemic factors are placed in the immediate context of the pandemic. She deconstructs the inherent inequalities embedded in the mantra of 'social distancing'. Such pandemic protocols of maintaining distance disproportionately impact the already disenfranchised and build on uncomfortable associations with untouchability and pollution avoidance.

Dhananjay W Bansod, Pradeep S Salve and Suresh Jungari advance this argument by focussing on caste disparities in health care utilization in India. They argue that 'health' and 'health care' need to be distinguished. Factors outside the health sector play a key role in determining the health status of individuals and communities, such as the local standard of living, education, political enfranchisement, and access to basic minimum social services. A number of exogenous factors affect healthcare in any given society, including vernacular constructions of well-being which factor into the maximization of health care facilities (Jungari and Bomble, 2013). Their chapter focuses on health care utilization across different caste groups; and examines the factors affecting health care utilization among SC/STs compared to other social groups in India. The centrepiece of analysis is The National Family Health Survey-4 (NFHS-4). The paper also explores women's health indicators such as ANC4+, Adverse Pregnancy Outcomes (APO), child health, and low birth weight. Using empirical evidence, Bansod et al. have established that caste disparities factor into utilizing health care facilities.

Exploring beyond health care utilization, **Arindam Roy** outlines gendered health inequality within the households. He asserts that households, no matter how defined, have been constructed through a feminist epistemology as the primary site of women subjugation. Roy departs from the popular discourses on gender inequality by analyzing health care inequalities caused by systemic neglect, perpetrated by patriarchal households, of girl children from the time of their births (Sen and Ostin, 2012). The chapter proposes that the status of women in the household needs to be understood beyond economic deprivations, and needs to concentrate on girl child morbidity status to make sense of her secondary position within the household.

Similarly, **Smritima Diksha Lama** looks at the well-being of tea plantation workers in Darjeeling, in the Western Himalayas, a centre of quality tea production in the world. She highlights that despite the high quality and retail value of Darjeeling tea, the workers are largely excluded from benefiting (Besky, 2014). Based on fieldwork, she argues that a crucial aspect of their social precarity is inaccessibility of proper healthcare. Through an analysis of gender, she establishes a correlation between sociogenic factors and health. She observes that the social determinants of health play a definitive role in unequally distributing health outcomes.

Crossing the Himalayas, **Bamdev Subedi** discusses socioeconomic disparities in accessing health care services in Nepal. He points out that despite impressive progress in some health indicators in the past decades, equitable access to quality health care services remains elusive. Dalits, ethnic minorities, and the poor sections fall far below the national average. Based on village fieldwork conducted in Southwest Nepal, Subedi examines disparities among three major caste/ethnic communities (Brahmin/Chhetri, Adivasi/Janajati, and Dalits) in access and utilization of health care services. Based on his empirical findings, he argues that Dalits are increasingly utilizing health post services, which are the local outlets of government health care services. He notes that Dalits rely more on local health traditions, since individual expenditures are too high for western healthcare. He also suggests that the quality of traditional medicine, on which the underprivileged groups mostly rely, needs to be improved, along with their own knowledge of traditional medicines.

Last, **Chandani Liyanage** profiles the social epidemiology of chronic kidney disease with uncertain etiology in Sri Lanka. She illustrates persistent inequalities among agricultural communities in a dry zone of Sri Lanka, the country which is ranked best in South Asia regarding health indicators. Chronic Kidney Disease of uncertain etiology (CKDu) has become a critical health hazard in dry zone areas in Sri Lanka since the 1990s, adversely affecting agricultural communities. The disease was first identified by local health care providers by accident. Liyanage argues that structural violence and agricultural modernization are causal factors for the emerging disease (Bourguignon, and Farmer, 2004). She bases her arguments on fieldwork carried out in two breakout areas in a dry zone, and explains how CKDu reinforces persistent inequalities among agricultural communities there. She highlights the social stigmatizing practices around CKDu. When communities are labelled as 'CKDu hot spots', it impacts adversely on victims, which reinforces intergroup inequalities (de Silva 2012).

Chapter 14
Inequality and Exclusion in Access to HealthCare: Learning from the Pandemic

Sanghmitra S. Acharya

Abstract Inequality is historically known to impact negatively on poverty reduction and economic growth. It is also known to accentuate inequality and perpetuate differentials in access to resources providing health, education and employment opportunities. Therefore, inequality of any nature and form needs to be examined, evaluated and addressed to initiate and propel positive changes. Endemic poverty, unemployment, lack of sanitation and safe drinking water; and effective healthcare determine as much as produce inequalities. The labyrinth of social relations and institutions often result in the exclusion of certain social groups on the basis of identities like gender, caste, ethnicity, region and religion. This perpetuates inequality induced marginalization and discrimination affecting access to services, goods and resources which restrict knowledge acquisition and skill development. Social exclusion, however, does not necessarily equate to poverty. Although, there is a strong correlation between socially excluded groups and high levels of poverty which influence health and its correlates. In this unequal world, there are 'privileged' and 'underprivileged' groups whose status is determined by the conducive environment for propensity to access resources and avail opportunities. A discussion on inequality in the global and national context, and how inequality affects access further perpetuating exclusion, is imperative at this time when the pandemic COVID-19 has opened new dimensions of deliberation. This paper explores the prevailing inequalities and their impact on access to healthcare in general, and vulnerabilities of people engaged in works related to cleaning and cremation.

Keywords Inequality · Poverty reduction · Unemployment · Social exclusion · Cleaners

S. S. Acharya (✉)
Centre of Social Medicine and Community Health, School of Social Sciences, Jawaharlal Nehru University, New Delhi, India

© The Author(s), under exclusive license to Springer Nature Singapore Pte Ltd. 2022   275
S. S. Acharya and S. Christopher (eds.), *Caste, COVID-19, and Inequalities of Care*,
People, Cultures and Societies: Exploring and Documenting Diversities,
https://doi.org/10.1007/978-981-16-6917-0_14

Introduction: Recognizing an Unequal World

The unequal world is the function of lopsided resource distribution. The poorest 40% of the world's population accounts for five per cent, while the richest 20% accounts for three-fourths of world income. About 0.13% of the world's population controlled a quarter of world's assets, the richest 20% accounting for 77% of total private consumption as against just 1.5% by the poorest fifth. The world's 2,153 billionaires have more wealth than the 4.6 billion people who make up 60% of the planet's population. Countries where inequality has grown, are home to more than two-thirds (71%) of the world population (United Nations, 2020). However, income inequality has declined in most countries of Latin America and the Caribbean and in several African and Asian countries over the last two decades. Despite progress in some countries, income and wealth are increasingly concentrated at the top. The share of income going to the richest one per cent of the global population increased in 46 out of 57 countries from 1990 to 2015. The bottom 40% earned less than 25% of income in all 92 countries (United Nations, 2019). Differential access is evident in the priorities in spending set by different countries. Japan prioritizes the entertainment sector to spend US$ 35 billion. Europe spends US$ 105 billion on alcoholic drinks, US$50 billion in cigarettes and US$ 11 billion in ice cream. Cosmetics in the United States are prioritized at US$ 8Billions. The world spending amounts to US$ 400 for narcotic drugs and US$ 780 for military. As compared to this spending, the additional cost to achieve universal access to basic services in all developing countries is US$ 7 billion for education; US$ 9 billion for water and sanitation; and US$ 15 billion for reproductive health (HDR, 2018). Therefore, exclusive sectors-alcohol, cigarettes, cosmetics, for instance, are prioritized over education and health nationally and globally. This also reflects on the attention given to the privileged versus underprivileged populations. It is evident who wants luxury and lifestyle consumer goods and who needs basic services. Such planning strategies by the governments are known to perpetuate inequality and poverty often leading to exclusion and discrimination (Sen, 1992; Kabeer, 2000).

Understanding Inequality as Privilege and Disadvantage

Against this backdrop of global trends, some questions become pertinent. What is inequality? Why do inequalities exist? How is it connected to privilege and disadvantage? In simple terms inequality means unequal access to resources which create a gap between privileged and underprivileged groups because some people and the groups they belong to are disadvantaged (or underprivileged) as compared to the others; have poorer or no access to resources than others; experience disadvantage and have poor access due to their group identity. This influences access to wealth and health and the most important correlates employment, education. The disadvantaged position leads to prejudicial treatment and deliberate denial of access causing lack of material benefits and basic necessities, possession of assets and humiliation. This labyrinth is often interconnected and engages with marginalization, undermining equality and equity. Thus, marginalization may be explained as the treatment of a person or group as insignificant or peripheral through the process of making a group or class of people less important or relegated to a secondary position. This labyrinth includes:

EXCLUSION: keeping someone/some groups out; they are deliberately not included.

DISCRIMINATION: unjust or prejudicial treatment of different categories of people, especially on the grounds of race, age, sex, or disability.

DEPRIVATION: lack of material benefits considered to be basic necessities in a society; being kept from possessing assets, enjoying, or using services, resources and opportunities.

HUMILIATION: to reduce (someone/some groups) to a lower position in one's own eyes and/or others' eyes.

Most disadvantaged or underprivileged population groups are poor, and most privileged groups are non-poor (IIPS & ICF, 2017; NCDHR, 2019). Often the 'misery' of the underprivileged or disadvantaged is often explained by the demographic characteristics and the limited nature of resources.

The literature on why these inequalities persist, or even widen, in spite of the increases in overall educational levels, remains poorly developed. Educational credentials exclude the marginalized groups due to the prejudiced preconceived notions of 'sub-standard'. Hence, educational systems conceived by the privileged elites often put impediments that support excluding the subordinate groups from higher education (Jadhav, Mosse, & Dostaler, 2016) due to economic as well as social reasons. This is significant in the light of privatization, making higher education economically inaccessible, and socially difficult to access by the underprivileged. Food productivity has increased since independence (Patnaik, 2008), though the storage facilities have played havoc with the grains.

In India, there has been a steady decline in decadal growth of population from 24.80% in 1971 to 17.64% in 2011. Infant Mortality Rate (IMR) has declined from 165 per 1000 live births in 1950–55 to 53 in 2005–2010. Crude Birth Rate has almost halved from 43.3 during the same year to 23.1 during 2005–2010. Crude Death Rates (CDR) dropped from 25.5 to 8.3 during the same period. Fertility too declined from 5.9 to 2.73 (MoHFW, 2015). Literacy has also improved in the last five decades (Fig. 14.1). Despite these positive changes, some people have access to resources and services while others do not have or have partial access. It is this realm of resources allocation and access, that determines the level of poverty. Redistribution of resources to deficit regions and the creation of an enabling environment for the deprived populations to access the resources and services is what constructs the relationship between development and inequality, rather than population size or growth.

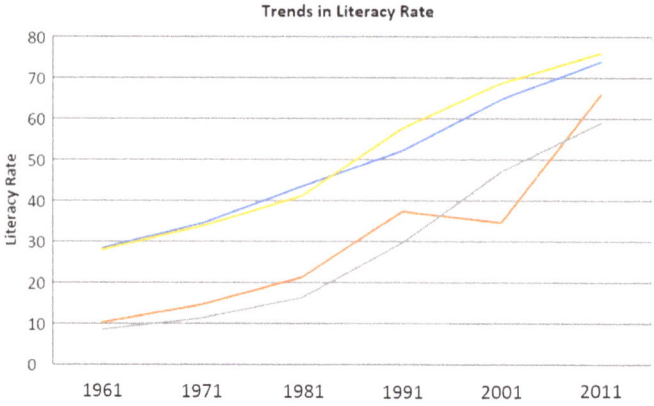

Fig. 14.1 Trends in literacy rate. *Source* RGI (2011)

Wealth and Income Inequality

Wealth and income reflect on economic propensity which influences access to resources and determines inequality and exclusion. As stated earlier, among those who are poor, the majority also belong to the socially disadvantaged. About 11% among SCs are in the highest wealth quintile as compared to about 27% in lowest. wealth quintile. Similarly, among the STs, the share is 5.5% in the highest and 46% in the lowest wealth quintile. It is remarkable that a little over 10% underprivileged castes (SCs) as against about 36% privileged castes (others) are among the highest wealth quintile. In contrast, about 28% SCs compared to about 10% others are in the lowest wealth quintile. Within castes, the highest differences are among privileged castes—and growing—and the least wealth differences are to be found among SCs. This is evident from the National Family Health Survey 2015–16 (NFHS-4).

It is noteworthy that among OBCs and STs too, the top 10% cornered most, around 52% of wealth in 2012. Among the top 10% of SCs, the share of their wealth increased by three percentage points to 46.7% by 2012. The privileged caste households earned nearly 47% more than the national average annual household income. The top 10% within these castes owned 60% of the wealth within the group in 2012. The wealthiest one per cent among them grew their wealth by nearly 16 percentage points to 29.4% by 2012. The wealth and income gap are large and growing across all castes. Since 1991 when the structural adjustment programme was ushered, till 2016, in the 35 years, the share of wealth held by the top 10% has increased 24% points to 55% (Bharti, 2018).

Marginalized caste groups such as the Scheduled Castes (SCs) and Scheduled Tribes (STs) earn much less than the national household income average of Rs. 113,222. The SC and ST households earned 21% and 34%, respectively, less than the national average. The OBC households fared better but still earned 8% or Rs 9,123 less than the annual Indian average. In contrast, among privileged caste groups,

Brahmins earned 48% above the national average and non-Brahmin privileged castes, 45%. Restating her position as one of the most unequal countries, India has the top 10% population controlling 55% of the total wealth, recording an increase from 31% in 1980. Others (non-Hindu, non-Muslim groups and those who do not fall under the SC, ST and OBC categories) were found to be the richest group, though they make for only 1.5% of the country's population. They earned an annual income of Rs 242,708, twice the annual household income average in India (Bharti, 2018). This was evident almost a decade earlier in the works of Attewell and Madheswaran (2007), Deshpande and Newman (2007) and Borooah et al. (2014). All their research supports the inference that marginalization of the underprivileged caste groups is a pivotal factor which restricts access to resources causing inequality. Beteille (1969) observed 'Caste, kinship or family, either or all these can hamper economic progress if they impose restrictions', much earlier.

Inequality and poverty among rural households in India were studied using household monthly per capita consumption expenditure data of nearly 20,000 households by Borooah et al. (2014). It examined whether inequality and poverty in India were induced by caste, or whether distributional and deprivation outcomes are 'caste blind' and entirely determined by the attributes of the individual households. The central inference drawn was that households' outcomes with respect to their position on the distributional ladder, or with respect to their chances of being poor, are dependent on their caste. The Scheduled Castes (SCs) and Scheduled Tribes (STs) vis-à-vis the privileged caste groups, experience lived reality of subordination, humiliation and subservience in everyday life in modern India. The study explored human development, inequality, poverty, education, child malnutrition, health, employment, wages, gender, and access to public goods and established that the privileged caste Hindu households perform far better compared to the SC, ST, and Muslim households because of the differential access to resources and services which support better outcomes. More recently, the relationship between happiness and the social group to which one belongs, was examined. Findings corroborate the thesis of subordination, subjugation, powerlessness and consequent exclusion of those who belonged to the 'underprivileged groups' (Borooah, 2020).

A large proportion of the existing poverty is explained by inequality induced discrimination (Attewell & Madheswaran, 2007; Borooah et al., 2014). The Rangarajan Committee[1] was assigned the task to revisit the Tendulkar Panel's formula for estimation of poverty. The new poverty line put the number of poor at 363 million in 2011–12 as against 270 million estimated by the Tendulkar Panel. Those spending less than INR 30 in rural areas and INR 47 in urban areas were to be considered as poor. By the new estimates, the number of poor declined from 455 million in 2009–2010 (Table 14.1).

---

[1] Expert Group to Review the Methodology for Measurement of Poverty, also known as the Rangarajan Expert Committee, was set up by the then Planning Commission to review the poverty levels indicated by its predecessor, the Tendulkar Expert Committee that yielded very low rural and urban poverty lines.

Table 14.1 Shifting load of poverty by different measurements

Poverty measurement methodology	Poor as % of India's population	NOTE
C Rangarajan Committee	29.5 (N = 363 million)	Expenditure of Rs. 47 a day (urban) and Rs. 30 a day (rural)
Suresh Tendulkar Committee	21.9 (N-270 million)	Expenditure of Rs. 33 a day (urban) and Rs. 27 a day (rural)
World Bank[a]	21.2	US$1.25 a day per person on purchasing power parity of INR 18.75
World Bank[b]	12.4	US$1.90 a day per person on purchasing power parity of INR 28.5

Source Planning Commission (2012)
[a]https://www.business-standard.com/article/economy-policy/world-bank-poverty-estimates-are-poorsays-government-115102100056_1.htm
[b]https://povertydata.worldbank.org/poverty/country/IND

Such persisting inequalities are known to produce exclusion and discrimination, denying access to resources, opportunities and services which augment incomes, wealth and social position. It is imperative to understand inequality as a trigger for exclusion and discrimination affecting the well-being of population. Health as an important constituent of well-being merits understanding.

Inequality and Health: The Interconnect

Health is an important component of well-being. Inequalities in income and educational attainment contribute to health inequality. Analysis of inequalities in health and health systems provides a key insight for making societies more inclusive. More than a quarter (26–29%) of people in the lowest income segment and lower social position do not avail care they need due to costs compared to 8–14% of people with the highest income level and higher social position. Households in the bottom income quintile (where populations with low social position are located) are more likely to incur catastrophic health spending (Solar, 2010: Pampel et al., 2010). Inequality and health are significantly associated with mortality. The slope in the relationship between socioeconomic status (SES) and health shows that each level of the hierarchy exhibits less morbidity and mortality than lower levels (Adler et al., 1994, 1999; Marmot, 2015). Studies document that the slope is characterized by a threshold, usually around the median for income, where additional increases in SES have a diminished effect in reducing morbidity and mortality rates (Kitagawa & Hauser, 1973; Wilkinson, 1986; Williams, 1990). Even though overall mortality rates have been declining, socioeconomic differentials in mortality have been widening in recent decades. Comparing data from the 1960s to those for the late 1970s and 1980s, U.S. studies reveal that income and educational differentials have widened over time (Williams and Collins, 1995; Thorat, 2007; United Nations, 2020). Similarly, widening socio-economic differentials in mortality have been observed in England, Wales, France, Finland, Norway, and the Netherlands (Department of Health & Social Security, 1980) and in other parts of the world (Mackenbach et al., 1989; Kunst & Mackenbach, 1994; Solar & Irwin, 2010; Borooah et al., 2014, 2015; Lynch, 2017).

Social Exclusions and the Health Gap

Social exclusion is a denial of access to resources, opportunities, and services due to some group-based attributes such as ethnicity, race, caste and religion, rather than the status of an individual such as joblessness, social protection, differently abled, delinquent, widowed, single motherhood etc. Basis of exclusion is perpetual, unlike status. Therefore, exclusion necessarily is permanent and not transient. A jobless person can get a job, social protection can be received, differently abled can get some support. But members of a race, ethnicity and caste group remain with the groups always. Discrimination is defined as the distinction between people on the basis of disability, gender, sexual orientation, age, religion etc., leading to levels of inequality which impair social functioning of individuals (Kabeer, 2000; Shah, et al., 2006; Thorat, 2002). Discrimination against groups, can be social, economic, personal or political. An explanation regarding the difference and relationship between social exclusion and discrimination, would be in order here. Discrimination refers to preferential treatment of some over others. But once it is systematically practised against some groups, it metamorphoses in social exclusion. Social exclusion is more intense than discrimination. It implies discrimination in absolute terms, complete denial of access to resources, opportunities and services.

The notion of social exclusion is an expression first developed by Rene Lenoir (1974) based on labour market discrimination examined by Becker (1971). Social exclusion is also defined as 'discrimination against culturally defined groups' (de Haan, 2007). It occurs when some groups are discriminated against, because of the prejudice, and are perceived to be inferior (Darity, 1998), or are disliked by those who have 'a taste for discrimination' (Becker, 1971). Inferiority is often attributed to genetics (DNA) or group-based cultural norms, both of which have no empirical basis as group characteristics and amount to 'blaming the victim' (Darity, 1998). It is not an individual sentiment, but a reflection of a collective (dis)interest against and apathy towards the excluded group (Thorat, 2007, 2018; Borooah, 2020). It is institutionalized through rules of social behaviour. It is also reflected in 'unfavourable inclusion' (Sen, 2000) where certain identified groups are forced to engage in some inferior (polluting, demeaning and low paid) activities, while kept away from better (profitable, socially desired and high paid) activities.

Health is influenced by social exclusion and inequality (Wilkinson, 1990; Adler et al., 1994; Krieger, 2000; Marmot, 2015; Acharya, 2020). By ensuring access to quality care, through prevention and public health policies, health systems play a key role in improving health outcomes. Health systems can contribute to reducing inequalities if they enable access to services based on needs rather than the ability to pay. Access to health resources is materialized through the availability of resources and personnel. Denial of access to resources consequent of exclusion due to social identities is evident in access to health care resources too as all other resources.

Poverty, Social Exclusion and Ill-Health

Poverty and social exclusion are often taken for granted while considering ill-health effects (Narayan, 2018; Nayar, 2007). Social exclusion in health refers to the complete denial of access to health resources and services, such as the refusal of being treated at a hospital. In Indian context it is practised on the basis of caste and untouchability due to which some groups and individuals are denied the rights and opportunities which others enjoy. Discrimination against certain groups occurs in most societies. In India, caste is the unique feature lending itself as a formidable axis for exclusion and discrimination. Caste is synonymous with low socio-economic status and poverty. In the identification of the poor, Scheduled Caste and Scheduled Tribes and in some cases the Other Backward Castes may be considered as socially disadvantaged groups who have a higher probability of living under adverse conditions and are thus prone to ill-health (Acharya, 2017; Diwakar, 2015; Kumar, 2019). The health status and utilization of services by such groups give an indication of their social exclusion as well as an idea of the linkages between inequality and health (Banerji, 1982; Nayar, 2007). Caste, income and regional inequalities determine health (Baru et al., 2010). The Scheduled Tribes and Scheduled Castes in poor wealth quintiles are at a greater disadvantage in all indicators of health as compared to other groups (Acharya, 2017; Narayan, 2018; Raushan & Acharya, 2019).

Government Efforts to Reduce Health Inequalities

Governments are responsible for reducing inequality in health by addressing medical errors and enhancing safety. They are expected to provide healthcare, ensure access to quality care for vulnerable populations, and regulate health care markets for equitable access. They are also expected to support the acquisition of new knowledge to nurture the health care workforce; develop and evaluate health technologies and practices; monitor health care quality; inform healthcare decision makers, and convene stake-holders from across the health care system to address health inequalities. Therefore, the New Agenda for Health includes social determinants of health.

   As a signatory to the Alma Ata Declaration in 1978, revitalizing primary health-care was seen as inevitable in order to meet these challenges. The role of the government in influencing population health is not limited to the health sector. Intersectoral connections across sectors, viz, transport, agriculture, employment and education,

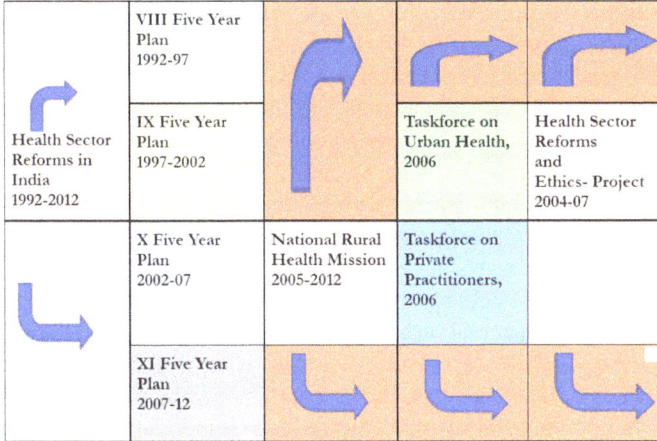

Fig. 14.2 Strategies of the Health Sector Reforms in India. *Source* Author

besides the health systems become relevant. The government's role in ensuring a healthy population across social groups, and protecting the public's health equitably across social groups become pertinent. The health sector reforms ushered in the early 1990s during the Eight Five Year Plan, lead to the launch of many schemes and programmes for the purpose. The National Rural Health Mission (NRHM) was initiated in 2005 with two task forces being set up for urban health and private practitioners (Fig. 14.2). Subsequently, the schemes and strategies were subsumed under the National Health Mission.

Ensuring Healthy Lives?

The Sustainable Development Goal 3 aims to achieve universal health coverage, and provide access to safe and effective medicines and vaccines for all—leaving no one behind. However, the challenges faced in doing so have been many in the last one year ever since the unprecedented pandemic has overstressed the already burdened health system in India. Economic deprivation in a large segment of the population, especially socially excluded, generally results in poor access to healthcare. Poor educational status leads to non-utilization of scanty health services and increase in avoidable risk factors especially the underprivileged. The current pandemic has only strengthened the health inequalities. One of the major concerns has been the low access of socially marginalized and underprivileged populations to health services.

It is evident from the NFHS-4 data that in India, STs and the SCs are most deprived of basic health facilities. The SCs and the STs have to travel longer to reach a health facility, and most of them are not able to meet the provider as compared to 'others'. It is noteworthy that the difference, however, is reducing, yet the gap between privileged and underprivileged persists (Fig. 14.1).

Since the persistent gap continues, it is evident that, while there has been an overall improvement in health indicators, the current policies have failed to achieve the expected outcomes among the underprivileged groups (Diwakar, 2015). Similar reflections are evident from the Janani Suraksha Yojana (JSY) initiated in 2005 under the National Rural Health Mission (NRHM) for improving the Maternal Mortality Rate (MMR) by promoting institutional delivery. The scheme is often used to measure the level of access to maternal and child health. The financial incentives provided to mothers for institutional delivery and institutional care during delivery was instrumental in improving maternal and child health among the Dalits (Diwakar, 2015; Behara & Acharya, 2020). Women from underprivileged groups face greater problems in accessing healthcare than those from among the privileged caste groups (Fig. 14.3). While financial barriers emerge as an important factor for nearly one-fifth of the women from the underprivileged groups, availability of the care providers affects 45–46% underprivileged women as compared to 42% from privileged groups. Distance from the health facility as a problem in accessing health facilities needs to be seen in the light of the socio-physical layout of the settlements. About 33% SCs and 42% ST women experienced distance as an obstruction to access care as opposed to less than a quarter of women from the privileged groups. Exclusion on the axes of space in addition to financial strength is clearly reflected.

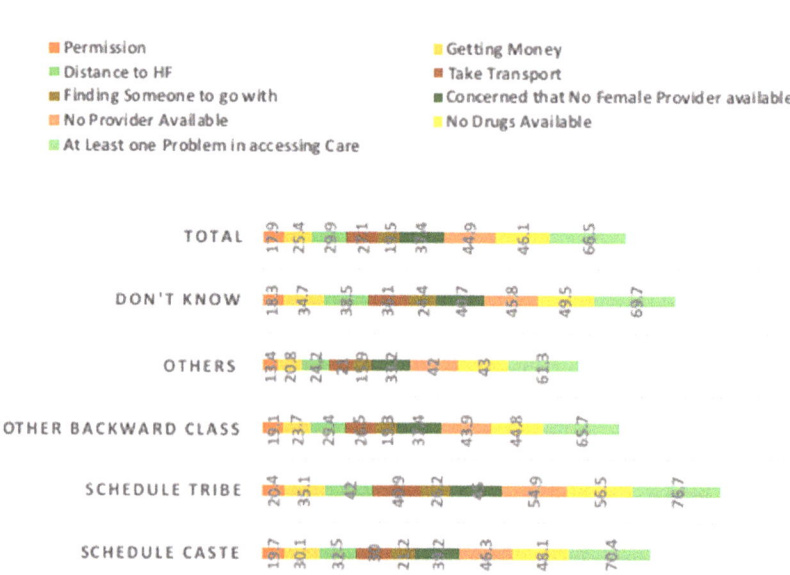

Fig. 14.3 Problems in accessing health 2015–16. *Source* IIPS & ICF (2017). Table 11.21, NFHS 4, 2015–16

Pandemic Lessons for Health Equity

The COVID-19 spread globally in a short span of time of less than two months lead the World Health Organization (WHO) to pronounce it as a health emergency on 30 January, 2020, the same day when India reported its first case. An interesting similarity is that the measures instituted to contain the outbreak at both the time points— 1918 and 2020, roughly 100 years apart, include 'social distancing' measures like isolation, quarantine, masks, hand washing, staggering rush hour to reduce crowds in the public spaces and transport systems- despite the technological advancements which the medical sciences have achieved since then. Lockdown at the national level, however, did not appear as a measure at the earlier time point. The pandemic has been used, in this paper, to illustrate the vulnerabilities of three disadvantaged groups- the migrant workers in the informal sector; dead body handlers in the cremation grounds; and the cleaners. These groups are stark examples of both social and economic disadvantages, because most of them hail from underprivileged communities and have restricted or no access to resources for improving their education, skills and employability.

Migrant Workers in the Informal Sector

The workers in the informal sector are largely migrants who adopted various cities as their '*karmbhoomi*' and dedicated their lives to build those cities by contributing their labour. They felt orphaned when the lockdown version 1.0 was announced. There were 562 active cases and the death toll was 13 (Ministry of Health & Family welfare, 2020). The 'city lights' which fueled their dreams and propelled them to toil to achieve them and aspire for more, the lockdown halted their lives with a jolt which threw them off the track. Their aspirational journeys were derailed on that fateful night, which gave them a few hours to prepare for it. The alternative perhaps was to block and restrict movement in the hotspots, rather than the country-wide lockdown.

The lock down version 1.0 required to give sufficient time to the people to plan their lives. Consequent to the lockdown, the work units shut down rendering most migrant workers in the informal sector, both jobless and homeless. The landlords were not willing to let them stay in their rented dwellings for the fear of non-payment of rent in the light of lost jobs; and the associated uncertainty with it. Therefore, as they left their homes in distress, access to food, shelter and sanitation facilities became dismal. While different states announced financial assistance, adverse stories compel us to think about the ways in which the state announcements were being executed. If people were allowed to disperse, rather than herded together without much support, the spread of infection would have been minimal, since till then, much of the transmission was associated with international travel.

Containing the streams of migrant workers within the cities became unmanageable in the absence of a robust plan by the end of the version 1.0. Employers were unsure of the ways in which their units will recover from the loss incurred due to four lockdowns and, therefore, were not able to engage with their employees. Govt strictures that employers must pay the wages during the period of lockdown had little logic especially when the state itself was reluctant in waiving off many such taxes. It had little logic and the workers had little choice than to say goodbye to their respective cities which they made their homes.

The trains needed to ply to bring the workers home, before they had contracted the infection in the herded spaces where they were lodged. But by the time the government decided to launch—'*shramik special*'—one wonders why 'special trains' when we already have the largest railway network in the world? What needed to be stipulated is the restricted capacity may be 1/3 or even 1/4 of the total, and would have saved many lives. As regards the 'special' trains, there certainly was nothing special about these trains! Why was that fanfare done to the trains carrying the migrant workers? Expenditure incurred on those events could have been put to a better use— ensuring that the tickets were available without hassles, for example. If *Vande Bharat* could be launched for international travellers to bring them back home, regular trains were the answer for the internal travellers. Once in the home state, more than the quarantine centres (QCs), home quarantine could have relieved the additional burden on already sagging public health. The initial fear and forceful taking away to and confining in the quarantine centres also stigmatized the plausible cases, which most likely went underground. Especially when the QCs needed more support, both in terms of infrastructure and personnel.

Cleaners

Much has been documented about workers in the informal sector, especially migrants and their experience of inequality in access to resources in the cities they chose to make their home. In this 'war' against COVID-19 a lot has been said about the 'frontline' workers—the doctors, and the nurses. In this 'armament-less war', the most neglected have been the cleaners—those who collect, transport and dispose waste, clean toilets, drains and sewer mostly manually; and work in the hospices. They continued to work while the world was 'staying home', yet their 'frontline' visibility was clouded by the prejudicial treatment by the others. From hospice to public spaces, domestic dwellings, offices and institutions, as 'essential services providers', they continued working without Personal protection Equipment (PPE). Despite the need for their vocation, provisioning of protective gear has been far from real for them even before the pandemic forced the voices for the PPE to be heard. The concern for their condition was tabled way back in 1949 through Scavengers' Living Conditions Enquiry Committee headed by BN Bavre; and subsequently other committees (Scavenging Conditions Enquiry Committee, 1960; and Customary Rights to Scavengers, 1969) headed by NR Malkani, reiterated their appalling conditions. It was only in 1994 that the National Commission for Safai Karamcharis came into existence and since then, has been responsible for executing many recommendations of the earlier committees. But much still remains to be done, especially in the light of COVID-19.

The cleaners provide an essential public service we all rely on. But it costs them their health, safety and dignity. They are mostly employed by the railways, urban local bodies and institutions of all kinds, both public and private. Their jobs are mostly in the informal economy without basic labour protections or rights, making them the most vulnerable workers. They are the backbone of the waste management system of the country. Yet, they have no, or very little social security, available only for those in the formal sector employment. They face rampant discrimination, but still keep our cities clean. They are enveloped in the conditions that expose them to debilitating infections, injuries, social stigma and even death from toxic gases and pit collapses. Now, they are also at risk of exposure to COVID-19 from handling unmarked medical and contaminated waste. Those in the hospices have been exposed to as much viral load as other frontline workers. But safety gears for them had a lower priority in the light of shortage. These are systemic problems which emanate from the caste-based society which relegates the cleaning occupations to specific caste groups positioned at the lower levels of social strata. Their historical deprivation has marginalized them allowing poor propensity. Inevitably, this has become the justification of their continuance of working with minimal support if any. While nearly half of them do not have any protective gear, only few of them are able to use them because they do not fit well and are heavy to use (Acharya, 2018). They obstruct more than support working.

A petition was filed by the Municipal *Safai Kamgar* and the Delhi Commission for *Safai Karamchari* on 8 May, 2020, pointing that the cleaners were exposed to hazardous material and gases. In the absence of protective gear, men were using handkerchiefs, and women their *sari pallav* or *dupatta*, in place of a mask. They were not even paid their wages for months. The Delhi Municipal Authority and the Delhi Government Health Department categorically stated that the WHO guidelines to deal with the COVID-19 pandemic were strictly followed to ensure protection of the cleaners. But despite that, not only their exposure continues, but also their enumeration in terms of work and exposure to COVID-19 remains unrecorded. There is no official documentation of their getting infected as well as affected. Many of them have been infected, exposing their families and communities to the spread of COVID-19. In fact, there is no record of the cleaners in the country, other than that collected by NGOs like Safai Karamchari Abhiyan (SKA) and Jan Sahas. The last census (2011) collected data on types of toilets which was used to estimate the number of cleaners as about seven lakh which was gross underestimation as compared to the NGOs including the project on sanitation workers undertaken by Dalberg Advisors which placed the number between 5–7 million.[2] Therefore, generating data on these crucial workers, particularly so during the health emergency which we are facing at the present.

---

[2] Dalberg Advisors (2017). Understanding Indian sanitation workers, and finding solutions for their challenges. https://dalberg.com/our-ideas/understanding-indian-sanitation-workers-and-finding-solutions-their-challenges/.

'Masaan' Workers

Those engaging in the actual act of handling the corpse for consigning them to the 'holy flames' belong to the Dom community, one of the lowest in the caste hierarchy. They are the traditional corpse-burners. They work in the heat; grey ash, to which the burnt bodies are reduced; and look impoverished and undernourished defying all efforts to prove otherwise. They often wrap a bright orange scarf (*gamchha*) around their head, and wear a black thread around the neck, pronouncing proximity to the Eternal One! Doing this work calls for attuning themselves to the smell of the burnt flesh, flames and smoke, amidst wailing of the loved ones. To endure this, their natural instinctive bent is towards the intoxicants such as cannabis (*ganja*), and liquor, often locally brewed. They emanate a mix of odours containing flashes of all these and the sweat. The cremation workers in at Manikarnika Ghat, the largest open-cremation site on the banks of the Ganga are the epitome of deprivation, disadvantage and perpetuated exclusion with minimal intergenerational mobility. The workers at various cremation grounds across the country have been working without being equipped even with the proper protective gears, leave alone the PPEs (Kumar, 2021). Most of them start working early in life. Due to the nature of work and the hazards involved, they take to alcohol consumption too early. The profession is inherited from the forefathers. While only the men of the community work, the women remain behind the confines of their homes. The work is tedious and was aggravated during the second wave of COVID-19. It was round the clock for nearly a month. Most of the handlers work for *maaliks*—the richer and influential Doms, who hire the poorer and vulnerable ones often on the work basis. The *maaliks* command the function of the cremation grounds. During the COVID-19 surge in April–May, 2021, transactions for cremation brought them fortunes which they perhaps had not earned ever before. Like always, they interacted directly with the families, bargained on the amount and cost of the wood to be used. In normal times it ranges from Rs 6,000–12,000. During the second wave, much like the private sector hospitals, many cremation *maaliks* enlivened the saying 'make hay while the sun shines' charging two to three times more money. The handlers got nothing in addition to their usual wages. In normal times too, they get a fraction of what the *maaliks* earn. To supplement their earnings, they are (and they were during COVID too) forced to sieve the ashes swept into the river from the cremation ground, to scavenge for gold and silver jewellery on the dead bodies. They often swim and dive for hours irrespective of weather, to earn some more. This way of additional earning is treated better than the heat of the burning bodies. (Iyengar, 2017). During the surge in the death due to COVID-19 during April–May this year, the burning of the bodies was incessant. The cremation workers have been working extra hours, almost round the clock because the pyre had to be readied for the next corpse. They were getting no or at best an hour or two of sleep.[3] Even in normal times they are woken up in the nights by their employers,

---

[3] Based on an informal discussion at Lodhi Road Crematorium with a worker handling the corpses on 26 April 2021.

often treated badly with the use of abusive language including manhandling.[4] It is noteworthy that while the relatives of the dead people were all masked and wore gloves, most of the cremation workers handling the bodies were without either of the two protective gears.

It is noteworthy that the persons at the airport are screened with respect while the migrant labourers are sprayed with disinfectants queuing them up in the herd with their hands up as the criminals. And what about the persons engaging in sanitation, waste picking and garbage collection, its transportation and disposal? Their work allows them very little option to wash hands as frequently as per the government advisories, and stay at home. Some institutions decided to stop the sanitation workers from door-to-door collection of garbage on their premises, but had to withdraw the order within a day. Most of them are migrants and are employed by urban local bodies and private firms. Most of them are poor and hail from Dalit communities and live-in squatters and slums where availability and storage of water itself is a concern. Their plight is twofold- they deal with garbage and filth, are exposed to viruses, bacteria, poisonous gases and are also vulnerable to accidents; and have little that they can do to practice the kind of personal hygiene being propagated. For them bathing is needed, hand washing is not enough to do away with the lingering stench of the filth from which they eke out their livelihood. More importantly, they need to use the masks and the gloves for their work even without the COVID-19 scare. In times of this crisis, they are all the more necessary for them. They are hardly seen using these basic safety gears, forget about the more sophisticated one which such workers in other countries are supplied with. Is it because they overwhelmingly come from Dalit communities, while the medical professionals do not, and the lives of the cleaners are perceived less valuable than the doctors?

Like the cleaners, data on cremation ground workers are also not available through official data sources. In the absence of any data, invisibility becomes inevitable and any intervention remains elusive. As these special workers continue to work during these testing times while others 'stay home', their exposure to risks has been immense. This also provokes the mind to consider what has been packaged under the phrase 'Social Distance'.

Terminological Inequalities: 'Social Distance' and 'Infection Safe'

The term 'social distancing' evolved during the 1918 Spanish Flu, which infected about 500 million persons and killed about 20–50 million people as documented in the pandemic history, the *Pale Rider* by Laura Spinney (2017). This term has been largely used by epidemiologists, to convey physical distance between socially connected people. Most of them, situated in western hemisphere, are unaware of

---

[4] Based on the narrative from cremation workers at Nigambodh Ghat. Delhi on 6 May 2021.

the social distancing which is practised in the Indian sub-continent given the hierarchical structure of our society. Since social stratification is endemic to South Asia,
the term appears appropriate for the nations who do not experience and practice it.
In our case, it categorically has to be stated as 'contagion distance'—keeping away
from the infection, to differentiate from 'social distance' which we practice fairly
much, given the graded inequalities entrenched in our society. No person affected
with coronavirus is 'socially untouchable'. The 'untouchability'—need to maintain
'contagion distance'—is caused due to infection. The need is, therefore, to get protection from the infection, thus '*infection safe*'. We in India practice 'social distancing'
fairly widely since long, and in a context which makes the phrase highly discriminatory. We are socially distant from, and critical of, each other on the basis of religion,
caste, region, language, ethnicity, colour, age, residence, gender, economic status
etc., despite the Constitutional safeguard professing otherwise. Taking cognizance
of this, the World Health Organization (WHO) replaced the phrase by 'physical
distance' from 20 March 2020.

Addressing the health needs is urgent and non-negotiable. However, in unequal
India, this may be the most difficult task even when it is made to believe that the
disease does not discriminate. We need to remember strictly what the system and its
elements do.

Containment Measures

As evident from the government's own admission, in the National Health
Profile 2019, the public spending on health was just 1.17% of the Gross Domestic
Product, although striving to increase it to more than 2.5%. This pandemic is the
apt time to mend the long-drawn mistake of continued inadequate share of GDP for
health. A major proportion of health expenditure is borne by households as out-of-
pocket expenditure (OOPE) in India. The already precarious incomes of the workers
considered here makes them helpless in want of resources. This situation has aggravated tremendously, twofold, as a worker in hazardous conditions and inadequate
provisions; and as an affected person. Therefore, since this pandemic is not a disease
caused by lifestyle habits or socio-cultural reasons, the need is that medication is
necessarily subsidized. The mechanism to regulate these services from hoarding
and black market needs to be stipulated and put in place. Access to vaccines for
all; and vaccination has to be free of cost, in the public sector. Across the world
vaccination has been promoted by the state without the citizens having to pay for it.
With budgetary allocations having been done for the purpose, the onus rests on the
government.

Nudges and Boosts

Of late the nudge theory[5] has been used among the health professionals to help them decide on various issues including hand hygiene. The same can be applied to improve hand hygiene and use of masks for the COVID safety protocol, among the cleaners (or conservancy), informal sector migrant and cremation workers to decrease the work-associated infections. This, however, has to be alongside the employers and the state. An enabling environment needs to be created for making a more thought-out decision for the allowance of the nudge for the purpose devised. It also provides the scope to undo the wrongs done historically to the communicates which provide these sets of workers. This is likely to widen the opportunities for these communities and their workers. Emanating from psychology and behavioural economics, 'nudge', are interventions which 'direct people in a particular direction while preserving their freedom of choice' with a fiscal component (Thaler & Sunstein, 2008). In contrast, 'boosts' aim to nurture people's capability to make their own choices, and to exercise their own agency. Building on this distinction, relevant support from the employers and the stare will be imperative. It can also be used for the implementation of the regulatory mechanisms for provisioning healthcare service to people in general and to these workers in particular (Ralph Hertwig & Till Grüne-Yanoff, 2016).

Conclusion

The Goal 10 of the SDGs is to reduce inequality within and among countries. It aims to empower and promote the social, economic and political inclusion of all, irrespective of age, sex, disability, race, ethnicity, origin, religion or economic or other status; ensure equal opportunity and reduce inequalities of outcome, including by eliminating discriminatory laws, policies and practices and promoting appropriate legislation, policies and action in this regard; formulate and implement policies, especially fiscal, wage and social protection policies, and progressively achieve greater equality. Development indicators at aggregate level have improved in last decade or so. Poverty has declined indicating improvement in well-being indicated through improved infant and maternal mortality. Literacy, access to drinking water and sanitation facilities have also improved; and the houseless population has decreased for the country as a whole. However, the disaggregated data on different social groups tell a different story. Rate of improvement for SC and ST has been slower than the 'Others' who have benefitted more than the excluded groups due to inequalities which have continued historically.

Health should be perceived as an investment and receive greater budgetary allocation. Education, safe water and sanitation need priority. Therefore, monitoring health

---

[5] The 'nudge' concept was popularized in the 2008 through the book' Nudge-Improving Decisions About Health, Wealth and Happiness' authored by the behavioural economist Richard Thaler and legal scholar Cass Sunstein, University of Chicago.

inequalities across social groups is essential for achieving health equity. Health inequality monitoring requires health data disaggregated by relevant inequality dimensions such as demographic, social, economic, geographical factors in order to identify health differentials between population sub groups. Disaggregated data provide evidence on who is being left behind and informs equity-oriented policies, programmes and practices. Data on COVID-19 too needs to be collected and disaggregated by social groups to reflect on the inequality and exclusion experienced by some groups. Global Inequality Report 2020 observed that addressing inequality is a matter of political choice. Therefore, India must increase its public expenditure on health; and provide data disaggregated by social groups in addition to space, gender and age. Else, even the pandemics of such severity, will not be able to salvage the 'illness' we are suffering from.

To ensure healthcare access among the vulnerable populations is the prerogative of the State since the financial burden of curative care is higher among lower income groups, most of whom are Dalits. There is evident association of low health status with poor, women, rural, tribal, scheduled castes and even minority groups. Therefore, the need is to revisit policy environments and implementation regimes to ensure health equity through socially conscious public health systems.

References

Acharya, S. S. (2017). Health equity in India: An examination through the lens of social exclusion. *Journal of Social Inclusion Studies, 4*(1), 104–130.

Acharya, S. (2018). Health equity in India: an examination through the lens of social exclusion. *Journal of Social Inclusion Studies, 4*(1), 104–130.

Acharya, S. S. (2020). 'Population-poverty linkages and health consequences: Understanding global social group inequalities'. *CASTE: A Global Journal on Social Exclusion, 1*(1), 29–50.

Adler, N. E., Boyce, T., Chesney, M. A., Cohen, S., Folkman, S., Kahn, R. L., & Syme, S. L. (1994). Socioeconomic status and health. The challenge of the gradient. *American Psychologist, 49*(1):15–24.

Adler, N. E., & Ostrove, J. M. (1999) Socioeconomic status and health: what we know and what we don't. *896*, 3–15. https://doi.org/10.1111/j.1749-6632.1999.tb08101.x. PMID: 10681884.

Attewell, P., & Madheswaran, S. (2007). Caste discrimination the Indian Urban labour market-evidence from the national sample Survey. Caste and economic discrimination. *Economic and Political Weekly, 42*(41).

Banerji, D. (1982). *Poverty, class, and health culture in India*. New Delhi, India: Prachi Prakashan.

Baru, R. V., Acharya, A., Acharya, S., Shiva Kumar, A. K., & Nagaraj, K. (2010). Inequalities in access to health services in India: Caste, class and region (Co-authored with R Baru, et al) *Economic and Political Weekly, 45*(38), 18–24.

Becker, G. S. (1971). *The economics of discrimination*. University of Chicago Press.

Beteille, A. (1969). *Castes: Old and new, essays in social structure and social stratification*. Asia Publishing House.

Bharti, N. K. (2018). *Wealth inequality, class and caste in India, 1961–2012*. Paris School of Economics. World inequality Database. World Inequality Lab. Paris. November 20.

Borooah, V. K., Diwakar, D., Mishra, V. K., Naik, A. K., & Sabharwal, N. S. (2014). 'Caste inequality and poverty in India: A re-assessment. *Development Studies Research. An Open Access Journal, 1*(1), 279–294. Publisher Routledge.

Borooah, V. K., Diwakar, D., Mishra, V. K., Naik, A. K., & Sabharwal, N. S. (2015). *'Caste. Discrimination and Exclusion in Modern India.*

Boroaah, V. K. (2020). A quantitative analysis of regional well-being: Identity and gender in India, South Africa, the USA and the UK (Routledge Studies in Development Economics).

Darity, W. A. (1998). Persistent disparity: Race and economic inequality in the United States since 1945. Myers, Samuel L. Cheltenham, UK: E. Elgar Pub. ISBN 1-85898-658-3. OCLC 37315423.

de Haan, A. (2007). *Reclaiming social policy-globalization.* Palgrave MacMillan.

Department of Health and Social Security. (1980). *Inequalities in health: Report of a research working group (The Black Report).* Department of Health and Social Security.

Deshpande, A., & Newman, K. (2007). Where the path leads—The role of caste in post-university employment expectations. *Caste and Economic Discrimination. Economic and Political Weekly, 42*(41).

Diwakar, G. D. (2015). 'Caste, health and discrimination: Understanding policies and programme implementation in India.' *Journal of Social Inclusion Studies, 2*(1), 43–58. https://doi.org/10.1177/2394481120150103.

IIPS and ICF. (2017). *National Family Health Survey (NFHS-4), 2015–16*: India. International Institute for Population Sciences (IIPS) and ICF. India. Mumbai: IIPS.

Iyengar, R. (2017). A day in the life of a corpse-burner. https://www.livemint.com/Leisure/rbcQ3K 5FhR8fTddOmV8UGM/A-day-in-the-life-of-a-corpseburner.html.

Jadhav, S., Mosse, D., & Dostaler, N. (2016). 'Minds of caste—Discrimination and its affects' anthropology today Vol 32 No 1, February 2016. *Guest Editorial Column.* print ISSN 0268–540X online ISSN 1467–8322 available online at www.wileyonlinelibrary.com/journal/anthhttps://doi.org/10.1111/1467-8322.12221..

Kabeer, N. (2000). Social exclusion, poverty and discrimination towards an analytical framework. *IDS Bulletin, 31*(4):83–97. https://doi.org/10.1111/j.1759-5436.2000.mp31004009.x.

Kitagawa, E. M., & Hauser, P. M. (1973). *Differential mortality in the United States: A study in socioeconomic epidemiology.* Harvard University Press.

Krieger, N. (2000). Discrimination and health. In L. Berkman & I. Kawachi (Eds.), *Social epidemiology* (pp. 36–75). Oxford University Press.

Kumar, K. (2019). *Patterns of discrimination between sub-castes among Dalits-understanding the consequences on access to resources, services and opportunities in Sonbhadra District, UP.* Ph.D. thesis submitted to Centre of Social Medicine and Community Health, School of social Sciences, Jawaharlal Nehru University, New Delhi.

Kumar, P. (2021). Shocking apathy: Workers at cremation ground made to work without protective gears. *Times Now News* 15 April. https://www.timesnownews.com/videos/times-now/india/sho cking-apathy-workers-at-cremation-ground-made-to-work-without-protective-gears/94901.

Kunst, A. E., & Mackenbach, J. P. (1994). International variation in the size of mortality differences associated with occupational status. *International Journal of Epidemiology., 23*(4), 742–750. [PubMed: 8002188].

Lynch, J. (2017). Reframing inequality? The health inequalities turn as a dangerous frame shift. *Journal of Public Health (Oxf), 39*(4), 653–660. https://doi.org/10.1093/pubmed/fdw140. PMID:28069990.

Mackenbach, J. P., Stronks, K., & Kunst, A. E. (1989). The contribution of medical care to inequalities in health: Differences between socio-economic groups in decline of mortality from conditions amenable to medical intervention. *Social Science and Medicine, 29*(3), 369–376. [PubMed: 2762863].

Marmot, M. (2015). *The health gap: The challenge of an unequal world.* Bloomsbury.

MoHFW. (2015). *Performance audit of tribal subplan, MHRD, MoHFW, Min of ayush report of auditor and comptroller general.* Union Government CIVIL. Report No 33 of 2015 (Performance Audit).

MoH & FW. (2020). *Annaul report 2019–2020.* https://www.india.gov.in/ministry-health-and-fam ily-welfare-6.

Narayan, N. (2018). *Health care access among vulnerable populations in Delhi metropolitan city: Examining explanation of social discrimination.* Ph.D. Thesis submitted to Centre of Social Medicine and Community Health, School of social Sciences, Jawaharlal Nehru University, New Delhi.

Nayar, K. R. (2007). Social exclusion, caste & health: a review based on the social determinants framework. *KR Nayar. Indian Journal of Medical Research, 126*(4), 355–363.

NCDHR. (2019). Discrimination based on work and descent and untouchability: Global profile and a common framework to eliminate the practice, Asia Dalit Rights Forum. In *Amnesty International, The Inclusivity Project. National Campaign for Dalit Huma Rights, Delhi.*

Pampel, F. C. P. M. K., & Denney, J. T. (2010). Socioeconomic disparities in health behaviors. *Annual Review of Sociology 2010, 36*, 349–370. https://doi.org/10.1146/annurev.soc.012809.102529.

Patnaik, U. (2008). Theorizing poverty and food security in the era of economic reforms. Globalization and the Washington Consensus: its influence on democracy and development in the south. In G. Lechini (Ed.), *Buenos Aires: CLACSO, Consejo Latinoamericano de Ciencias Sociales.* ISBN 978–987–1183–91–3 Disponible en: http://bibliotecavirtual.clacso.org.ar/ar/libros/sursur/lech/12patna.pdf.

Planning Commission (2012). *Planning Commission Report 2012.*

Ralph Hertwig, R., & Till, G.-Y. (2016). Nudging and boosting: Steering or empowering good decisions. *Perspectives on Psychological Science* 1 –14. sagepub.com/journals.Permissions.nav. https://doi.org/10.1177/1745691617702496 www.psychologicalscience.org/PPS [accessed Jun 09 2021]. Available from: https://www.researchgate.net/publication/319023957_Nudging_and_Boosting_Steering_or_Empowering_Good_Decisions. https://doi.org/10.1177/174569161770 2496.

Raushan, R., & Sanghmitra, S. A. (2019). Morbidity and treatment- seeking behaviour among scheduled tribe in India: A cross-sectional study'. *Journal of Social Inclusion Studies SAGE Publications, 4*(2) 1–16 (2019). http://journals.sagepub.com/home/sisagepub.in/home.nav. 10.1177/2394481118818594.

René, L. (1974). *Les exclus: un français sur dix.* [The Excluded: One French Person out of Ten]. Seuil.

RGI. (2011). *Census of India, 2011.* Office of the Registrar General & Census Commissioner, India Ministry of Home Affairs, Government of India.

Sen, A. (1992). *Inequality reexamined.* Oxford University Press.

Sen, A. (2000). *Social Exclusion: concept, application, and scrutiny.* Harvard University Social Development Papers No. 1 Office of Environment and Social Development Asian Development Bank. https://www.adb.org/sites/default/files/publication/29778/social-exclusion.pdf.

Shah, G., Mander, H., Thorat, S., Deshpande, S., & Baviskar, A. (2006). *Untouchability in rural India.* Sage Publications.

Solar, O., & Irwin, A. (2010). A conceptual framework for action on the social determinants of health. *Social Determinants of Health Discussion Paper 2* (Policy and Practice) World Health Organization Geneva.

Spinny, L. (2017). *Pale rider: The spanish flu of 1918 and how it changed the world.* Public Affairs.

Thorat, S. (2002). Oppression and denial: Dalit discrimination in the 1990s. *EPW, 37*(6), 123–126.

Thorat, S. (2007). Thorat committee report-caste discrimination in AIIMS editorials. *Economic and Political Weekly, 42*(22), 141–145.

Thorat, S., & Madheswaran, S. (2018). 'Graded caste inequality and poverty: evidence on role of economic discrimination'. *Journal of Social Inclusion Studies.* https://doi.org/10.1177/239448 1118775873.

United Nations. (2019). *The sustainable development goals report 2019.* United Nations.

United Nation. (2020). *The world social report 2020: Inequality in a rapidly changing world.* Department of Economic and Social Affairs World Social Report.

Wilkinson, R. G. (1986). *Class and health: Research and longitudinal data.* Tavistock Publications.

Wilkinson, R. G. (1990). Income distribution and mortality: a 'natural' experiment. *Sociology of health & illness, 12*, 391–412.

Williams, D. R. (1990). Socioeconomic differen-tials in health: a review and redirection. *Social psychology quarterly, 53*, 81–99.

Williams, D. R. & Collins, C. (1995) US socioeconomic and racial differences in health: patterns and explanations. *Annual Review of Sociology, 21*, 349–386 Published by: Annual Reviews Stable https://www.jstor.org/stable/2083415.

Chapter 15
Caste Disparities in Health Care Utilization in India

Dhananjay W. Bansod, Pradeep S. Salve, and Suresh Jungari

Abstract Health and healthcare need to be distinguished from each other. Besides health care arrangements, many other factors outside the health sector play a key role in determining the health status of individuals and communities such as standard of living, education and access to basic minimum social services. A number of factors affect the evolution of health care arrangements in a society. They include its cultural understanding of ill health and well-being, the extent of socio-economic disparities, reach of health services, quality and cost of care. Health is a prerequisite for human development and is an essential component for the well-being of mankind. The health problems of any community are influenced by the interplay of various factors including social, economic and political. The study aims to assess the disparities existing in health and health care utilization across different caste groups and examine the factors affecting health care utilization among the SCs/STs as compared to other social groups in India. The National Family Health Survey-4 (NFHS-4) has been used for analysis. Bivariate and Decomposition analysis have been carried out to capture the Caste disparities in health and health care utilization in India. To explore the health disparities, we have considered women's health indicators such as four-plus ANC, and adverse pregnancy outcomes (APO) and for child health, full immunization and low birth weight was considered. Overall, the study concludes that there are caste disparities while unitizing the health care facilities. Therefore, efforts must be put in bringing health equity across different caste groups in India.

D. W. Bansod (✉)
Department of Public Health & Mortality Studies, International Institute for Population Sciences, Mumbai, India
e-mail: dhananjay@iipsindia.ac.in

P. S. Salve
Population Research Centre (PRC), JSS Institute of Economic Research, Dharwad, Karnataka, India

S. Jungari
Department of Public Health & Mortality Studies, International Institute for Population Sciences, Mumbai, India

Keywords Caste disparities · Immunization · Low birth weight · 4+ ANC ·
Adverse pregnancy outcomes

Introduction

India is one the most populous countries in the world, with a diverse population.
However, India is facing severe persistence of some social problems. The caste
stratification, discrimination and exclusion of Scheduled Castes (SCs) and Scheduled
Tribes (STs) population from formal employment, unequal distribution of resources,
assets, health inequalities are major challenges. The five-year developmental schemes
were also not achieved in reducing the caste-wise income inequalities in India. There
are more illiterate among poor, SCs and STs than non-poor, non-SC and non-ST (RGI,
2011). About 28% SC and 50% STs are in the lowest wealth quintile as against less
than 10% of high caste Hindus (IIPS & ICF, 2017).

Social scientists argue that the existence of the caste system posed an adverse
effect on economic development of the country resulting in stronger caste disparities
in health and education attainment. Most of the studies attempted using the data of
National Sample Survey Organization (NSSO) to prove the existence of economic
and income inequalities among different caste groups in India with different method-
ological approaches (Deshpande, 2006; Bakshi, 2008; Hnatkovska et al., 2012). A
study conducted using NSSO data found that caste-based discrimination causes 15%
lower wages for SCs and STs as compared to other social groups with equal quali-
fication. Further, study points SCs and STs worker are discriminated against both in
the public and private sectors, but the discrimination effects are larger in the private
sector, this may be due to the affirmative action like providing reservation to SCs
and STs in Government and public sector jobs (Madheswaran & Attewell, 2007).

The pilot study conducted by Indian Institute of Dalit Studies (IIDS) in 2002
(Thorat et al., 2003) found that inter-caste differences in employment rates and wage
earnings among casual wage labour, particularly in farm activities entailing similar
manual skills, therefore, seem to be unrelated to productivity. Further, qualitative
part of the study found the reason for discrimination in labour market showed that
employers belonging to upper castes prefer hiring workers belonging to their own
castes or upper castes, resulting in restrictions on the hiring of the SC labourers for any
work or selective works. Caste sympathy towards people of one's own caste turned
out to be one of the main reasons for preferential treatment accorded to labourers by
the higher-caste employers.

Recently, research on caste inequalities in income, economic status and health
acquired significant momentum in India. Particularly explaining the Caste-based
inequalities in income, wealth, education, health and assets (Borooah, 2005;
Bhaumik & Chakrabarty, 2006; Thorat, & Newman, 2007; Zacharias & Vakulabharanam, 2011; Jungari & Bomble, 2013; Jungari, & Chauhan, 2017; Acharya (this
volume). Indeed, the historical tradition of social division through the caste system
created a social stratification along with education, occupation and income lines

that has enormously contributed to widening the health inequalities continued into modern India.

The Health Survey and Development Committee's recommendations, popularly known as Bhore committee, 1946, have paved the way for future health policies and systems that have evolved (Ma & Sood, 2008). Implementing the recommendation for three-tier health care systems to provide preventive and curative healthcare, the Bhore committee could foresee the currently existing decisiveness in the health care system. The above recommendation was made to ensure the accessibility of primary care to all individuals irrespective of their socio-economic conditions (Chokshi et al., 2016). However, the under-performing public health system helped in the evolution of private health care providers (Chokshi et al., 2016). The private health care system further pushed the public health care system in the corner leading to a health care disparity across various socio-economic groups (Costa & Diwan, 2007). Despite substantial improvements in health indicators, there lies inequality in India's health care utilization (Joe et al., 2010). Health care inequalities can be seen in various socio-demographic aspects such as; gender inequalities (Patel & Chauhan, 2020; socio-economic inequalities (Ali & Chauhan, 2020; Srivastava, Fledderjohann, & Upadhyay, 2020b); urban–rural inequalities (Singh, 2013); poor-non-poor inequalities (Pande & Yazbeck, 2003), and caste inequalities (Bora, Raushan, & Lutz, 2019; Jungari & Chauhan, 2017; Bamdev Subedi (this volume). Furthermore, health inequalities could be seen in various sub-populations such as; older population (Srivastava, Chauhan, & Patel, 2020a), infants (Kumar et al., 2020), children (Arokiasamy et al., 2013), women (Jungari & Chauhan, 2017; Arindam Roy (this volume).

Immunization has been noted to be the most cost-effective measure to achieve a decline in childhood mortality and morbidity (Dutta & Agarwal, 2018). Despite achieving health and medical advancement, children in India still suffer from various vaccine-preventable infectious diseases (Debnath & Bhattacharjee, 2018). India launched the Expanded Programme on Immunization (EPI) in 1978 to tackle vaccine-preventable diseases. The programme further got a boost in 1985 and was expanded as the Universal Immunization Programme (UIP). When launched, UIP was to be implemented in all the districts of the country by 1989–90 in a phased manner. Furthermore, to strengthen the UIP, it became part of the Child Survival and Safe Motherhood programme in 1992. Since 1997, immunization has been an essential component of the Reproductive and Child Health (RCH) programme. It is currently one of the critical areas under the National Rural Health Mission (NRHM) since 2005. Under the UIP, the Government of India (GoI) provides vaccination to prevent seven vaccine-preventable diseases: Diarrhoea, Haemophilus influenzae type b (Hib), Hepatitis B, 'Diphtheria, Pertussis, and Tetanus', Measles, Polio, and Tuberculosis. Despite the progress of more than 40 years in providing immunization coverage, there remain inequalities in the immunization among children by their socio-economic and demographic characteristics (Bettampadi et al., 2021; Srivastava, Fledderjohann, & Upadhyay, 2020b; Khan & Saggurti, 2020; Barman & Dey, 2017).

As reported by the various National Family Health Survey (NFHS) reports, the immunization coverage has increased from 20% in 1992–93 to 36% in 1998–99, and further from 44% in 2005–06 to 62% in 2015–16. Previous studies noted that there are disparities in child immunization by caste (Mathew, 2012; Prusty & Kumar, 2014; Shrivastava et al., 2015), religion (Mathew, 2012; Shrivastava et al., 2015), household wealth (Mathew, 2012; Debnath & Bhattacharjee, 2018; Khan & Saggurti, 2020; Srivastava, Fledderjohann, & Upadhyay, 2020b), parental education (Mathew, 2012; Khan & Saggurti, 2020; Srivastava, Fledderjohann, & Upadhyay, 2020b), sex of the children (Mathew, 2012), order of the children/parity of the mother (Debnath & Bhattacharjee, 2018; Mathew, 2012), place of residence (Mathew, 2012; Srivastava, Fledder Johann, & Upadhyay, 2020b), region (Prusty & Kumar, 2014; Srivastava, Fledderjohann, & Upadhyay, 2020b), unequal access to antenatal care facility (Shrivastava et al., 2015; Debnath & Bhattacharjee, 2018), and place of delivery (Shrivastava et al., 2015).

Present Study

Despite considerable research on issues pertaining to caste-based inequalities in health in recent times, there is wider scope to understand the various dimensions of caste-based health inequalities and inequalities in utilization of health care services in India. This study aimed at examining the caste-based disparities in health and health care utilization across the different caste groups. Further, the study also examines the factors affecting health care utilization.

Data and Methods

The present study used National Family Health Survey (NFHS)-4, conducted in 2015–16, is the fourth round in the NFHS series that provides information on various indicators of population, health, fertility, mortality, nutrition status of women and children and health care utilization in India. All four NFHS surveys have been conducted under the stewardship of the Ministry of Health and Family Welfare (MoHFW), Government of India. MoHFW designated the IIPS, Mumbai, as the nodal agency for all of the NFHS surveys. ICF provided technical assistance through the DHS (Demographic and Health Surveys) Programme, which is funded by USAID. Assistance for the HIV component of the survey was provided by the National AIDS Control Organization (NACO) and the National AIDS Research Institute (NARI), Pune.

Sampling

Decisions about the overall sample size required for NFHS-4 were guided by several considerations, paramount among which was the need to produce indicators at the district, state/union territory (UT), and national levels, as well as separate estimates for urban and rural areas in the 157 districts that have 30–70% of the population living in urban areas as per the 2011 census, with a reasonable level of precision. A subsample of 15% of households was selected for the implementation of the state module, in addition to the district module. In the 15% of households selected for the state module, a long questionnaire was administered that included all the questions needed for district level estimates plus additional questions for the topics listed above. To achieve a representative sample of 15% of households, NFHS-4 conducted interviews in every alternate selected household in 30% of the selected clusters. In all, 28,586 Primary Sampling Units (PSUs) were selected across the country in NFHS-4, of which fieldwork was completed in 28,522 clusters. The NFHS-4 sample is a stratified two-stage sample. The 2011 census served as the sampling frame for the selection of PSUs. PSUs were villages in rural areas and Census Enumeration Blocks (CEBs) in urban areas. PSUs with fewer than 40 households were linked to the nearest PSU. Within each rural stratum, villages were selected from the sampling frame with probability proportional to size (PPS). In each stratum, six approximately equal substrata were created by crossing three substrata, each created based on the estimated number of households in each village, with two substrata, each created based on the percentage of the population belonging to SCs and STs.

Within each explicit sampling stratum, PSUs were sorted according to the literacy rate of women aged 6+ years. The final sample PSUs were selected with PPS sampling. In urban areas, CEB information was obtained from the Office of the Registrar General and Census Commissioner, New Delhi. CEBs were sorted according to the percentage of the SC/ST population in each CEB, and sample CEBs were selected with PPS sampling. In every selected rural and urban PSU, a complete household mapping and listing operation were conducted prior to the main survey. Selected PSUs with an estimated number of at least 300 households were segmented into segments of approximately 100–150 households. Two of the segments were randomly selected for the survey using systematic sampling with probability proportional to segment size. Therefore, an NFHS-4 cluster is either a PSU or a segment of a PSU. In the second stage, in every selected rural and urban cluster, 22 households were randomly selected with systematic sampling.

Independent Variables

Age of the mother, educational attainments, wealth quintiles, place of residence, and Caste.

Dependent Variables

Low birth weight of child, full immunization, four-plus ANC, and adverse pregnancy outcomes.

Statistical Analysis

Descriptive statistics, bivariate and multivariate techniques have been used for the analysis purpose. In multivariate analysis, decomposition method has been applied for understanding the disparities in health and health care utilization between SCs/STs and non-SCs/STs.

Blinder-Oaxaca Decomposition

Oaxaca (1973) developed a regression-based decomposition method to measure the inequality among groups. The Oaxaca decomposition partitions the variation in an outcome into two parts. The Blinder-Oaxaca decomposition technique is a useful method to explain the intergroup differentials in outcome variables using a set of predictors. Originally, this technique was used to decompose the labour market outcomes between different groups such as sex and race. However, the same method could also be used to study intergroup differences in any outcome variable (Oaxaca, 1973; Owen et al., 2008).

The differences of health care utilization of child as well as mother between SCs/STs and non-SCs/STs are due to different characteristics, which affects the health care utilization of child as well as mother.

The conventional Blinder-Oaxaca decomposition is based on two linear regression models that are fitted separately for the groups A and B: (A = SC/STs, B = Non-SC/STs)

$$Yk = Xkk + ek \tag{15.1}$$

And

$$Yk = Xk\ k + ek \tag{15.2}$$

Results

Table 15.1 depicts the status of full immunization of children aged 12–13 months by different social caste groups in India. The analysis shows that about two-thirds of children received full immunization irrespective of the residential areas. Similarly, SCs and other caste groups have received full immunization. For instance, 64% of children belonging to SCs residing in rural areas received full immunization as compared to the children residing in urban areas (63%). The place of residence has variation in receiving full immunization when considering the ST children. More than half (55%) of ST children who are residing in rural areas received full immunization compared to the 65% of their counterparts. The wealth status of the household plays an important role in child immunization. The results revealed that slightly more than half (53%) of the children with the poorest wealth quintile received full immunization irrespective of the caste groups in India. The full immunization subsequently increases with the advancement of the household's economic condition except for children belonging to STs. About seventy per cent of children belonging

Table 15.1 Percentage of full immunization of children age 12–23 months by socio-economic characteristics and caste groups in India

Variables	Full immunization						Total
place of residence	SC	CI	ST	CI	Others	CI	Total
Urban	62.73	60.76; 64.71	64.71	62.28; 69.89	64.31	63.37; 65.27	64.11
Rural	63.83	62.76; 64.89	55.06	53.57; 56.55	62.06	61.40; 62.73	61.56
Wealth							
Poorest	56.25	54.51; 57.99	50.15	48.13; 52.17	52.34	51.04; 53.64	52.97
Poorer	63.76	61.87; 65.65	59.04	56.30; 61.78	60.05	58.81; 61.29	60.87
Middle	67.60	65.62; 69.59	63.58	60.02; 67.14	63.70	62.51; 64.89	64.61
Richer	69.08	66.78; 71.38	67.89	63.15; 72.63	66.87	65.72; 68.02	67.32
Richest	70.10	66.95; 73.26	66.66	60.22; 73.10	70.37	69.19; 71.55	70.22
Educational attainment							
No education	55.93	54.21; 57.65	47.33	45.12; 45.12	50.67	49.52; 51.81	51.49
Incomplete primary	68.39	64.88; 71.90	58.31	53.54; 63.09	61.96	59.58; 64.33	63.02
Complete primary	62.32	59.26; 65.38	59.71	54.86; 64.56	57.62	55.56; 59.6	59.13
Incomplete secondary	67.54	66.05; 69.02	64.13	61.81; 66.46	66.44	65.58; 67.31	66.46
Complete secondary	68.03	64.58; 71.49	64.45	58.39; 70.50	69.58	67.99; 71.17	69.02
Higher	69.38	66.07; 72.68	62.14	55.72; 68.56	71.60	70.25; 72.94	70.89

to SCs and other caste groups with the richest wealth quintile received full immunization compared to the children belonging to STs (67%). Similarly, the educational attainment of women/mothers has an increasing trend for full immunization of children with the advancement in educational attainment. Altogether, 51% of children with full immunization whose mothers had no-education compared to the 71% with higher educational attainment. The similar results have been observed for social caste groups. More children belonging to the other caste groups (72%) received full immunization with higher educational attainment as compared to SCs and STs children at 69% and 62%, respectively.

The per cent of low birth weight among children with different social caste groups are presented in Table 15.2. Surprisingly, results show that overall low birth weight was found to be higher among children residing in the urban areas compared to the rural areas. Total 14% of children are born with low birth weight in rural areas compared to 15% in urban areas. Likewise, a similar trend has been observed for SCs and children belonging to other castes. Whereas, 18% scheduled tribe children residing in urban areas had low birth weight compared to the children residing in the rural areas (15%). Low birth weight is found to be higher among the children

Table 15.2 Percentage of low birth weight of children by socio-economic characteristics and caste groups in India

Variables	Low birth weight						Total
Place of residence	SC	CI	ST	CI	Others	CI	Total
Urban	16.35	15.70; 16.99	18.08	16.74; 19.41	15.01	14.69; 15.32	15.41
Rural	14.06	13.72; 14.39	14.73	14.28; 15.19	13.24	13.04; 13.45	13.64
Wealth							
Poorest	11.23	10.75; 11.70	13.93	13.33; 14.53	10.47	10.13; 10.81	11.41
Poorer	15.73	15.11; 16.34	16.03	15.16; 16.91	13.26	12.89; 13.63	14.25
Middle	16.16	15.48; 16.85	15.90	14.72; 17.07	15.19	14.80; 15.58	15.47
Richer	17.71	16.88; 18.55	19.36	17.64; 21.08	15.81	15.42; 16.21	16.33
Richest	14.47	13.43; 15.50	13.38	11.32; 15.43	14.14	13.74; 14.53	14.16
Educational attainment							
No education	11.98	11.51; 12.45	13.80	13.17; 14.44	10.92	10.63; 11.22	11.65
Incomplete primary	16.25	15.04; 17.46	15.94	14.45; 17.42	14.38	13.63; 15.12	15.09
Complete primary	15.49	14.50; 16.48	12.80	11.33; 14.27	14.45	13.82; 15.08	14.56
Incomplete secondary	16.61	16.08; 17.13	17.23	16.42; 18.04	15.58	15.28; 15.87	15.97
Complete secondary	15.64	14.43; 16.86	18.20	15.99; 20.40	14.52	13.97; 15.07	14.92
Higher	13.14	12.06; 14.23	12.26	10.29; 14.24	13.49	13.02; 13.95	13.39

belonging to the STs followed by SCs as compared with children belonging to other caste groups in both the areas. Considering the wealth quintile, surprisingly low birth weight among children increases with the advancement of household wealth status and decreases among the richest wealth quintile. For instance, 11% of children were born with low birth weight in the poorest wealth quintile which increased to 16% among children belonging to the richer wealth quintile. Similarly, all castes have an increasing trend in the low birth weight with wealth quintile. However, more ST children were born with low birth weight compared to the national figure. More or less 14% of children in all caste groups were born in low birth weight in the richest wealth quintile in India. About 11% of children were born of low birth weight among mothers who did not receive any education. Percentage is higher for STs children where 14% of children were born with low birth weight whose mothers were uneducated compared to their counterparts (SC—12% and Others—11%). Surprisingly, results are more or less similar to the wealth quintiles of households. Where the low birth weight among children increases with the advancement of educational status of mothers. For instance, 18% of STs children were of low birth weight whose mothers completed secondary education compared to their counterparts (SCs—16% and Other 15%).

The results of 4+ ANC by social caste groups in India are presented in Table 15.3. Overall, 52% of women residing in the urban areas received 4+ ANC as compared to the 32% in rural areas. When considering the difference is social caste groups; about one-thirds of women residing in rural areas received 4+ ANC irrespective of the caste groups. Four plus ANC visits are more among the women who belong to the other caste groups as compared with SCs/STs women in both the residential areas. The 4+ ANC have a positive association with the wealth quintile of the household which is reflected in the increasing trend of the result. For instance, only 17% of women in the poorest wealth quintile received 4+ ANC compared to the 61% of women in the richest wealth quintile. The similar pattern is observed for the women belonging to different social caste groups. At the same time there are considerable differences when we compare the estimates between the social caste groups. For instance, 14% of other caste group women with the poorest wealth quartile received 4+ ANC compared to the SCs (17%) and STs (23%). The utilization of the 4+ ANC increased with the advancement of the wealth status of the household. Sixty-one per cent Other caste women in the richest wealth quintile received 4+ ANC compared to only 14% those in the poorest quintile. Likewise, the results are more or less for other caste groups also. When we consider the richest wealth quintile, more or less 60% of women received 4+ ANC in other castes and SCs. On the other hand, 56% STs women in the richest wealth quintile receive 4+ ANC compared to the SCs (60%) and other caste women (61%). Surprisingly, more than one-fifths (23%) STs women with no-education received 4+ ANC compared to the 19% of SCs and 17% of other caste groups. With the advancement of education attainment the difference remained more or less same among the social caste groups except the higher educational attainment group. Where, 63% of other caste group women utilized 4+ ANC compared to the SCs (56%) and STs (58%).

Table 15.3 Percentage of 4 plus ANC by socio-economic characteristics and caste

Variables	ANC 4+ visits						
Place of residence	SC	CI	ST	CI	Others	CI	Total
Urban	49.82	48.95; 50.70	47.46	45.73; 49.19	52.50	52.06; 52.93	51.75
Rural	30.89	30.45; 31.34	30.90	30.30; 31.49	32.52	32.24; 32.80	31.91
Wealth quintile							
Poorest	16.68	16.12; 17.24	22.89	22.16; 23.61	14.09	13.70; 14.47	16.65
Poorer	33.50	32.70; 34.30	36.15	35.00; 37.30	28.85	28.35; 29.35	30.99
Middle	44.51	43.59; 45.44	45.80	44.20; 47.40	40.66	40.13; 41.20	41.97
Richer	51.42	50.33; 52.52	49.91	47.73; 52.08	50.23	49.69; 50.77	50.44
Richest	60.22	58.77; 61.66	55.59	52.59; 58.60	61.05	60.49; 61.60	60.78
Educational attainment							
No education	19.13	18.56; 19.70	22.71	21.94; 23.47	17.24	16.88; 17.60	18.58
Incomplete primary	36.90	35.32; 38.49	33.34	31.43; 35.25	31.71	30.72; 32.69	33.25
Complete primary	30.65	29.39; 31.92	32.39	30.33; 34.45	30.64	29.81; 31.47	30.83
Incomplete secondary	44.88	44.18; 45.58	41.62	40.56; 42.67	45.27	44.87; 45.67	44.83
Complete secondary	50.43	48.76; 52.10	48.55	45.69; 51.41	52.28	51.50; 53.06	51.76
Higher	56.25	54.65; 57.84	57.84	53.44; 59.41	62.51	61.85; 63.17	61.34

The adverse pregnancy outcomes by different caste groups are presented in Table 15.4. About one-fifth of women have adverse pregnancy outcomes in India. STs women (19%) residing in urban areas have less adverse pregnancy outcomes compared to women belonging to SCs (22%) and other castes (21%). The results are more or less same by wealth quintile. For instance, 20% of STs women in the poorest wealth quintile have adverse pregnancy outcomes compared to 22% women from SCs and other caste groups each. The results are more or less similar for other wealth quintile categories also. Such as 16% of STs women with the richest wealth quintile have adverse pregnancy outcomes compared to the 22% women of SCs and 19% of other caste groups. Educational attainment does not make much changes in the adverse pregnancy outcome of women by the social category in India. At the outset, the results depicted that 19% of women with no-education have adverse pregnancy outcomes compared to the 21% among SCs and 22% of other caste groups. Similarly, the STs women have lower adverse pregnancy outcomes irrespective of the educational attainments compared to the STs and SCs categories. In the higher educational attainment about 17% scheduled tribe women have adverse pregnancy outcome which is comparably lower than the SCs (22%) and with other caste groups (19%).

Table 15.4 Per cent of adverse pregnancy outcomes with various caste groups

Variables	Adverse Pregnancy Outcomes (APO)						
Place of Residence	SC	CI	ST	CI	Others	CI	Total
Urban	21.59	20.87; 22.31	18.73	17.37; 20.09	20.68	20.33; 21.04	20.76
Rural	21.84	21.43; 22.24	18.87	18.36; 19.39	21.57	21.32; 21.81	21.28
Wealth	**SC**		**ST**		**Others**		**Total**
Poorest	21.73	21.10; 22.36	19.57	18.87; 20.27	22.26	21.80; 22.73	21.56
Poorer	22.77	22.05; 23.48	18.45	17.51; 19.39	21.92	21.46; 22.37	21.69
Middle	20.04	19.29; 20.78	19.08	17.81; 20.36	21.61	21.16; 22.06	21.05
Richer	22.72	21.80; 23.64	17.08	15.43; 18.72	21.15	20.71; 21.59	21.25
Richest	21.63	20.41; 22.85	15.59	13.39; 17.79	19.39	18.94; 19.84	19.56
Educational attainment	**SC**		**ST**		**Others**		**Total**
No-education	21.11	20.51; 21.71	19.11	18.38; 19.85	22.07	21.68; 22.47	21.37
Incomplete primary	22.73	21.34; 24.12	19.5	17.85; 21.15	23.2	22.29; 24.10	22.5
Complete primary	23.15	21.99; 24.32	16.19	14.55; 17.83	23.03	22.26; 23.79	22.35
Incomplete secondary	21.88	21.30; 22.46	19.17	18.32; 20.02	20.93	20.60; 21.26	20.98
Complete secondary	21.44	20.06; 22.81	19.1	16.84; 21.36	21.57	20.93; 22.21	21.41
Higher	22.01	20.68; 23.35	16.95	14.68; 19.22	18.72	18.19; 19.26	19.13

Decomposition Analysis

Result of decomposition for full Immunization among children aged 12–23 months shows the contribution of explained effect in explaining the gap in average z score of full immunization for SCs/STs and Non-SC/STs population in India (Table 15.5). The average of natural log of full immunization among children age 12 to 23 months was 0.63 for non-SCs/STs and 0.58 for SCs/STs, thus the non-SCs/STs and SCs/STs gap of 0.052 meant that the full immunization is more by six per cent among non-SCs/STs children than the SCs/STs children.

The negative contribution indicates that the determinants were narrowing the gap between the SCs/STs and Non-SCs/STs population. In particular, wealth and educational attainment were the most important factors explaining the gap in the SCs/STs and Non-SCs/STs. The socio-economic and demographic predictors can explain up to 72.2% of the total variation in full immunization. The z score contribution in full immunization by age of mother (1.77%), wealth quintile (58.11%), and educational attainment (20.10%) are the major contributing factor, while negative contribution by

Table 15.5 Decomposition for full immunization of children (12–23 months) among SC/STs and general castes

Contributing factors	Coef	Level of significant	95% CI	% Contribution
Caesarean delivery				
Differential				
Prediction_ Non-SCs/STs	0.632	***	(0.626, 0.38)	
Prediction_ SCs/STs	0.580	***	(0.573, 0.587)	
Difference (Non SCs/STs–SCs/STs)	0.052	***	(0.043, 0.061)	
Explained				
Age of mother	0.001	***	(0.000, 0.001)	1.77
Place of residence	−0.004	***	(−0.006, −0.002)	−7.79
Wealth quintile	0.030	***	(0.026, 0.035)	58.11
Educational attainment	0.011	***	(0.008, 0.013)	20.10
Total	0.038			72.20
Unexplained				
Total	0.019			36.32

***$P < 0.01$, **$P < 0.05$, *$P < 0.10$

the place of residence (−7.79%) tends to narrow the difference in full immunization in SCs/STs and non-SCs/STs population.

Result shows the contribution of the explained effect in explaining the gap in average z score for low birth weight between SCs/STs and Non-SCs/STs (Table 15.6). The gap between non-SCs/STs and SCs/STs is −0.010 meaning the low birth weight is found to be less among non-SCs/STs children than the children belonging to SCs/STs.

In low birth weight, −73.77% of the total gap could be explained with the help of the characteristics included in the analysis while the rest remain unexplained. The contribution of age of mother (7.93%), to the explained variance. The negative contribution by the place of residence (−12.77%), wealth (−61.05%), and educational Attainment (−7.88%) tend to narrow the differences in low birth weight between non-SCs/STs children and children belongs to SCs/STs.

The result reveals that the difference between non-SCs/STs and SCs/STs is 0.043 indicates non-SCs/STs women are more likely to go to health care facilities for four-plus ANC visits than the SCs/STs women (Table 15.7). The socio-economic and demographic predictors could explain up to 178.1% of the total variation in more than four ANC visits to the health care facilities. The z score contribution in four-plus ANC visits can be seen by place of residence (10.8%), wealth quintile (118.7%), and educational attainment (50.3%) to the explained variance of 178.1%, while negative contribution by age of mother (−1.6%) tend to narrow the difference in more than four ANC visits between SC/STs and Non-SC/ST women.

Table 15.6 Decomposition for low birth weight of children among SC/STs and general castes

Contributing factors	Coef	Level of Significant	95% CI	% Contribution
Caesarean delivery				
Differential				
Prediction_ Non-SCs/STs	0.138	***	(0.136, 0.140)	
Prediction_ SCs/STs	0.148	***	(0.145, 0.150)	
Difference (Non SCs/STs–SCs/STs)	−0.010	***	(-0.013, −0.007)	
Explained				
Age of mother	0.000	***	(0.000, 0.000)	7.93
Place of residence	0.001	***	(0.000, 0.002)	−12.77
Wealth quintile	0.006	***	(0.004, 0.008)	−61.05
Educational attainment	0.001	***	(0.000, 0.002)	−7.88
Total	0.007			−73.77
Unexplained				
Total	−0.016			168.96

$^{***}P < 0.01$, $^{**}P < 0.05$, $^{*}P < 0.10$

Table 15.7 Decomposition analysis for 4+ ANC visit to the health care facilities of pregnant women among SC/STs and general castes

Contributing factors	Coef	Level of significant	95% CI	% Contribution
Caesarean delivery				
Differential				
Prediction_ Non-SCs/STs	0.389	***	(0.386, 0.391)	
Prediction_ SCs/STs	0.345	***	(0.342, 0.349)	
Difference (Non SCs/STs–SCs/STs)	0.043	***	(0.039, 0.048)	
Explained				
Age of mother	−0.001	***	(−0.001, −0.001)	−1.63
Place of residence	0.005	***	(0.004, 0.006)	10.83
Wealth quintile	0.052	***	(0.049, 0.054)	118.66
Educational attainment	0.022	***	(0.020, 0.023)	50.25
Total	0.077			178.11
Unexplained				
Total	−0.041			−95.27

$^{***}P < 0.01$, $^{**}P < 0.05$, $^{*}P < 0.10$

Table 15.8 Decomposition analysis for Adverse pregnancy outcome among SC/ST and general castes

Contributing factors	Coef	Level of significant	95% CI	% Contribution
Caesarean delivery				
Differential				
Prediction_ Non-SC/ST	0.213	***	(0.211, 0.215)	
Prediction_ SC/ST	0.208	***	(0.205, 0.211)	
Difference (Non-SC/ST–SC/ST)	0.005	***	(0.001, 0.008)	
Explained				
Age of mother	0.000	***	(−0.001, 0.000)	-9.97
Place of residence	0.001	***	(0.000, 0.002)	13.25
Wealth quintile	−0.002	***	(−0.004, 0.001)	-35.33
Educational attainment	0.001	***	(−0.001, 0.002)	11.05
Total	−0.001			−21.01
Unexplained				
Total	0.010			217.37

$^{***}P < 0.01$, $^{**}P < 0.05$, $^{*}P < 0.10$

There is no difference as such for adverse pregnancy outcomes among women whether she belongs to non-SCs/STs or SCs/STs community (Table 15.8). The socio-economic and demographic predicators can explain up to −21.01% of the total variation in adverse pregnancy outcome (APO). The Z score contribution in the APO by different background characteristics. The place of residence (13.25%) and educational attainment (11.05%) are the major contributors in explaining the variance of −21.0%, while negative contribution by the age of mother (13.3%) and wealth (−35.3%) tends to narrow the differences in APO between SCs/STs and Non-SCs/STs women.

Discussion

The study aimed to examine the Caste group differences in Health and Health care utilization and equity in India's healthcare using a large-scale demographic survey. The study considered two-child indicators (Full immunization and low birth weight of child) and two indicators of women (Four+ ANC and Adverse pregnancy outcome) to assess the Caste differences. The results revealed that considerable caste differences were found in the full immunization of children. Children from SCs and STs communities have had less per cent of full immunization than other caste groups.

Some of the past studies conducted in different parts of the country also reported similar results (Ali & Chauhan, 2020; Kumar & Gupta, 2015).

This indicates children born in the SCs and STs communities are disadvantaged against protecting life-threatening diseases due to incomplete immunization. Hence, there are higher infant and child mortality levels among SCs/STs (Shrivastwa et al., 2015; Vishwakarma et al., 2020). Government efforts must focus on achieving universal child immunization, not leaving any community children behind. Special efforts also needed to reach out to the tribal children in remote and hilly areas. The health equity approach in achieving immunization is also important to address the immunization gaps among various Caste groups in India.

There has been ample evidence of a rapid increase in the utilization of maternal health care services, particularly antenatal services in India, after the initiation of Janani Suraksha Yojna (JSY) under the flagship programme of National Health Mission. However, the current study found that as far as four-plus ANC visits are concerned, there is a gap in various Caste groups. SCs and STs women received less than four-plus ANC visits than the other caste groups women. The rapid improvements in ANC services' utilization patterns have not contributed to bringing the utilization gap to a close. Hence, there is a need to relook at the problems and issues facing SCs and STs women while utilizing the ANC services. Several published studies have pointed out that the health care providers are often absent from the duty in the remote and tribal areas that may lead to less utilization of essential health services among the tribal population (Mavalankar, 2016; Narain, 2019). Pregnant women having four or more ANC visits are able to detect any possible pregnancy complications. Previous literature confirms that there is a greater need for the health equity approach in addressing the provider side's problems and issues in increasing health care use (Acharya, 2020).

Study results show that caste differences in children's low birth weight, education, and residence place are also significant predictors of low birth weight of children. The higher prevalence of low birth weight of children among several weaker sections of the population with higher levels of low birth weight is not a good indicator of the overall health status of mother and child and development of any country. Past studies also provided evidence of the higher and unacceptable prevalence of children's low birth weight among disadvantaged groups of populations such as SCs, STs, and OBC (Kader & Perera, 2014; Jungari & Chauhan, 2017). One of the well-known risk factors of children's low birth weight is the poor nutritional status of the mother (Khanal et al., 2014).

Therefore, interventions must be targeted from adolescent girls to pregnant women for improving the nutrition status. Interventions during pregnancy also need to be intensified by providing diverse food supplements to pregnant women through the Anganwadi centres. Community-level interventions to educate the people about the importance of healthy girls and women to have healthy babies will have benefits in the long run.

Furthermore, the study also used the decomposition analysis for the robust examination of disparities in health status and utilization of health care services among the various Cast groups. The results confirmed the existence of disparities in the utilization of health services among various caste groups, with the higher disadvantage happening with the SCs and STs Caste group populations. The Other Caste group population had a good advantage in all the services utilization. Over the period of time India has been able to narrow down the gap in utilization of health care services among various Caste group populations. However, the desired level of equity in healthcare is not achieved, leaving a considerable population being left out with a higher burden of infant and child morbidities and mortalities. It is also evident that women with low education attainment and belonging to rural areas have higher chances of disadvantage in utilizing MCH services. Therefore, efforts must be put in to increase the education and wealth status of SCs and STs.

The study results further confirm that SCs and STs Children and women are at a greater disadvantaged position; hence, several efforts must be undertaken to improve the health status with a health equity approach. Understanding local health issues and undertaking various health interventions with an equity approach may help in increasing the utilization patterns of various health services. Further, availability, accessibility and affordability are important predictors of utilization of maternal health care services. Hence, the government and health care providers must focus on increasing the availability, affordability and accessibility of MCH programmes concerning the disadvantaged caste groups.

More robust research is needed to understand the factors affecting maternal health care services within different Caste communities so that specific targeted interventions can be possible. Undertaking qualitative research in specific communities and geographical areas will help in assessing the specific reasons for under-utilization of MCH services. Some of the studies also must be conducted with health care providers to understand issues from the provider's perspectives. Future research should also be undertaken to examine the issues in implementing various schemes for pregnant and lactating women.

Conclusion

Overall, the study concludes that Caste disparities exist while utilizing the health care facilities in India. The degree of disparities varies with different health care indicators and by different socio-economic underline factors such as place of residence, wealth and educational attainment of women. To eliminate the disparities between SCs/STs and non-SCs/STs population while utilizing the health care facilities, government efforts should focus on equalizing the educational attainment among the women who belong to SCs/STs at par with non-SCs/STs women. Over time India has been able to narrow down the gap in utilization of health care services among various caste group populations. However, the desired level of equity in healthcare is not achieved, leaving a considerable percentage of the population being left out with a higher burden of infant and child morbidities and mortalities. Therefore, efforts must be put into bringing health equity across different caste groups in India.

To achieve the Sustainable Development Goals (SDGs) in maternal and child health, India must address the Caste-based disparities within the county. Until and unless reducing the Caste-based disparities in health care utilization, there is no meaning in achieving SDGs targets.

References

Acharya, S. S. (2020). Population-poverty linkages and health consequences. *Caste/a Global Journal on Social Exclusion, 1*(1), 29–50.

Ali, B., & Chauhan, S. (2020). Inequalities in the utilisation of maternal health care in rural India: Evidences from national family health survey III & IV. *BMC Public Health, 20*(1), 1–13.

Arokiasamy, P., Jain, K., Goli, S., & Pradhan, J. (2013). Health inequalities among urban children in India: A comparative assessment of empowered action group (EAG) and south Indian states. *Journal of Biosocial*.

Barman, S., & De, P. (2017). Socio-economic inequality of child immunization in the Eastern and North-Eastern States of India. *Demography India Special Issue*, 16–26.

Bakshi, A. (2008). Social inequality in land ownership in India: A study with particular reference to West Bengal. *Social Scientist*, 95–116.

Borooah, V. K. (2005). Caste, inequality, and poverty in India. *Review of Development Economics, 9*(3), 399–414.

Bhaumik, S. K., & Chakrabarty, M. (2006). *Earnings inequality in India: Has the rise of caste and religion based politics in India had an impact?*

Bettampadi, D., Lepkowski, J. M., Sen, A., Power, L. E., & Boulton, M. L. (2021). Vaccination inequality in India, 2002–2013. *American Journal of Preventive Medicine, 60*(1), S65–S76.

Bora, J. K., Raushan, R., & Lutz, W. (2019). The persistent influence of caste on under-five mortality: Factors that explain the caste-based gap in high focus Indian states. *PloS One, 14*(8), e0211086.

Chokshi, M., Patil, B., Khanna, R., Neogi, S. B., Sharma, J., Paul, V. K., & Zodpey, S. (2016). Health systems in India. *Journal of Perinatology, 36*(3), S9–S12.

De Costa, A., & Diwan, V. (2007). 'Where is the public health sector?' Public and private sector healthcare provision in Madhya Pradesh, India. *Health Policy, 84*(2–3), 269–276.

Debnath, A., & Bhattacharjee, N. (2018). Wealth-based inequality in child immunization in India: A decomposition approach. *Journal of Biosocial Science, 50*(3), 312–325.

Deshpande, S. (2006). Exclusive inequalities: Merit, caste and discrimination in Indian higher education today. *Economic and Political Weekly*, 2438–2444.

Dutta, A. K., & Aggarwal, A. (2018). Newer development in immunization practices. *Indian Journal of Pediatrics, 85*(1), 44–46.

Hnatkovska, V., Lahiri, A., & Paul, S. (2012). Castes and labor mobility. *American Economic Journal: Applied Economics, 4*(2), 274–307.

International Institute for Population Sciences (IIPS) and ICF. (2017). National Family Health Survey (NFHS-4), 2015-16: India. Mumbai: IIPS.

Joe, W., Mishra, U. S., & Navaneetham, K. (2010). Socio-economic inequalities in child health: Recent evidence from India. *Global Public Health, 5*(5), 493–508.

Jungari, S., & Bomble, P. (2013). Caste-based social exclusion and health deprivation in India. *Journal of Exclusion Studies, 3*(2), 84–91.

Jungari, S., & Chauhan, B. G. (2017). Caste, wealth and regional inequalities in health status of women and children in India. *Contemporary Voice of Dalit, 9*(1), 87–100.

Kader, M., & Perera, N. (2014). Socio-economic and nutritional determinants of low birth weight in India. *North American Journal of Medical Sciences, 6*(7), 302–308

Khan, N., & Saggurti, N. (2020). Socioeconomic inequality trends in childhood vaccination coverage in India: Findings from multiple rounds of National Family Health Survey. *Vaccine*.

Khanal, V., Zhao, Y., & Sauer, K. (2014). Role of antenatal care and iron supplementation during pregnancy in preventing low birth weight in Nepal: Comparison of national surveys 2006 and 2011. *Archives of Public Health, 72*(1), 1–10.

Kumar, P., & Gupta, A. (2015). Determinants of inter and intra caste differences in utilization of maternal health care services in india: Evidence from dlhs-3 survey. *International Research Journal of Social Sciences, 4*(1), 27–36.

Kumar, P., Patel, R., Chauhan, S., Srivastava, S., Khare, A., & Patel, K. K. (2020). Does socio-economic inequality in infant mortality still exist in India? An analysis based on the National Family Health Survey 2005–06 and 2015–16. *Clinical Epidemiology and Global Health, 9,* 116–122.

Ma, S., & Sood, N. (2008). *A comparison of the health systems in China and India* (Vol. 212). Rand Corporation.

Mathew, J. L. (2012). Inequity in childhood immunization in India: A systematic review. *Indian Pediatrics, 49*(3), 203–223.

Mavalankar, D. (2016). Doctors for tribal areas: Issues and solutions. *Indian Journal of Community Medicine: Official Publication of Indian Association of Preventive & Social Medicine, 41*(3), 172.

Madheswaran, S., & Attewell, P. (2007). Caste discrimination in the Indian urban labour market: Evidence from the national sample survey. *Economic and Political Weekly*, 4146–4153.

Narain, J. P. (2019). Health of tribal populations in India: How long can we afford to neglect? *The Indian Journal of Medical Research, 149*(3), 313.

Oaxaca, R. (1973). Male-female wage differentials in urban labor markets. *International Economic Review, 14*, 693–709.

Owen, O'., Eddy, D., Wagstaff, A., & Magnus, L. (2008). Analyzing health equity using household survey data: A Guide to techniques and their implementation. *WBI Learning Resources Series.*

Pande, R. P., & Yazbeck, A. S. (2003). What's in a country average? Wealth, gender, and regional inequalities in immunization in India. *Social Science & Medicine, 57*(11), 2075–2088.

Patel, R., & Chauhan, S. (2020). Gender differential in health care utilisation in India. *Clinical Epidemiology and Global Health, 8*(2), 526–530.

Prusty, R. K., & Kumar, A. (2014). Socioeconomic dynamics of gender disparity in childhood immunization in India, 1992–2006. *PLoS One, 9*(8), e104598.

Registrar General of India. (2011). *C-8 Educational Level by Age and Sex for Population Age 7 and Above.* Registrar General & Census Commissioner of India. Ministry of Home Affairs, Government of India. https://censusindia.gov.in/2011census/C-series/C08.html.

Shrivastwa, N., Gillespie, B. W., Kolenic, G. E., Lepkowski, J. M., & Boulton, M. L. (2015). Predictors of vaccination in India for children aged 12–36 months. *American Journal of Preventive Medicine, 49*(6), S435–S444.

Singh, P. K. (2013). Trends in child immunization across geographical regions in India: focus on urban-rural and gender differentials. *PLos one, 8*(9), e73102.

Srivastava, S., Chauhan, S., & Patel, R. (2020a). Socio-economic inequalities in the prevalence of poor self-rated health among older adults in India from 2004 to 2014: A decomposition analysis. *Ageing International*, 1–18.

Srivastava, S., Fledderjohann, J., & Upadhyay, A. K. (2020b). Explaining socioeconomic inequalities in immunisation coverage in India: New insights from the fourth National Family Health Survey (2015–16). *BMC Pediatrics, 20*(1), 1–12.

Vishwakarma, M., Shekhar, C., Dutta, M., & Yadav, A. (2020). Gaps in infant and child mortality among social groups and its linkages with institutional delivery and child immunization using census and National Family Health Survey (2015–16). *Journal of Public Health, 28*(3), 293–303.

Thorat, S., Mahamallik, M., & Panth, A. (2003). *Labour market and occupational discrimination in rural areas.* Indian Institute of Dalit Studies (IIDS), New Delhi.

Thorat, S., & Newman, K. S. (2007). Caste and economic discrimination: Causes, consequences and remedies. *Economic and Political Weekly*, 4121–4124.

Zacharias, A., & Vakulabharanam, V. (2011). Caste stratification and wealth inequality in India. *World Development, 39*(10), 1820–1833.

Chapter 16
Reflections on Gendered Health Inequalities within Households

Arindam Roy

Abstract The present paper views anatomical and epidemiological differences among gender have led to the differential proclivity of diseases among gender. The risk of cervical cancer or ovarian cancer or breast cancer is rather high among women, whereas vulnerability to testicular and prostate cancer is more common among men. But this gender-driven epidemiological occurrence has nothing to do with the differences in life expectancy or morbidity status among genders. This new approach has unravelled the structured inequality embedded in a given society to deconstruct the fatalistic explanation of the morbidity status of women. According to this approach, women's proclivity to fall prey to recurring ailments or morbidity is biological. A Feminine Mystique is constructed to domesticate her and the patriarchal discriminatory values, which have been feeding into a girl child to make her a docile subject, have their invariable impact on her health outcome. The paper identifies household as the fountainhead of discrimination against women. It also engages with 'gender inequality in health' as a whole new approach to uncover women's vulnerabilities within household.

Keywords Household economy · Women · Vulnerability · Gender inequality in health · Health outcomes

Introduction

The household, no matter how it is defined, has been considered in the feminist epistemology as the primary site of women subjugation. There is mushrooming of literature on the appropriation of women's unpaid labour in the household economy. The present paper, however, intends to make a departure from the popular discourses on gender inequality by casting some light on gender inequality in health, caused due to systematic and systemic neglect of a girl child since her birth by the patriarchal households. The differential health outcome between genders, which is mooted by

A. Roy (✉)
Department of Political Science, The University of Burdwan, Burdwan, West Bengal, India

the gender inequality in health approach in recent times, is nothing new. In fact, it has been with us for centuries, but it is mostly overlooked and rationalized as fait accompli by equating it with gender differences in health.

The present paper views that the above approach is a biassed one. The anatomical and epidemiological differences among gender have led to the differential proclivity of diseases among gender. For example, the risk of cervical cancer or ovarian cancer or breast cancer is rather high among women, whereas vulnerability to testicular and prostate cancer is more common among men. But this gender-driven epidemiological occurrence has nothing to do with the differences in life expectancy or morbidity status among genders. This new approach has unravelled the structured inequality embedded in a given society to deconstruct the fatalistic explanation of the morbidity status of women. According to this approach, women's proclivity to fall prey to recurring ailments or morbidity is biological. It can be explained by the very nature of upbringing of girls in a given society, which is substantially constructed by patriarchal values. It is the invisible dictum of patriarchy, carried forward by generations of docile women folk, which has structured the very texture of the household concerned. If a girl child is at all allowed to appear on this earth, she is being taught to withstand a life-long journey of compromise, starting from sharing meals with her male sibling to education and the way of life. A Feminine Mystique is constructed to domesticate her (Friedan, 1963). The patriarchal discriminatory values, which have been feeding into a girl child to make her a docile subject, have their invariable impact on her health outcome.

Unlike the gender differences in health outcome which require further scientific innovations, the gender inequality in health, which is by and large socially and cultur-ally constructed, demands immediate policy intervention. Therefore, the need of the hour is to look at the status of women in the household beyond the economic depri-vation and to concentrate on her morbidity status to make sense of her secondary position within the household. The paper has the following sections: Sect. 1 identi-fies household as the fountainhead of discrimination against women; Sect. 2 'Gender Inequality in Health' presents a whole new approach to uncover women's vulner-abilities within households; Sect. 3 mainly highlights the nature of the study and methodology; Sect. 4 mainly deals with the findings of the study, and finally Sect. 5 presents a concluding observation.

Household as the Fountainhead of Gender Discrimination

Household is generally couched as a place of love, warmth and intimate rela-tions. However, it is also known as a site of intense competition, egocentrism, subor-dination, domestication and indoctrination. The feminist scholars of all hues have endorsed it in their deliberations. Gender inequality, the perennial embarrassment of humanity, originates in the household. However, the above definition obfuscates the subtle difference between household and family. Though households and fami-lies are conceptually different, they do overlap in practice. Scholars are divided in conceptualizing the term 'household' for its supposed intersection with family and kinship group. Hence, a clarification is necessary to proceed with further discussion on households. Indonesian Demographic Health Survey, 2007 defined a household 'as a person or a group of persons, related or unrelated, who live together in the same dwelling unit and share a common source of food' (Dommaraju and Tan, 2014).

Drawing on survey or census data, demographers are usually focussing on the same dwelling unit, common provision of food from a common granary or using a common hearth or cooking pot or identifying the same person as the head of households in defining a household. Whereas the economists consider households as a production-consumption unit with shared labour and economic resources, the anthropologists identify kinship and lineage as the major components of households. However, defining a household this way often ignores the importance of local complexities and nuances of households usually exhibited in social relationships or external networks. As per the US Census Bureau, notwithstanding the interchangeability of the usage of these terms, there is a marked difference between household and family. Based on the classification made by the US Census Bureau, a household can be defined as an institution where one or more persons live in the same house, apartment, or condominium but may or may not be related to each other, and a family is one where two or more persons living in the same room are bounded by birth, marriage or adoption. Therefore, families are bound to be households, but not the other way round. The 2010 Federal Census has counted 116.72 million households across America, of which 77.54 million households are categorized as families and the rest 39.18 million households as 'non-family households' (Thomas, 2012).

The present paper is mainly referring to family households. It explores the gender discrimination in households as non-family households are more mechanical, where staying together has instrumental rationality. It is in the household where several discriminatory patriarchal values and constructions have been systematically infused into girl's psyches. Interestingly, here women play the key role for facilitating patriarchy. Several studies have demonstrated that the status of women, especially their vulnerabilities, is not determined by the patriarchy alone, rather they are very much determined by the 'intra-household differentials in women status' or their autonomy within the households. Economically speaking, women have been exploited within the household by robbing off their labour. Driven by a typical outdated 'breadwinner/homemaker' binary, the relentless toil is undertaken by the womenfolk in the name of the domestic choir has never been acknowledged and remained mostly unacknowledged, let alone getting paid for it. It is because of the sexual division of labour and the gendered role of discharging domestic care work duly backed up by social norms, the burden of domestic work falls disproportionately on women.

However, this burden is not confined to the homemakers alone. The working women, who have been perennially stretched between domestic needs and professional requirements, have to bear the brunt. Apart from the domestic and professional workloads, women within the households have to shoulder a huge invisible mental load, which has mostly remained unacknowledged. Brigid Schulte, the author of *Overwhelmed: Work, Love and Play When No One Has the Time* (Schulte, 2015) in an interview, has nicely encapsulated the otherwise neglected source of work-related vulnerability in the following words: 'It's all of the stuff that you have to keep in your mind. It's just an explosion of details and logistics and planning and organizing and making appointments and remembering the appointments and getting people to the appointments, remembering birthdays, doing the 'kinwork' […] keeping the ties, the family and bonds of friends, keeping those strong…' (Gross, 2020).

Economists have argued in favour of accounting for the women labour in the domestic choir. The International Labour Organization (ILO) has come out with some startling statistics to demonstrate the magnitude of economic deprivation of women in the benign garb of the domestic choir. As per the ILO report entitled, *Care Work and Care Jobs: For the future of Decent Work*, the time spent on unpaid care work is tantamount to 16.4 billion hours per day, of which women contribute to more than three fourths (76.2%) of the total. The said report has come to this conclusion based on the time-use data consisting of both the paid and unpaid care works representing 66.9% of the world's working-age population from 64 countries (ILO, 2018). In India, women, on an average, spend 351.9 min/day on unpaid work vis-à-vis an average of 51.8 min/day by men.

However, the present paper argues that gender discrimination is highly structured and extended beyond economic deprivation. Women are not only deprived econom- ically within the household by being roped in several non-remunerative domestic drudgeries but also subjected to systematic and systemic neglect that leads to serious health hazards including morbidity among women vis-à-vis men. Though often gone unnoticed, it is brazenly rationalized as the fallout of the woman's anatomy. However, in reality, it is the outcome of the very process of the upbringing of the girl child within the household. Unlike those households where the girl child is not welcome and a female foetus is meant for termination, the status of a girl child in other so-called liberal households is no better either. There are a number of examples where some girl children who are fortunate enough to be allowed to come on this earth, albeit willy nilly, have to live a life with a benign sense of neglect embedded within house- holds. Gender discrimination starts inside the mother's womb as reflected in several national and international reports. For example, WHO in its 2011 report has shown an overall picture of dwindling sex ratio at birth in Asia. The average biological sex ratio at birth, as reported by WHO, is 106 boys for every 100 girls, which was even more miserable in Eastern, South and Central Asia (Di Cesare, 2014). Apart from sex-selective termination of foetus or abortion in case of late realization, the girl child who manages to appear on this earth, escaping the embedded son-preference preva- lent in the society, has to bear a life-long saga of sacrifice and compromise. From sharing of food to the choice of school, a girl child has been taught from her very childhood to withstand preferential treatments which she has to undergo throughout her life vis-à-vis her male sibling.

The neglect is not confined to sharing of food or educational preferences alone, even medical attention is also badly tilted towards the male sibling. For example, vaccinations, access to healthcare and household health care expenditure are mostly reserved for the male child. Consequently, a girl child who manages to survive braving preferential treatments within the household develops several avoidable gynecolog- ical disorders, in addition to malnutrition, at the time of puberty due to the sheer apathy of the womenfolk in the household. Several socio-cultural and religious constructions and taboos have been invoked in households to legitimize the deprivation of the adolescent girl child from getting proper medical attention. Consequently, a sizable section of girl children has succumbed to several avoidable diseases and contributed to the 'missing women' category.

The proclivity of women to fall prey to recurring illness is not a matter of mere biology, but very much an offshoot of the systemic neglect and apathy of the patriarchal households. The above-mentioned vulnerabilities that women have to face within the households mostly happen during the normal situation on a day-to-day basis. However, the situation gets further worsened for women when households encounter any disaster or calamity. Be it natural disasters like flood, tsunami, earthquakes or vector-driven epidemics, women have to suffer the most. Though disasters have a more or less equal primary impact on the affected section, the long-lasting secondary impact varies widely in terms of gender, class, and so on. For example, our experiences demonstrated that women and marginal sections have to face the wrath of disaster more than their male and upper-class counterparts. However, it should be mentioned that the affected sections, like women and marginal sections, are not mutually exclusive. In fact, in real life situations, these categories do overlap and make the classification almost impossible as women and class keep intersecting each other.

The ongoing pandemic of COVID-19 and its unprecedented impact on the lives of the common people in general and women in particular may be a case in point. The pandemic has exacerbated the already existing disproportionate workloads of women within the household. The imposition of lockdown and other legal-administrative measures in the wake of the outbreak of the pandemic have not only brought the economy into a grinding halt but have also transformed our very worldview. The socio-cultural ambience has undergone a sea change as the entire humanity has been forced to confine themselves indoors with serious repercussions for women. The sudden closure of schools and other educational institutes and introduction of work from home schedules has quadrupled the workloads for women, who have been struggling hard to balance work and home fronts. Being the primary caregiver, both formally at work and informally at home, women are more likely to be exposed to the risk of contamination of the lethal virus of COVID-19. Moreover, the global economic downturn due to the sudden outbreak of the pandemic has its debilitating impact on the livelihood of the millions of people in the global South, who are forced to lead their life in utter penury (World Health Organization, 2020). Further, such economic hardship has resulted in rampant domestic violence and strained inter-family relationships with women at the receiving ends.

Ironically, the lockdown measure, which was imposed to protect people from the aggravation of virus, has eventually endangered the life of women by trapping them into domestic ambience with abusive partners, parents or family members or sexual predators. This increased risk of gender-based violence during the pandemic has been christened by *UN Women* as the 'shadow pandemic' (Guidorzi, 2020). The sudden spurt of cases of domestic violence during lockdown has validated the above point. For example, a Singapore-based women's rights organization, the Association of Women for Action and Research (AWARE), has reported that there has been a 137% spike in the cases of domestic violence in Singapore since the beginning of lockdown in March 2020 (Nanthini and Tamara, 2020).

In the following section, an attempt will be made to go beyond the typical economic interpretation of women subjugation within the household, and venture into a rather unexplored terrain of health and nutrition.

Gender Inequality in Health: An Overview

The gender inequality in health approach has brought home an altogether new perspective to gender inequality by interrogating the prevailing fatalistic perception of women's health i.e. 'biology is destiny' embedded in households. It problematizes the intriguing coupling of nature and nurture which, in effect, has determined the tenor of morbidity and vulnerability in human beings. As an important determinant of health, gender has confounded the apparent biological dimensions of vulnerability. In feminist literature and policy discourses, many factors have been identified for the secondary status of women vis-à-vis men with their obvious impact on the overall health outcome. These include; firstly, there are several prejudiced constructions and practices about women's health within households and communities; the second important factor is the variability of exposures and vulnerabilities of women to disease, disability and injuries; and thirdly, the gender biases in health systems and biassed health research are also held responsible for the secondary status of women vis-à-vis male (Sen and Ostlin, 2012). Fourthly, intersectionality is also considered as a critical issue of gender, which may lead to 'multilayered discrimination'. It uncovers the multiple locations and variations of marginalization, the process of subject formation and differentiation and systems of domination in a given society (Iyer et al., 2012).

It operates at three different levels: 'the multi-dimensional way in which power operates and subjectivity, subjection and social location are subsequently constructed; the different levels at which interactions occur; and the differing degrees and forms of penalty and privilege between social locations and subjects' (Hankivsky, 2011). However, this approach is not free from biases. Unlike the mainstream research in health, which normally overlooks the importance of gender in the variability of health outcome by conflating sex and gender in empirical methods, the gender inequality approach over-emphasizes the vulnerability of women as the only victims of gender inequality, leaving behind the male vulnerability. Hence, at the very outset, a few conceptual riddles need to be straightened up. First, there is a general tendency of treating women vulnerability as fait accompli of women, which is interrogated by the gender inequality in health approach; secondly, all sorts of differences in health outcome between men and women should not be bracketed as patriarchal constructions as gender differences in health outcome are sometimes biological and sometimes, they are a heady concoction of sex and gender.

Before we figure out gender inequality in health within households, a distinction between gender differences in health and gender inequality in health deserves some space here. Though often these two terms are considered identical, there is a subtle distinction between them. The gender differences in health are considered as a normal phenomenon, born out of biological differences. The chromosomal variation, to be more specific, leads to anatomical differences between men and women and their resultant vulnerability to different diseases. For example, the sex chromosomes (46 XX versus 46 XY karyotypes) are held responsible for the developmental differentiation in anatomy and physiology of men and women and the resultant differences in health outcome (Snow, 2012). Accordingly, we find that women are more prone to the risks of haemophilia, ovarian deformities, cervical cancer and so on because of XY karyotypes whereas vulnerabilities like testicular and prostate cancers are more common to men because of XX karyotypes (Snow, 2012). Hence, the gender difference in health has to be understood as a normal outcome of the biological constitution and should not be meddled with other issues, even if that involves further scientific innovations. The very biological logic behind such difference shuns any policy intervention whatsoever.

On the other hand, gender inequality in health is conceptualized as differential health outcomes between men and women which are socially and culturally constructed. It is deemed as one of the many ramifications of the deeply rooted structural inequality against women in a given society, which requires serious policy intervention. Since gender has the potential of determining the structural location of women and men in society and their subjective experiences, the persistence of gender biases within communities will have their invariable impact on health outcome. The nuances of gender constructions, especially the way it shapes the behavioural pattern of women folk in a given society, can be explained in a better way if we draw on the life cycle perspective study. The life cycle perspective is a newly applied methodology in social science research that claims to have presented a nuanced overview of different facets of a woman's life starting from very birth to death. The present paper in the light of a popular health programme, i.e. RCH in the district of Burdwan, West Bengal (India), intends to investigate whether the dismal health outcome in the district has anything to do with patriarchal gender constructions within households and suggests a few possible ways to plug the policy shortcomings.

The Study

The study in the light of a flagship health programme, initiated by the Government of India i.e. Reproductive and Child Health (RCH) in the district of Burdwan, West Bengal (India), intends to investigate whether the dismal health outcome in the district has anything to do with patriarchal gender constructions within households. The study was ethnographic in nature, which had been conducted in two blocks of opposing political affiliations in Burdwan district. The basic objective of the study was to explore how gender intermeshes with several other social markers like religion, cultural values etc. to the disadvantage of women's health in particular and women empowerment in general.

Methodology

The choice of Burdwan district as the universe of study was based on the following reasons: first, the district represents the pluri-cultural mosaic of the country; secondly, Burdwan is among a few advanced districts in West Bengal which has a wider network of health service providers; thirdly, the district has been considered as the epicentre of Left mobilization in West Bengal that came into the limelight for socialist experimentations with land reform, land redistribution and avowed pro-poor stand. To further investigate the relationship between gender and health, two blocks from Burdwan district viz. Bhatar and Memari were selected.

Here, the rationale behind choosing the aforesaid blocks was to explore the impact of political mobilization on gender sensitization. The selected blocks represent two opposing political trends with Memeri I being considerably pro-Left and Bhatar being significantly non-Left. Memari-I block is known for its long and rich legacy of Left mobilization and socialist experimentations such as land reform, land redistribution as the left coalition had controlled the block along with the state for more than three decades. Primarily rural in nature, the Bhatar block under consideration has been a stronghold of Congress despite strong Left mobilization across the district. Even in the 1977 assembly election, which was a watershed in the history of West Bengal, when Left Front stormed into power with an overwhelming majority, Bhatar remained as a glaring exception with a stronghold of Congress. Bhola Sen of Indian National Congress had survived the Left ascendancy, and managed to garner a comfortable margin of 56.52% and continued to function as the MLA till 1982. In the Assembly election of 1982, he lost to CPM leader Syed Md. Masih. Though the Left Front was able to retain this assembly constituency for five consecutive elections (1987, 1991, 1996, 2001, 2006), the opposition had a considerable support base in this constituency with an average of 40% vote share in all the previous elections (District Panchayat Election Officer & District Magistrate, 2008).

Since reproductive health is the public health programme, which is administered in the private domain, a mere quantitative method is not sufficient to garner intimate information regarding reproductive health. A total sample of three hundred (300) households from the above two blocks had been selected for primary survey. From each selected block, 150 households were divided in three categories, of which 50 households comprised of Muslim and 50 of Scheduled Caste, Scheduled Tribe and Other Backward Class whereas 50 comprised of General category respectively. The receivers/beneficiaries were mainly the cross-section of people (representing both the sexes drawn mainly from the above categories). However, such a survey would not have approximated the scenario if the deliverer's perspective had not been incorporated. Since the health sector in India is marked by medical pluralism, mere data from the biomedical deliverer is not enough to understand the complexity of the health sector. Hence, the study had gathered information through in-depth personal interview and personal narrative from three sets of health deliverers present in rural India- biomedical professionals (doctors, health workers, para-medical staff and village-level workers); a group of medical practitioners who are not directly engaged in state health delivery mechanism, but cater to the people under study (RMP-Registered Medical Practitioners); and quacks, religious medical men like *Ojhas* and *Tantriks*. As a technique of data collection, the study relied mainly on both quantitative and qualitative methods, especially focussed group interview and narrative analysis, to grasp the intricacies of gender dimension in health outcome.

Findings

The study has classified the respondents into two sections, i.e.,- receivers and deliverers, to garner the complex information regarding gender discrimination within households. The present section has cherry picked a few revealing narratives generated in course of the field study to validate our argument.

Receivers' Perspectives

Here respondents are mainly the cross-section of people, representing both the sexes drawn mainly from the Muslim, SCs, STs and general castes. In the study, we have encountered several popular narratives of disapproval of health programmes, especially reproductive health initiatives under RCH programme, like contraception, menstruation hygiene, prenatal and postnatal care of mother and children smack of gender prejudices. Rojina Bibi, 53, a housewife and mother of six children exclaimed: '*Contraception is by nature antithetical to Islam. Children are the greatest endowment of Allah. To terminate a baby in the womb is tantamount to a great sin. It is against the will of almighty Allah!*' Here religious sentiment is infused among the women folk through the socialization process to rob them of their right to decide about their family and its size. Similar kind of conviction was echoed in the words of other respondents as well and that is not confined to Islam alone.

Even among Hindus, similar indoctrination persists, as was evident in the words of Monmon Das, 38, a primary school teacher and mother of one child, who has lamented the abortion of her first issue: '*I still regret the decision of the doctor to abort my first issue on health ground. The doctor later explained that the abortion was a medical exigency as my pregnancy had developed serious complications. Despite explanations, I think that I had committed an unpardonable sin*'. An interesting narrative of Hamida Begum, 33, a housewife, educated till standard eight, would be relevant here to mention as to how gender discrimination determines the health-seeking behaviour: '*I can remember those days of my pregnancies. I had been reeling under the spell of melancholy and bad mood for no apparent reasons. Sabnam was only two years old then and was totally dependent upon me. My mom-in-law seldom took her for a stroll when I was busy cooking our meal. My husband Akram, 32, was also not much of help. He was busy with his job and hardly offered any help. Even when he tried to help me, my mom-in law started howling as if he did something forbidden. Besides, my mom-in law along with other elderly members of the family put continuous pressure on me for a son. I used to visit the nearby dargah once a week for prayer. Thanks to Allah that finally Anwar came to my life and saved me from repeated pangs of child bearing.'*

The above narrative of Hamida was indicative of multiple vulnerabilities of women where patriarchal values, male dominance and religious-cultural practices in the said situation appear to be mutually constitutive and reinforcing. Another narrative, generated in the course of survey, deserves special mention here, which demonstrates how social customs and practices are invoked to deprive women of adequate medical attention. Interestingly, here women themselves act as the agency of patriarchy. Tania Bibi, a housewife aged 28, from Debipur village, made a comment on health-seeking behaviour, which is indicative of dominant cultural perception regarding women's health: *'Now-a-days it has become a fashion to visit a doctor. In our times, we did not visit doctors so frequently. After all, we come into this world as women. So we must learn to suffer. Seeing a doctor for mere abdominal pain in those days (menstruation) is a luxury!.'*

Similarly, cultural factors, especially shared beliefs, myth and taboos play a determining role in shaping women's health-seeking behaviour, which, in turn, determine the fate of a given health programme. Generally, in a given society, patriarchal values sneak in through the socialization process. The innumerable customs, myths, shared beliefs and taboos exist in every society on pregnancy and newborn, which are customized by the patriarchy. For example, nutritional deficiency is one of the major factors behind the perennial vulnerability of women. Interestingly, in the society under study, we find that patriarchy has indoctrinated its women folk of ideal womanly behaviour where they are expected to abide by a host of discriminatory behavioural practices as normal. A girl child is taught about this difference from her very infancy and is instructed to follow a code of conduct which includes among others that girls should not eat in the first place, and they should give lion's share to the male siblings, etc.

Consequently, a girl child, who has been suffering from perennial nutritional deficiency, would fall prey to a host of avoidable ailments by the time she reaches her adolescence. The patriarchal indoctrination is so encompassing that women who are basically involved in the kitchen are considering such discriminatory allocation of food and practice of giving male members precedence over girl child as absolutely normal. A few such puzzling narratives emerged out of discussion, which are indicative of gender discrimination, that have an impact on women health outcome: Madhuri Mukherjee, 42, housewife and a mother of two said: *'we as women have lot of responsibility. We cannot take our food with other family members. As mistress of the family, we make sure that male folk of the family must be fed first. We female members should take our meal afterward. It brings prosperity to the family'*. Similar sentiment was echoed by Ruksana Begam, 41, a village level health worker: *'we often taught mothers not to discriminate among the children in food allocation. But tell me how a housewife can accept a meal before other members of the family.'*

In addition, adolescent girls are also taught not to discuss intimate physical issues with others and utmost secrecy has to be maintained during menstruation. Namita Sen, 30, a school teacher and mother of two children has encapsulated the above fact in her own words: *'I can recollect my adolescent days. My mother always remained tense for no reason. She endlessly advised me what to do and what not to do in those days. My mother taught several such nitty gritties so that my behaviour would not generate unnecessary 'attention'. I was taught how to wash my undergarments and how discretely they should be dried up. Even my mother had adequately sensitized me about the uneasiness and lower abdominal pains, the normal symptom of menstruation cycle so that I may not complain about it in public.'* The patriarchal indoctrination, especially the shame of one's own body, is so comprehensively instilled among the women folk that their behaviour patterns including the health-seeking behaviour bear indelible mark of it. This indoctrination starts at the very early stage where the girl is taught that she is different from her male siblings. Hence, she should 'behave' the way she is expected to behave. The ideal behaviour of a girl, though widely varies from society to society, includes almost everything from food habits, toilet training, lingerie etiquette and so on.

One narrative in this context deserves special mention. The RCH programme is replete with examples where cultural factors play a determining role. The RCH programme was conceived to address a number of issues, and among others, one important issue is RTI. Under the programme, awareness generation among the adolescent girls is given utmost priority. Most of this problem is generated due to ignorance about sexual hygiene, fear of social stigma and sanction. On being asked why he had refused ANC and PNC for his wife, One Aminur Molla, a marginal worker aged 38, with secondary education, said:

Yes, I am aware of the ANC and PNC. But how can I send my pregnant wife to the health centre, which is always overcrowded. She had to wait for long hours in such an embarrassing state (pregnant state) just to get some free boris (Tablets)! We strongly believe in the grace of Allah and leave it to the hands of Allah. No matter what the problem might be, Allah will bail us out.

The above narrative speaks of underlining patriarchal sanctions, which deter women from availing public health measures since they are not compatible with the patriarchal value system. The patriarchal social structure sanctioned the public appearance of pregnant women. Sometimes, cultural and religious sanctions are also imposed to ensure patriarchal domination. For example, a fear of evil air was often instilled to restrict women folk within the four walls of the family. Our study further revealed a similar presence of patriarchy, which acted as a powerful deterrent for the women to realize their health needs. For example, family planning was treated as an absolute male prerogative. Women were never consulted. In case of permanent family planning, instead of vasectomy, the IUD measures for women like cooper-T were generally adopted. In the course of discussion on family planning, one Amina Bibi, aged 32, a mother of two, has come out with such life experiences: *I can distinctly recall those restless afternoons and sleepless nights when Sakila was only 9 months old. An unknown fear of imminent danger haunted me. I had lost my body weight at an alarming rate. I was always in a bitter mood, and it changed erratically and without any reason. I kept on requesting my husband to take protection. But he did not care about it. The elderly of my family and my mother-in law had refused to give any importance to my ill-health, and kept on insisting for a baby boy for retaining family lineage. Thank Allah that I could give a baby boy or else I would have to suffer the pangs of child bearing for many more times. Finally, Aynul was born and my husband took me to a private hospital for ligation.*

Deliverers' Perspectives

The above narratives and comments from the receivers have been validated by similar narratives of the deliverers. This section provides a brief overview of the deliverer's perspective. Sometimes gender construction is so encompassing and stifling that in some societies the issue of reproductive health is considered a taboo. Hence, these are rarely discussed in public, let alone asking for remedies. Even parents feel embarrassed to share the basic physiological information with their daughter. Consequently, they rely upon some half-baked information leading to several gynecological problems including infertility. One MBBS doctor, from the area under study, has cast some light on it by sharing his experiences: '*I have encountered a good many cases of Reproductive Tract Infection (RTIs), which were usually cloaked in the garb of casual ailments. Ailing women and their male accomplice usually hide their actual problem in fear of stigma and social sanction. But the suppression of the disease only aggravates its intensity. Timely detection of these gynecological cases may save them from deadly RTIs. I personally counsel them to bring such cases to the notice of the doctors immediately*'.

Gender construction is so pervasive in the area under study that creating awareness about sexual hygiene, prenatal and postnatal cares etc., which come under the fold of RCH programme, has suffered serious setbacks. Cloaked in the garb of an apparent nonchalant attitude, the health-seeking behaviour of the people in the universe under study bears the mark of a strong gender prejudice as it is evident in the words of a health worker of Bhatar block hospital: *We always try to educate the women folk, especially those who could not afford sanitary napkin, as to how they could go for some cheap homemade alternatives like cotton pads. We teach them how to make this piece of cotton hygienic and safe for the next use. But in most cases, the rural women either avoid our suggestion or do not care much. Even those who abided by our prescription often kept those cotton pieces in such places where secondary infection was only obvious. Moreover, rural women often wash the cotton pads in contaminated water, leading thereby to several reproductive tract infections like itching, white discharges, and so on. They are always haunted by the fear that they might be caught by someone drying up those things... They are taught to maintain utmost secrecy in drying up those things.*

Here, ignorance about sexual hygiene was not the only reason for the attrition to the RCH programme, gender construction in association with cultural factors like taboo, fear of stigma and embedded inhibition all work in unison in shaping health-seeking behaviour of the people. Sometimes, even myths are constructed to maintain gender expectations. For example, one health councillor of Memeri Block Hospital had shared a very interesting myth regarding menstruation, which could have played spoilsport for the government sponsored RCH programme. '*I had encountered one of the most debilitating myths regarding menstruation in one of our awareness generation camps on sexual and menstruation hygiene. When I was interacting with the villagers and making them aware of possible ways as to how they could maintain hygiene with homemade cotton pads, one of the participants from that village questioned the feasibility of maintaining hygiene. She said that our suggestion of washing and drying up the cotton pads for re-use was not applicable since they did not have a discreet and hygienic place to dry up those pads. She said that she was always apprehensive of the possibility that somebody would have seen those pads or come in physical contact with them when they were put on the sun or come in proximity of the foul air emanating from it. Any such incident would affect the health of her husband or prospective husband in case of adolescent girls. So deeply lodged was the myth among the village women that they preferred dark and humid and unhygienic corners of the room for drying up cotton pads, instead of out in the sun. Consequently, most of the women were suffering from fungal infections like itching, white discharges etc.*'

Similarly, in our study, we found that women who were suffering from low haemoglobin rarely collected the freely distributed iron and calcium tablets. On being asked why they did not collect those tablets, most of the receivers said that they could not collect medicines due to some preoccupations. However, one village level health worker, in the course of our interaction, had given us the clue. He told us that women generally refused to take those medicines because that required pregnant women to be physically present at the sub-centres. Sabina khatun, one ASHA worker, 27, narrated her personal experience: '*we were sent to a village which was reported to have the lowest in terms of medicine intake. To get into the roots as to why free tablets remain unutilized, we had interacted with the residents of that village. But no one actually expressed the truth. But one saddik mullah, 71 ruefully expressed 'how could we send our women to collect free boris in that stage. The public appearance of pregnant women, you know, with their swollen belly attracts unwelcoming male gaze*'.

Since the Indian health sector is marked by a purported trend of medical pluralism, the deliverers of health services here include the people who do not fall directly within the ambit of public health mechanisms like the religious medical men. In our study, we had interviewed such religious medical men to understand the role of magico-religious factors in the overall health-seeking behaviour of women folk in the area under study. However, these religious medical men, unlike their popular stereotyping; come out with several liberating health messages. But owing to the deep seated religious-cultural values system nurtured by the patriarchy households, as evident in the area under study, they were compelled to invoke religious symbolism like pani pora, maduli, tabiz and so on. One Hafesaheeb, a Muslim religious medical man from the area under study, had candidly narrated: '*most of the people coming to me for health relief are women and they suffer so much because they have ignored the basic principles of good health on the pretext of family values. I usually give them one or two tabiz (religious pendant) and tell them to take a few health precautions like, drinking adequate water, taking regular baths, maintaining personal and sexual hygiene, wearing washed clothes for better result. No religious medicine can do miracle healing, until and unless the basic sense of hygiene is maintained. At best, I can only pray to the almighty Allah for the patient's speedy recovery. But so deep was the conviction about the miracle healing among the women folk in the area that they refused to subscribe to any rational idea. Hence, as a survival strategy, I provide them willy nilly a few such things like tabiz, pani pora in the name of Almighty so that they follow our health instructions.*'

Similar sentiment was echoed by an ojha, Rajan, 38, from the area under study. He told us that '*the people who used to come to me are very superstitious in nature. Though I know it pretty well that their ailments have their roots in their typical unhygienic lifestyle, I seldom speak out the truth as I fear losing my customers*'.

The above narratives, generated in course of the study, have underscored the multidimensional nature of women vulnerability nurtured within the households.

Conclusion

Hence, household is the central locus of women's disempowerment. It is instrumental in structuring and institutionalizing inequalities against women. Taking a popular public health programme i.e. RCH as an example, the paper with the help of an ethnographic study has uncovered how households instilled patriarchal discriminatory values among women folk, leading to multiple vulnerabilities for them including gender inequality in health. Though woman empowerment is often posited as the smart solution to undo the century old history of injustices, unlike a mechanical process of change, it demands a thorough revamping of the role perception of women vis-a-vis men in a given society in addition to other concrete measures of ensuring their rights and capacity. Several modalities have been offered to ensure women empowerment which include, among others, women's access to resources, changes in legal status, changes in social status, ensuring women's role in political decision making and so on. However, being the prisoners of homogeneity, policymakers usually treat the issue of women empowerment as a mere policy straightjacket to be applied uniformly and uncritically across the societies.

For these reasons, the traditional conceptualization of women empowerment needs to be interrogated on the following grounds: first, women empowerment has no uniform pattern across societies as it is contextually determined. Hence, we need to keep 'sociology of space' in mind in addressing the variability of empowerment. Secondly, women are not just one group among various disempowered subsets of society (the poor, ethnic minorities, and so on); they are a cross-cutting sub-category of individuals that overlaps with all these other groups. Thirdly, unlike a host of other marginal groups, household and interfamilial relations are the fountainhead of discrimination perpetrated against women. Fourthly, women empowerment requires the transformation of those institutional structures that support patriarchy. Fifthly, women as a social category intersect with a host of interlocking social vectors like ethnicity, class, religion and so on, leading to multi-layer discrimination. Consequently, several attempts in the direction of women empowerment end up being futile exercises. Hence, discarding one approach of women empowerment and replacing it with another is not the solution as each and every approach contains some element of truth. Therefore, a holistic method, integrating many and varied approaches of empowerment, is the need of the hour. Here 'the acquisition of critical awareness about the structure of discrimination, exploitation and oppression in which one is placed' or what is popularly known as 'conscientization' may be of much help.

References

Di Cesare, M. (2014). Women, marginalization, and vulnerability: Introduction. *Genus, 70*(2–3). https://doi.org/10.4402/genus-637.

Dommaraju, P., & Tan, J. (2014). Households in contemporary Southeast Asia. *Journal of Comparative Family Studies, 45*(4), 559–580. https://doi.org/10.3138/jcfs.45.4.559.

Friedan, B. (1963). The feminine mystique. New York: W. W. Norton.

Gross, T (2020). Pandemic Makes Evident 'Grotesque' Gender Inequality In Household Work. www.npr.org/transcripts/860091230#:~:text=Pandemic%20Makes%20Evident%20'Grotesque'%20Gender%20Inequality%20In%20Household%20Work%20With,of%20child%20care%20and%20housework.%22.

Guidorzi, B. (2020). The 'Shadow Pandemic': Addressing Gender-based Violence (GBV) During COVID-19 in Pádraig Carmody, Gerard McCann, Clodagh Colleran, Ciara O'Halloran (eds.) COVID-19 in the Global South Book Subtitle: Impacts and Responses, Bristol University Press. Retrieved May 4th, 2021, from, https://www.jstor.org/stable/j.ctv18gfz7c.18.

Hankivsky, O. (Ed.). (2011). Health inequities in Canada: Intersectional frameworks and practices. UBC Press.

ILO. (2018). *Care Work and care jobs: for the future of decent work*. International Labour Office.

Iyer, A., Sen, G., & Ostlin, P. (2012). Inequalities and intersections in health: A review of the evidence. In *Gender Equity in Health: The Shifting Frontiers of Evidence and Action* (1st ed.,). Routledge.

Nanthini, S., & Tamara, N. (2020). Covid 19 and the Impacts on Women, S. Rajaratnam School of International Studies. Accessed March 05, 2021, from www.jstor.org/stable/resreo26875.

Schulte, B. (2015). *Overwhelmed: Work, Love, and Play When no one has the time*. Picador Usa.

Sen, G., & Ostlin, P. (2012). Gender as a social determinant of health: evidences, policies, and innovations. In *Gender Equity in Health: The Shifting Frontiers of Evidence and Action* (1st ed.). Routledge.

Snow, R. (2012). The Social Body. In Gender equity in health: The shifting frontiers of evidence and action (1st ed.). Routledge.

The Government of West Bengal: The Panchayat General Elections. (2008). District Panchayat Election Officer & District Magistrate.

Thomas, G. S. (2012). What the difference is between households and families. *The Business Journal*, dated 25th September, Accessed April 23, 2021, from. www.bizjournals.com.

World Health Organization. (2020). COVID-19 and violence against women. What the health sector/system can do. Accessed May 03, 2021, from, www.jstor.org/stable/resrep28231.

Chapter 17
Tea Plantation Workers and the Human Cost of Darjeeling Tea

Smritima Diksha Lama

Abstract This paper aims to highlight the precarity of plantation workers of Darjeeling, issues of inaccessibility to proper healthcare and inability to keep ill-health away. It draws from primary research carried out in two tea plantations of Darjeeling, West Bengal. Further, it also underlines the marginalized position of the women workers in the tea industry. Clinical factors are not the only cause of ill-health; rather there are social determinants of health such as means of livelihood, poverty, working conditions, accessibility, availability and affordability of and to basic services (housing, food security, water, sanitations, etc.) that play an important and definitive role. These in turn may influence the health choices of individuals while also leading to health inequalities.

Keywords Labour · Gender · Darjeeling · Tea plantations · Health

Introduction

Whenever one speaks of Darjeeling there is most definitely the talk of one of the three Ts namely, Tourism, Tea and Timber. The Darjeeling region has been cultivating, growing and producing tea for over 160 years. The establishment of the tea industry in Darjeeling was possible due to the enterprise of the then-superintendent Dr. Campbell who started the experimental growth of tea in 1840. Today there are 87 tea estates operating in Darjeeling. Darjeeling tea is considered to be the 'champagne of teas' and yet the tea estate workers, at the lowest rung of the employment hierarchy, toiling in the tea estates remain some of the poorest in the organized sector. They are most crucial in the tea chain being involved in the delicate art of hand-plucking the '*dui paat ek suiro*' (two leaves and a bud) which makes the perfect cup of Darjeeling tea.

Health is a complex phenomenon which is governed by both biological and socio-genic factors. While health condition is said to be biological in origin the disparities in health status between nations and between social groups are largely determined by

S. D. Lama (✉)
Freelance Researcher/Consultant in Public Health, Public Health Foundation of India (PHFI), Gurgaon, India

© The Author(s), under exclusive license to Springer Nature Singapore Pte Ltd. 2022   333
S. S. Acharya and S. Christopher (eds.), *Caste, COVID-19, and Inequalities of Care*,
People, Cultures and Societies: Exploring and Documenting Diversities,
https://doi.org/10.1007/978-981-16-6917-0_17

the way society is organized along economic, social and political axes. With scanty opportunities for education, inhuman living conditions, poor hygiene and health care facilities, the tea plantation labourers are made to 'bleed where no wounds exist'. The tea estate owners—big, medium or small, the trade union leaders and the elected representatives at the district, state and the national level tend to ignore these plights of the tea plantation workers despite their dependence on these workers as substantive vote banks. This indicates that the people's representatives have been found to be consistently lacking both in willingness and wherewithal to place the deteriorating condition of the tea workers before the respective legislative institutions. This kind of marginalization of the workers and/or their needs is also said to breed inequality (Baru et al., 2010; Rajbangshi & Nambiar, 2020; Acharya, this volume). The Plantation Labour Act (PLA, 1951) was enacted by the Government of India (GoI) for the tea producers/estate owners to abide by and provide the workers with housing, healthcare, water, sanitation facilities, rations and education for their children. However, empirical evidence from field data as well as literature suggests otherwise. Several decades after the act was passed, there is possibly no plantation in Assam and West Bengal with all provisions. And even if some provisions are provided by the owners, then the quality of the service is dismal.

Even availability of health services has been unequal in India which has been held responsible for widening the differentials in health outcomes. Inequalities in access to health care services have been attributed to factors like social identity, economic differentials and regional disparities. Most ill-health is not just caused by germs and infection rather it is caused by poverty, unemployment, unequal wages, patriarchy as well as a lack of basic necessities such as housing, proper food, water, sanitation, health services, etc. And as Loewenson (1992) states it is easy to get impressed by the visible signs of efficient production while driving through plantations. Moreover, what remains hidden from the view are the conditions of the workers and where ill-health, poverty feature in the balance sheets of plantation economies?

This chapter, therefore, endeavours to examine the human cost of Darjeeling tea. The tea workers being the backbone of a tea estate, bringing green leaves from bush to our cups, their health and well-being appear to be least discussed and of no prime concern to the producers as well as the state. This cost appears to be borne by none other than the workers' themselves leaving them vulnerable and marginalized.

Key Organizational Features of the Tea Industry

The key organizational features of the Indian tea industry which have a bearing on the socio-economic conditions, livelihood and health of the workers in the plantations are as follows:

Plantations have a vertical work hierarchy and this maintains the class distinction between the workers and the management. The feudal relations of production.

Majority of the labour force comprises women and is the only industry in the organized sector employing such a high proportion of female labour. The female workers are mainly employed in plucking of tea leaves (requiring delicate handling in order not to bruise the tea leaves) and in light maintenance work.

Historically, the plantations had a system of indentured labour wherein planters encouraged families rather than individuals to migrate to the plantations. And by encouraging families to migrate, they ensured that workers were cut off from the places of their origin and were settled in the plantations for purposes of future recruitment. This has led to generations of families being employed in the tea estates.

The casual workers in the estates are mostly recruited from within the workers' families settled in the estate. About one-third of the total labour force consists of casual labour in tea plantations. Kalyan (2012) in his study on Assam tea plantations has also referred to high casualization of workforce in the tea plantation structure especially in the hazardous and risk-prone jobs.

In comparison to other sectors, the rate of unionization is fairly high in the tea industry. But the effectiveness of these unions in securing and safeguarding the interests of the workers has not been very impressive. Their contribution in political mobilization is comparatively higher.

Wages of the plantation workers are lowest in the organized sector.

From Garden to Cup[1]

Tea has an immense network of people connected to it apart from the consumers alone. These are the growers, those who pluck, manufacturers, suppliers, brokers, sellers, traders and retailers, etc. supplying tea across the globe. Tea production is a combination of industry and agriculture since work related to green leaf is an agricultural activity while processing is an industrial activity. Figure 17.1 depicts this tea production phenomenon. Workers are engaged in the tea industry not only at the estate level but many earn their livelihood from ancillary activities associated with production, value addition and the marketing of tea. Tea is usually exported after primary processing in bulk form by garden mark and grade. This means that blending, final packaging and marketing—which are the most lucrative stages in the overall process—are mainly carried out by tea companies in the buyer countries (Van Der Wal, 2008). This implies that in the supply chain of packaged tea the maximum profits start accruing after the commodity passes through the farm gate and fetches the maximum at the various stages of value addition. Thereafter a very small proportion of the profits included in the retail price of tea goes to the tea-producing country. Instead, the workers, without taking into account the larger market benefits beyond the farm gate are condemned to a life of penury.

---

[1] The term 'garden' has been used instead of 'estate' because the workers perceive and call their 'workplace' as such. They see the transformation of the 'green (tea) leaves' to the final product/commodity packed in the boxes (for market) as relevant to 'their garden' instead of estate. The use of this term here is also associated with the general parlance of the term, easy to understand by the common people. The term 'garden' is also the traditional English term being used since the British times.

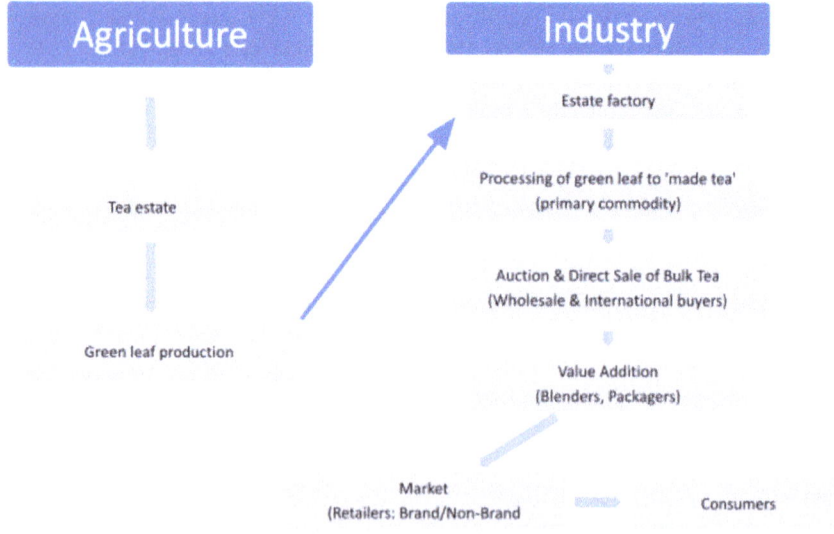

Fig. 17.1 Tea leaf activity from garden to cup. *Source* Developed by the author

An earlier study revealed through interviews with industry experts that the brand of Darjeeling tea is curated largely for international consumption as the companies aim for foreign exchange earnings rather than for domestic consumption (Lama, 2019). Darjeeling tea is sold in bulk in auctions or directly to private buyers as a 'commodity'. The 'brand' evolves only further down the supply chain when value addition is done in the form of blending and packaging by the companies. The finished brand of Darjeeling tea in the supermarket aisles or online stores majority of which are not sold by estate name. Despite, having various social justice markers such as Rainforest Alliance, Fair Trade and Ethical Tea Partnership indicate their ethical sourcing. Instead, it is sold under the brand of companies like Lipton, Unilever, Tata, Tetley, etc. These brands get the advantage of the faithful connoisseurs of the Darjeeling tea for its flavour, colour and '*terroir*'.[2] The wage labourers, however, rarely make it to the social scientific depictions of *terroir* food production (Besky, 2014a). This implies that while there is a discussion on tea, *terroir* and trade that is further supported by tags like Geographical Indications (GI), the workers toiling daily are not provided any further protection nor are their conditions of work discussed. Therefore, while Darjeeling is identified by its tea, the individual estates and the workers are lost by the time the tea is transported from the garden into our homes and various other 'tea serving' places.

---

[2] (Besky 2014a) Foods with *Terroir* or 'taste of place' is a concept associated with artisanal foods produced by small farmers and due to the Geographical Indication (GI) tag that Darjeeling tea received in 1999 its taste too is now associated with a place.

Social Realities of Tea Workers

Primary research was carried out by the author with the research design involving mixed methods as both quantitative and qualitative methods were used. The author obtained data from the field using a semi-structured interview schedule for the household survey of 200 tea estate workers (100 in each tea estate). In order to get a holistic understanding of the tea industry and its workers, the author conducted the survey in two types of plantations of which one was a traditional tea estate and the other was an organic tea estate. The sample population of this multi-sited study was primarily drawn from the permanent workers who are at the lowest level of the employee pyramid of the tea plantations as they are the most vulnerable and they make up most of the employees of a tea estate.

There are four categories of employees in a tea estate:

- Management: At the top of the employee pyramid
- Staff: White-collar office staff subordinate to the management
- Sub-staff: Supervisory watch and ward staff
- Workers (Field[3] and Factory): at the bottom of the employee pyramid subsisting on daily wages.

A plantation is characterized by a hierarchy at work and the largest bulk of the hierarchy, i.e. the daily wage worker is at the bottom and these workers at the plantations are categorized as:

- Permanent and Casual workers
- Factory and Field worker
- Male and Female worker.

The nature of their work is back-breaking, low paid and least secure. Injuries are common, along with water-borne and respiratory diseases as well as various other health hazards which are faced due to the exposure to insecticides and pesticides.

In the following section with the help of fieldwork data I attempt to outline the social disparities among the plantation workers by highlighting the conditions that can be understood to impinge upon their health and well-being. It discusses the socio-demographic profile, wage, work entitlements, socio-economic conditions and access to basic amenities as factors affecting health and livelihood of the tea plantation workers. The PLA (1951) ensures that the tea producers are to provide basic amenities to the plantation workers. However, empirical evidence from the field data suggests otherwise.

Some of the notable features that emerged are as follows:

---

[3] Field workers are the workers who are responsible for maintenance works in the estate and includes activities like sowing, weeding, spraying, mulching as well as the most important of all the plucking of the tea leaves.

Social Hierarchy

At the managerial level while it is rare to have a Nepali manager it was very much the case in Organic Tea Estate (TE) where the Nepali manager had been working as assistant manager in one of the other estates owned in Darjeeling by the same group. At Traditional TE as tradition has been in the Darjeeling hills the manager hailed from Rajasthan which is in North India. It has been seen in the past that the presence of Nepalis in the managerial post has been insignificant (Rasaily, 2003). This was also reiterated by the Executive Director at the Organic TE and said even today the practice is not very common as the owners feel that if a Nepali is kept at the highest post (managerial) in an estate then he will easily concede to the demands of the workers.

The workers, staff and sub-staff are all descendants of Nepali workers who had been brought by the British when they first opened tea estates in Darjeeling. It is noteworthy that in the tea estates, the personnel at higher positions of work hierarchy are mostly from outside the region. The local population is usually hired for positions at low and subordinate levels only.

Level of Education

Avenues of education are limited in tea estates as they are in remote and inaccessible locations with poor infrastructure which keeps the area underserved. Fifty per cent of the males and 37.9% of the female workers were educated up to class eight at the traditional estate and an equivalent percentage of 38.1% of women workers and 40.5% of the male workers were educated up to the same level in the organic estate. It was reported by the workers that they could not study further due to lack of educational institutions closer to where they were living as well as due to the abject poverty of their parents who were unable to educate them further. It was believed that there was a 'dearth of jobs' and studying further was pointless as 'plucking tea leaves does not require high education levels'. They could survive with their limited education. Thus, cost of education and lack of an educational facility along with the understanding that educational attainment will not get them a job proved to be the disincentives towards it. However, some workers were working hard to ensure their children receive education beyond primary school so as not to engage them in plantation. Plantation work requires hard work with very little returns and workers do not want the same for their children. While there is little scope for occupational and social mobility among tea estate workers, the above discussion indicates that workers desire for education to better the livelihoods of their children.

Workers' Ages

It was observed that the majority of the population in both the sites were in the age group of 31–50 years of age and were the second generation of workers. There were a few cases wherein there was an age discrepancy at the time of induction in the tea estate. These workers lamented that they would retire before they turned 60 since their year of birth was noted incorrectly at the time of induction. This indicated the vulnerability of the workers and the lack of any grievance redressal mechanism. When asked if the workers' union would be able to intervene on their behalf, it was reported that the union would hardly involve themselves in such cases and were mostly active during wage negotiations (which occur once every three years) or for garnering votes from the public for assembly and general elections.

> The union asks for a birth certificate as proof of age but we have no official document. They simply wash their hands off of our troubles and give excuses to not be involved when they have to struggle with our demands. They just call general meetings for the sake of it and to show that the union is concerned about workers' rights. (43-year-old male field worker)

Caste

With respect to caste, data suggested that it did not appear to play a big role in the everyday lives of the plantation workers or work conditions. Workers reported that some of them had made the effort of getting a caste certificate hoping to get some benefits. But for them it was just another paper as they did not know what to do with the certificates. In some cases, they had acquired one on being informed by neighbours or relatives who advised them to obtain caste certificates for at least their children if not themselves.

> I do not have a caste certificate but I got one made for my daughter who is in school thinking it might be of some use to her. They say it helps with college admissions and government jobs. (38-year-old female field worker)

Such instances indicate the aspirations of the tea workers who wish to do as much as possible for their children to have a better future. The next section brings attention to the status of the workers in Darjeeling. It examines their livelihood through wage, working conditions, entitlements and access to basic amenities.

Wages

Income is an important determinant of living standards and hence it also has implications on the workers' education, housing, health and health-seeking behaviour. Income in many ways determines their ability to access resources, opportunities and services and to prioritize their needs.

Table 17.1 Rates of daily wages

States	Years				
	1982–1983	1999–2000	2005–2008	2014[b]	2018[b]
Assam	8.90	37.60	58.50	94	137
West Bengal	9.90	34.80	58[a]	95 (90 in Darjeeling)	132
Kerala	12.20	66.17	72.26–89.78	216.53	321
Tamil Nadu	13.08	74.52	77–79	209.27	241

Source Tea Statistics 1982–1983, 1999–2000, 2005–2009; [a] 2008–2010; [b] Newspaper reports

It is important to note that the workers who pluck the leaves delicately so as to not pluck any more than 'two leaves and a bud' are considered as 'unskilled' workers. This paradox is an example of exploitative nature of the relationship between management and workers wherein the 'skill' of plucking goes unnoticed and most times unrewarded. Due to poor working conditions and emoluments, they are unable to meet their basic living costs (Banerji & Willoughby, 2019) or have a decent standard of living.

The tea pluckers receive a daily wage. This includes the piece rate, i.e. price paid to the pluckers based on weight of tea leaves over and above their daily task and is discussed in detail in another section. It is to be noted that the payment of wages to workers comprises both cash (daily wage, piece rate an annual bonus) and non-cash components (subsidised rations, protective gear, firewood, tea, housing, healthcare and primary education).

Table 17.1 indicates the wages of the tea plantation workers across the tea-producing states of India. In West Bengal and Assam tea workers' wages are determined by collective bargaining mechanism, the wages are not notified under the Minimum Wages Act (1948). While in Kerala and Tamil Nadu wages of the workers are notified by Minimum Wages Act (1948) preceded by tripartite consultation (Sarkar, 2016). However, Sarkar (2016) states that yet the wages are sub-optimal in the contemporary context and the implications is that despite being a part of the organized workforce the tea plantation workers remain in abject poverty and can be categorized as 'working poor'.

The average plucking workers are expected to complete in a day in Tamil Nadu is 25 kg/day and in Kerala it is 16 kg/day (Neilson and Pritchard, 2010). While in Darjeeling as per the interviews held with the management it was reported that during peak season in the traditional estate the workers have a task set at plucking up to 9 kg/day depending on the type of tea bush (China variety 7 kg/day; Clone 8 kg/day and Assam variety 9 kg/day). In the fair-trade certified organic tea estate visited the task for plucking was set at 8 kg/day irrespective of season. Hence, we see that there is a stark distinction between the north and south Indian tea plantations in terms of tasks assigned each day. This could also be explained by the fact that while Darjeeling tea involves a 'fine art' of plucking only the tips while the tea plucking in south allows for up to four to five big leaves below the tips as well.

The Labour Commissioner's report (2018) states that an unskilled agriculture worker in West Bengal receives Rs. 244 per day, a full-time unskilled worker engaged in Beedi leaf plucking is paid Rs. 243.76 (Rs. 6,338 monthly) while the Darjeeling tea plantation worker was being paid Rs. 132.50 per day. As per the latest newspaper reports, wages of tea plantation workers in Bengal from 1 March 2018 were increased to Rs. 150 per day. In the same year, from 1 September workers started receiving a wage of Rs. 176 per day. As of 1 January 2021, the wages have been increased to Rs. 202 per day. Yet, the Darjeeling tea plantation workers remain the lowest paid workers across industries within the state of West Bengal.

Workers remain unaware about how exactly their wages (received either weekly or fortnightly), bonuses or arrears are calculated. They trust the system but some lament and say things like:

> What can we do? I did not study after Class Eight, therefore, I do not have the capability to do such calculations or keep a track. Sometimes I even lose track of the number of days when I have taken leave. We are one community and we get by with the hope that we are not cheated as we put in a lot of hard work in the making of the tea. (56-year-old female worker)

In another interview with a young male worker in the organic tea it was revealed that workers also face issues in claiming retirement benefits. He said '*my father retired 2 years back and he is yet to get his retirement benefits. They keep asking for documents and make us go from pillar to post. My father laments whether he will be able to receive his money in this lifetime*'.

The argument given by producers for the low wages of the workers in the tea plantation has always been the rising cost of production. There is a disconnection between the market realization and the benefits to the workers. Since time immemorial owners of the tea estates have been complaining about falling tea prices and their inability to break even or accrue any profits. Thus, they absolve themselves from the responsibility of providing workers with some benefits. This has also been a major excuse for the producers to have kept the wages low as they project that the cost of production is higher than the market realization. Increasing production costs, high taxes and low labour productivity are said to be the causes for lack of profitability (Selvaraj & Gopalakrishnan, 2016). However, plantations must provide 'living wages'[4] to the workers rather than just subsistence wages.

Housing

In terms of housing, it is interesting to note that despite earning low wages, workers continue to work in the tea estates. This is perhaps because of the provision of housing

---

[4] In an interview with a stakeholder holding a managerial post at the organic fair-trade certified garden it was reported that the concept of 'living wage' has never been floated in the tripartite wage agreement meetings and that only the Fairtrade Labelling Organisation was working on deciding 'living wage'. The workers have always been said to be paid subsistence level wages which have remained below the minimum wage (for example, agricultural and/or beedi workers) within the state and/or outside.

as mandated by the PLA (1951) which ensures a roof over the workers' head. This leads to fixity of the workers and their dependent families within the estates and ensures the supply of labour to the estates. Besky (2017) and Makita (2012) have talked about '*fixity*' of the workers to the land. While on the one hand the workers are educating their kids so as to prevent them from joining plantation work on the other hand the workers are also tied to the land unable to give up their houses that have been in their family for generations. This marks the aspirations nurtured for the younger generation as much as the uncertainty of alternate occupation in the absence of adequate skill and training.

Plantation houses are inherited by the workers yet have no ownership rights (Besky, 2017). This practice, which ties jobs to houses across generations, extends colonially rooted forms of ethnic marginalization into the present. Although the houses are provided by the tea plantation, many workers presume that the house is owned by them. Whereas in fact it is only leased out to them till the time somebody from the same household is employed in the plantation. Therefore, it was important to understand the fixity of the workers to estate work. At both the tea estates when ownership of the houses was discussed with the workers majority of them understood that the houses are company-owned. In an interview with a female worker she exclaimed, '*all the houses are company owned. But they should give us the ownership rights especially since we have invested our bonus money or money from our savings for the upkeep and maintenance of the house. Had we depended on the management to improve the conditions of the houses we would still be living in dilapidated houses that have not been repaired for ages*'.

In some instances, the assumption of private ownership is probably made by the workers as they have invested in the upkeep and expansion of their homes and think of the houses as private properties. Focus group discussions with the male workers at the two estates also revealed that this understanding exists irrespective of the type of estate. The following quotes highlight this:

> The company hardly repairs the houses after so many years of working in the estate most of us still have semi-*pukka*[5] houses and whatever expansion and upkeep has been done has been done with our hard-earned money or our bonuses. How can we give up on our houses after investing so much? Will the management reimburse us if we vacate?

> Of course, it's private ownership after giving so many years to the plantation and after investing on the upkeep and expansion of the house, how can we give it back to the management. There will be somebody or the other who we will find to join the estate job if and when the time comes for retirement.

The next of kin of a retired worker is supposed to take up the estate job in order to keep the house within the family or vacate if there is no next of kin. A factory clerk said that the job in a tea estate was '*Badhyata ko kaam*' which translates to 'obligatory work'. He wanted to express the fact that he and his previous generations had been working in the estate when his forefathers moved to Darjeeling to join the tea estate and they were provided with housing. In order to keep the house within

---

[5] Semi-pukka refers to houses in which either the roof or the walls are made using durable materials such as cement, bricks, etc. while either of the two are made of thatch, bamboo, etc.

the family and due to lack of any other employment opportunity he had also joined the same line of work and quit his education after the tenth grade. This is an instance often repeated in many households in the tea estates wherein just to retain the houses any member of the house is convinced to join the plantation for work under *Badli* system.[6]

Another case in point was that of a graduate working in the estate as field labour. The reason provided was that there was no next of kin other than this son who could join the estate job as his father was retiring. They could not afford to move out of the estate housing, therefore, the graduate son had to join the work. Since his father had retired as a worker the management had to employ the son as a worker. The only perk that was promised to him due to his college degree was that within a year he would be promoted from field to the factory. Whereas it takes years of work in the field to be promoted and most field workers retire without ever being promoted. There is little else in terms of occupational mobility for the workers and they appear to be tied to the land as the houses are handed down from generation to generation and hence the familial tie with the house is difficult for them to break. It is this 'tying down' of the workers to the land that the producers of Darjeeling tea exploit for their own purposes. To some extent, they may be compared to a modern-day version of bonded-labour.

Water and Sanitation

Housing and the living conditions are known to affect the health of the worker. It was considered necessary to investigate the water and sanitation facilities available to the households as well as at the work sites.

More than half of the houses in organic tea estate, i.e. 70% had supply of water to their houses (either direct to home or public tap) and less reliant on spring water or '*dhara*'. While, in the traditional tea estate less than half of the houses, i.e. 43% had water supply and it was noted that they relied heavily on spring water. There was awareness among the workers to boil water before consumption as they said it would keep them disease-free. Both the study sites reported a high percentage of workers using boiled water for consumption.

> Earlier when we were kids, we hardly bothered about the treatment of drinking water. But with growing awareness and to avoid falling sick we have been using boiled water for our consumption. Obviously, if we boil water to such high temperatures, it should kill all germs. Yet my son had diarrhoea a few months back I suppose even if you do everything right sometimes sickness cannot be avoided. (39-year-old female worker)

> Most houses use boiling methods to treat water for personal consumption and we also carry the same at our work sites. But sometimes when we run out of water while working, we resort to drinking water from the springs and sometimes that too is not available especially during summer months when some springs dry up. (48-year-old female worker)

---

[6] The *Badli* (substitute) system was introduced wherein dependent members of the workers would replace the retiring workers.

This was a noteworthy case as we see that while the workers are careful about consuming boiled water at their homes the same cannot be said about the work sites. Thus, their work sites could make them vulnerable to water-borne diseases.

In order to understand why workers in the organic tea estate had greater access to water facilities than those in the traditional TE it was inferred from the key informant interviews that the public health engineering department (PHE) along with the plantation management had constructed water tanks across the estate. Piped water was provided to most houses or community taps were made in case pipeline could not be constructed directly to the workers' houses. Only a few houses, especially those in the farthest of villages within the organic tea estate relied on spring water. While in the traditional tea estate there was more of a problem with respect to water supply as many villages did not have piped water to their homes. There was no evidence of the PHE department having worked for the estate. It was reported that most of the houses that had piped water had managed to do so by coming together as a community or were reliant on the management of having made some provisioning of piped water. But the true source of this water supply was natural springs that are common across the region. It was also reported that they had difficulty in fetching water especially during the summer months as the natural springs would dry up. Thus, it is seen that there are differentials in easy accessibility to water (basic human need) which may not necessarily be due to the nature of the estates; rather an active part is played by the state and the estate management.

As regards the sanitary conditions, if we look at data on provisioning of toilet facilities among the estate workers, we see that there is a slight difference between the two estates. In the traditional estate there were 94% of worker households that had a toilet facility available and of the remaining that said they did not have toilets; they were sharing with another family. While in the organic estate there were 82% of the households that had toilet facility while the remaining who said they did not have any toilet facility meant they were either sharing or they resorted to open defecation. With the recent thrust of *Swachh Bharat Abhiyan*[7] one would think that the practice was expected to have completely vanished. But there were three per cent of the workers who had no option other than open defecation. In the organic fair-trade certified estate, toilets were being added in houses that did not have them and this was probably why 3% of the worker households reported to be practicing open defecation. The management emphasized that in collaboration with a local non-governmental organization (NGO) and from fair-trade premium funds the workers were being helped with the toilet construction. On discussion with the workers, it was reported that since 2012 up till 2014 toilets were being built for worker households with premium funds along with local NGO support. However only basic raw material was being provided, i.e. two bags of cement, a toilet pan, few iron rods and two tin sheets while the rest of the investment was to be made by the workers out of their pockets. In terms of manpower two workers from the estate were being provided

---

[7] *Swachh Bharat Abhiyaan* (Clean India Movement) was a campaign launched by the government of India on 2nd October 2014 and aimed to achieve its mission (open defecation free and improving waste management) by 2nd October 2019.

to help each household with the construction. However, the workers lamented that despite funding from two agencies (Fair trade and NGO), they were still expected to generate their own funds and hire masons to build a functional toilet.

Education and Occupational Mobility

As previously discussed, in the section on level of education, schooling facilities in the plantations are inadequate and due to these limited avenues, the future of the workers' children is at stake. Schooling is available only till the lower primary level. As a result, children of tea workers are sometimes forced to join the tea industry as unskilled workers with little education and no alternative employment opportunity. Education is a costly affair especially since the workers send their children outside of the estate once they are done with primary school. Some even send their children to private English-medium schools run outside of the estate. Due to such expenses (over and above living expenses) many workers in the tea estates supplement their wages with additional income by raising livestock (hens, pigs, goats, etc.), sometimes the dependents of the workers operate a corner shop, or a family member employed outside of the estate helps.

> My eldest son works in Siliguri in a hotel. He sends money back home regularly. This has enabled me to repair and maintain my dwelling. My daughter is also studying in an English medium school in Kurseong town. We would not be able to afford all these expenses without the additional income. I am satisfied with the fact that my children would not be dragged into this life of penury in the garden job. (38-year-old female worker)

Many of the estate workers aspire that their children may be well-educated so as not to be stuck in the estate as labourers due to the poor conditions of living and work. It was reported by many workers that '*although I may not be educated, I know the importance of education in today's day and age and encourage my children to study and learn*'.

> [...] since we are close to town there is a greater chance for one of us to move out of the estate and explore better work opportunities. My son has completed his schooling and speaks good English I am sure he can get a job in one of the several hotels in town. Many of us have also sent our kids to Darjeeling town to study and look for work as there are more opportunities there rather than being wasted in the estate. (40-year-old female worker)

It must also be stressed that there were a few cases where the children were enrolled in graduate programmes. However, this was more out of volition and self-help rather than any direct aid from the plantation owners or the government. It is doubtful whether such an experience could be replicated across the community yet such instances are indicative of the aspirations of the workers.

Contrary to such illustrations there were also families which were large and had just one working member as unemployment is also high in these isolated enclaves. The condition of the house spoke of their poverty. The family members appeared impoverished and undernourished. The unemployed, especially men, had drinking habits and this was an issue of concern for their working wives or other family members. This is also indicative of income inequality which could be embedded in social identity such as caste and ethnicity. While the workers gave politically correct responses regarding social identity, there are chances that such disparities were present. Families belonging to different social groups- caste and ethnicity, for instance, stayed in separate residential blocks. In the organic estate there was a village settlement named '*Sarkidhura*' and upon discussion it was ascertained that this labour line had been set up during the time of the British. *Sarkis* is considered to be belonging to the SC community among the predominantly *Nepali* population in the Darjeeling hills. Literature also corroborates that such residential segregation is likely to be an outcome of the erstwhile colonial arrangement (Chatterjee, 2003). About 90% of the workers are tribal, SC and OBC populations with origins in central Indian Plateau and Nepal. They are settled here for generations, but are still viewed as immigrants and suffer from social discrimination similar to that of landless farming population. There is a sense of indifference towards them. The geographical separation between the tea estates restricts cohesion among the workers. Geographical remoteness obstructs access to means to learn diversified skills, especially for the young children. There are periods when there is no active employment in the estates. Opportunities to enhance skill can be useful for such times (Kadavil & Chattopadhayay, 2007).

The pursuit of profit, the building of the tea empire and social apartheid together has created the tea plantation industry and the estate workers of Darjeeling as also elsewhere within the country. This tea plantation model was developed on the much maligned economic and social theory based on exploitation—of the land, environment and labour. Unfortunately, this plantation model has remained the same. This plantation model over the years has created a plantation culture of dependency and poverty among the plantation society. The children of the tea workers rarely get an opportunity to move out from the social and economic class they are born into.

In the previous sections of this chapter, it has been made amply clear that there exist social determinants of health and some of these have been discussed above as they appear to play out in the lives of the tea estate workers. The next section elucidates on this further by bringing into focus health conditions of workers as well as the availability, accessibility and affordability of healthcare in the tea estates. These are said to be important determinants for improving population health (Baru et al., 2010).

Health Concerns of Workers, Patterns of Provisioning and Utilization

Many scholars have postulated health as being socially produced. Some of the earliest studies in public health point out that health should not be merely seen from a medical perspective, i.e. only in the parlance of disease/illness and cure/prevention rather it should also be seen as a product of various social factors such as poor sanitary and

Table 17.2 Common health problems

Health problem	Reported symptoms
Eye pain/Headache	Watery eyes, headache and weak vision
Hand/Leg/Back pain	Aches and pains
Hypertension	Headache, high blood pressure and vomiting
Gastric	Gas, heartburn, indigestion and headache
Gout	Pain or swelling in joints
Gall bladder stone	Sudden pain in the right side of body and nausea

living conditions (McKeown et al., 1972). The pattern of ill-health and health services in the plantation sector is thus a useful focus of analysis in examining the human costs of production of Darjeeling tea and who bears them. Just as a tea bush needs continued care and maintenance so do the workers that spend all their time on the job bent over these tea bushes.

The health conditions of the workers were examined through reported illnesses from among the workers' households and the most commonly reported health problems can be seen in Table 17.2.

Data also suggested that *joro* (fever) was the most commonly reported illness and is said to be recurring in nature. This also indicates weak immunity which could be due to poor nutrition at the household level and also due to fatigue by working in harsh conditions irrespective of hail or sunshine. Most workers did not consider fever, cough and cold or even aches and pains as being health problems. This indicates an internalization of ill-health. This can also be seen in the following narrative that emerged from a focus group discussion with the women workers at the traditional estate.

> We are engaged in strenuous work on a daily basis and we depend on daily wages for our subsistence. We do not have time to consider minor aches and pains as health problems. Being poor is a curse and we in the tea estates are worse off as there is no access to doctors. The dispensary is run by a compounder who just hands out the same medicine for all complaints. Why does the company not employ a doctor? Even if they cannot give us a higher wage, they should at least provide us with good facilities.

It was reported by the compounder at the estate hospital that '*there is seasonality involved in the patterns of illness experienced by the workers. During the rainy season the most common complaints are diarrhea, fever, cold, typhoid and cough. There is also an increase in the number of workers with complaints of diabetes and hypertension. We also treat the children of the workers up to the age of 18 years. Winter months are relatively disease free but there are still cases of fever and pneumonia. Irrespective of season the workers often come with cuts and insect bites that they get while working. Earlier there used to be cases of tuberculosis among the tea estate workers but there have been no cases in the past two years*'.

A high percentage of workers also reported to have been dealing with low blood pressure. When asked to elaborate the workers reported feeling dizzy, experiencing fatigue and sometimes also feeling faint. This could be attributed to their poor diet lacking in nutrients as well as the hard work they put in everyday thereby making them feel weak and have a low blood pressure (also could signify anaemia). When probed further about their action taking it was reported that they did approach the estate hospital and/or dispensary and were provided with Vitamin syrup or tablets and asked to improve diet by including animal protein and lastly, they were asked to rest. However, such solutions are not conducive for the plantation workers as will be further discussed in the following section.

The diet could not be improved given the wages nor could they afford to 'rest' which would result in wage loss. It is also noteworthy that what was reported as 'low blood pressure' (the symptoms) could actually indicate anaemic conditions. However, it can be understood that the workers are unaware of the fact that their low blood pressure in fact indicates anaemia which is due to their poor nutritional intake. Gothoskar (2012) reports in her study that workers and their families often emphasize the fact that anaemia is endemic in tea estates. Thus, we see that despite feeling weak and tired the workers continued their work as they did not pay too much attention to their ill-health. This also signifies the importance of work over health for the workers in order to earn a living to be able to afford to eat.

A 40-year-old woman who has been a field worker for over a decade explained '*a while ago I developed an urinary tract infection. It used to burn when I urinated but I was ashamed to mention it to anybody and since I could not miss work, I suffered in silence for about a week. But then things got very tough for me as I could not even sit properly. I eventually had to skip work and visited the block health center. But the doctor who looks after such cases was not available. It was in vain that I went so far and also lost my day's wage*'. Also being financially constrained it has been seen that workers defer treatment despite the display of symptoms. Two women workers reported having poor eyesight due to which they had frequent headaches. The worker from Traditional TE had to traverse a long way for her eye check-up and she dreaded making the trip again as it was a costly affair. The trip along with her eye check-up had cost her Rs. 300 and she was dreading how much the spectacles would cost her if she decided to buy one. She also pointed out that it would be difficult for her to work in the field while wearing spectacles and so she chose not to wear spectacles. Also being the only earner in her household and sending her kid to school she said she could hardly make ends meet.

Literature corroborates that women workers sometimes delay seeking health care because the cost of being sick was substantial: a day's wage for non-permanent workers and half a day wage for permanent workers (Rajbangshi & Nambiar, 2020). Health systems are highly context-specific and there are no single set of best practices that are applicable to one and all. If we look at some of the causes of mortality especially in Traditional TE it was seen that there were two cases wherein the death had been caused due to fever.

> Fever is only an excuse for death in a tea garden. We are living in such difficult terrain it is difficult to take the patient to the hospital in time and the nearest hospital to us is the garden hospital that has no qualified MBBS doctor. Who do we turn to at the hour of need? (43-year-old male worker)

... my sister also worked in the estate along with me. She came down with a fever once and we thought it would go after running its course for a couple of days. But her condition started worsening after three days. We had shown the *jhakri* (traditional healer) but it did not help. We then approached the sub district hospital in town. She was admitted in the evening and at midnight she breathed her last. The blood reports also came the next day after her death but no cause of the fever was detected. You see, in our situation a simple illness like fever can also be deadly. But what can we do? We tried to avoid going to the hospital because the ambulance was not available since it's only for very serious patients. (27-year-old female worker)

A point to ponder upon in the above case is that in an era of technological and scientific advancements in all fields there are still cases of people dying due to simple illnesses like fever. Also, in such situations who decides the severity of the patients' conditions to be considered for availing the ambulance facility in the tea estate.

There was also the provision in the plantations for reimbursement of medical expenses for any medical condition that the plantation dispensary or plantation hospital is unable to provide or resolve. Upon inquiry the workers at both sites reported that some of their retired relatives (having passed his job to next of kin) faced many hurdles even in claiming their retirement benefits.

If we look at the above discussion on the reported illnesses and the dietary habits of the tea plantation workers, we are able to have a glimpse into the 'health seeking' as well 'health care seeking' behaviour among the plantation workers. It was observed that the workers were aware and worried whenever they experienced any discomfort regarding their health and to keep ill-health away, they always first approached the local traditional healer of their choice and when they could not be taken care of by the local healer, they approached the dispensary or garden hospital.

While a direct causality cannot be said to be occurring among the tea plantation workers in terms of their conditions of health and work especially if we look at the reported illnesses. However, it is noteworthy that an individual's health choices and health conditions are a result of their immediate environment as well as their socio-economic conditions. There is a multiplicity of health care institutions that are available for the workers but none provide a complete set of services. It was inferred from discussions held at both tea plantations that the conditions of ill-health were understood as being part of their occupation. Hence, it can be said that in terms of health conditions and provisions for health care there is still a long way to go for the tea estates to provide proper care to its workers. The workers are vulnerable not only because of the conditions in which they work but they also have no access to affordable and quality care especially in cases of emergency. Literature has repeatedly indicated that social determinants such as poverty, poor working conditions and poor social networks including unequal gender relations led to differences in health (seeking, promoting and care utilization) of an individual and increases inequities in health (Rajbangshi & Nambiar, 2020; Subedi, this volume; Acharya, this volume).

Tea Gardens Through a Gender Lens

With regard to gender composition there are more women than men employed as workers in the plantations. Since colonial times, planters exhibited an interest in women workers because of the long-term advantage of a self-reproducing and stable workforce (Bhadra, 2004). Most workers in the tea plantations are also accompanied by their family. Often, in the absence of employment in the tea estates, the family members engage in other employment such as, running a shop in the nearest town outside the tea estate, painting, masonry, etc.

In spite of the institution of labour laws and the PLA (1951), women workers have remained deprived and exploited. The main labour-intensive activities include harvesting, ploughing, sowing, watering, fertilizing, weeding, pruning, controlling pests and diseases by applying pesticides or herbicides. The plucking of the prized tea involves only 'two leaves and a bud' therefore, it involves fine plucking to make the orthodox variety of tea. The plucking of bigger leaves also leads to the supervisors reprimanding the worker. This is one of the reasons for the non-implementation of mechanized plucking. Workers are on their feet for hours at a time, with a basket slung over their backs holding harvested leaves irrespective of the weather conditions. The women workers complain of pain in their fingers, bruising in their nails, poor eyesight, body ache, etc. due to the constant plucking and nipping at the tea bushes for fine leaves. Alas their work goes unrecognized while their 'nimble fingers' are romanticized in advertisements on retail packages, brochures, etc.

The women workers are engaged in arduous and repetitive work which is considered unskilled and they subsist on daily wages. They are also faced with a double burden of work as they not only are engaged in economic work but are also engaged in household affairs. Arindam (this volume), in a discussion on gender inequality in health within households and beyond, reiterates that working women are constantly stretched between domestic and professional requirements. The same was also reported by the plantation workers as they had to toil both at home and at work. While the former is unpaid the latter barely suffices for their household's sustenance.

As can be understood from the following narrative that emerged from a focus group discussion with the women workers.

> We have become used to some discomforts regarding our health. Aches and pains are part of a plantation worker's life. As we get older these health problems become more evident especially eyesight weakness is a major problem among the pluckers. We do not even consider fever, coughs and colds as illnesses. Our constitution is probably weak as we have poor diets and we use most of our strength in doing our jobs. Once we return home, while the men can rest, women also have to bear the burden of housework.

Since colonial times women workers have been given preference as they brought along with them their families thereby ensuring a supply of labour for the tea estates. In spite of their contributions, women workers are consigned to the lowest rung of the employee hierarchy at the plantations. Their labour is cheap and abundantly available while the feudal relations of production still persist. Very few women workers are promoted to sub-staff level indicating a lack of vertical mobility for the women workers within the plantation. However, a positive of the fair-trade certification in the organic tea plantation has been that there were women who had been promoted to the level of supervisory staff from among the pluckers. They also were members of the Joint Body and took part in decision-making.

The tea plantation system—reinforced by social norms—traps women in the lowest paid jobs with the fewest benefits and amenities, working long hours plucking tea, on top of the unpaid care work they do at home. Therefore, women workers are marginalized on multiple fronts—casualization of the workforce, limited upward occupational mobility and political space in trade unions. They also remain both isolated and bound to the land despite poor working conditions and because of their gender (Banerji & Willoughby, 2019). There are reports of maternal and infant mortality being higher in the tea estates as compared to populations outside the estates (Gurung & Mukherjee, 2018; Koshy & Tiwary, 2011). There are various measures which the governments and concerned bodies have taken but the women workers in the tea estates are yet to experience the fruits of development. Hence, a very focussed determination is essential to bring the women workers in the tea estates at par with their counterparts in other sectors.

The Way Forward

Findings from the study have validated that the tea workers in Darjeeling are highly dependent on plantations for food, drinking water, housing, education and healthcare as has been pointed out in literature on tea plantations of India. Housing is sub-standard with inadequate facilities like water supply, toilets, etc. The interplay of factors like work, socio-economic conditions, access to basic amenities, education, etc. leaves the tea plantation worker vulnerable to ill-health. These multitude of factors not only influence their living standards but also lead to differences in their health (seeking, promoting and care utilization) behaviour. Thus, social disparities in health place the tea workers who are already disadvantaged with respect to their work and wage conditions in a more vulnerable position.

Darjeeling tea has always been marketed as an exclusive and luxurious product (Besky, 2014b). Darjeeling was developed and seen as a place of colonial leisure and still enjoys a 'distinctness' in the global market. However, the workers remain poor, isolated, neglected and voiceless. Several international certifications are being acquired by the tea plantation industry of Darjeeling at a huge cost to the planters/owners to attract the first-world buyers and for profitability. Certifications like Rainforest Alliance, Ethical Tea Partnership, Fair-trade, etc. (attracts premium price and market for the goods) are all part of a social justice movement that began in the global north to protect the interests of those engaged in production of goods in the global south while these goods are moved from the north to the south. Darjeeling is reported to have the largest number of estates with Fair-Trade certification of any state in India (Besky, 2008; Sen, 2018). One-third of the tea estates in Darjeeling are organic and Fair-Trade certified and yet wages of the workers remain much below the minimum wage received by the agricultural worker in the state of West Bengal. This contradicts the very idea of social justice-based market mechanisms like a fair trade.

It is, therefore, imperative to understand the workers' issues and problems and to have policy dialogue on improving the workers' conditions and provisioning. Efforts must be made towards development for the tea plantation workers by creating a sense of ownership either by granting land rights or through greater stakeholder participation. This would not only improve economic access but also ensure solutions for addressing the social disparities that exist among the tea workers. Hence, we need to re-orient economic activity towards human development rather than towards technological developments. There is a need to revisit the PLA (1951) as well as ensuring implementation of the Minimum Wages Act (1948) in Darjeeling's plantations. Although the scale and velocity of globalization has increased in the past few decades it would seem that so would the market of Darjeeling tea.

On 30th January a public health emergency was declared by WHO on 30th January 2020 and subsequent lockdown across states was declared on 24th March 2020 in India as a means to curtail the spread of the disease. This is said to have affected all walks of life including the plantation sector. In North India (including Darjeeling tea industry) a somewhat unique phenomenon is said to have occurred. Abraham and Madhavan (2020) have brought to notice that price of tea was the only commodity, from among the plantations, to have experienced an upswing in prices probably due to supply constraints resulting in higher demand for the commodity. This they explain was due to the cyclical nature of the price of tea, wherein, it falls during January to March with a steep rise in April (due to premium on first flush tea and price of which was higher than past two years) continuing through a few months till September. However, most of the popular articles highlighted revenue losses as reported by tea associations in the north, the majority of whose members are plantation owners (PTI, 2020; Zahan, 2020). The tea plantation owners, irrespective of the pandemic, have always bemoaned over the low return of profit and increasing labour and social costs. And it seems that they will continue to divert the public's attention away from the 'human cost' of tea (especially Darjeeling) that is renowned across the globe.

Acknowledgements I would like to express my gratitude to all the respondents who allowed me a glimpse into their lives and enabled me to carry out my doctoral research for which I was awarded the degree in July 2020 from Jawaharlal Nehru University, New Delhi.

References

Abraham, V., & Madhavan, M. (2020). Performance of the plantation sector during the COVID-19 Pandemic. *The Indian Economic Journal, 68*(3), 438–456.

Banerji, S. & Willoughby, R. (2019). *Addressing the human cost of Assam tea: An agenda for change to respect, protect and fulfil human rights on Assam tea plantations.* Oxfam. Retrieved December 15, 2020, from https://oxfamilibrary.openrepository.com/bitstream/handle/10546/620876/bp-human-cost-assam-tea-101019-en.pdf

Baru, R., Acharya, A., Acharya, S., Kumar, A. S., & Nagaraj, K. (2010). Inequities in access to health services in India: caste, class and region. *Economic and Political Weekly*, pp. 49–58.

Besky, S. (2008). Can a plantation be fair? Paradoxes and possibilities in fair trade Darjeeling tea certification. *Anthropology of Work Review, XXIX*(1).

Besky, S. (2014a). The labour of terroir and the terroir of labour: Geographical Indication and Darjeeling Tea Plantations. *Agriculture and Human Values, 31*(1), 83–96.

Besky, S. (2014b). *The Darjeeling distinction: Labour and justice on fair-trade tea plantations in India*. University of California Press.

Besky, S. (2017). Fixity: On the inheritance and maintenance of tea plantation houses in Darjeeling, India. *American Ethnologist, 44*(4), 617–631.

Bhadra, M. (2004). Gender dimensions of tea plantation workers in West Bengal. *Indian Anthropologist, 34*(2), 43–68.

Chatterjee, P. (2003). *A time for tea: Women, labour and post/colonial politics on an Indian plantation*. Zubaan, New Delhi.

Gothoskar, S. (2012). This chay Is bitter: Exploitative relations in the tea industry. *Economic & Political Weekly*. Vol. XLVII. No. 50.

Gurung, M., & Mukherjee, S. R. (2018). Gender, women and work in the tea plantation: A case study of Darjeeling Hills. *Indian Journal of Labour Economics, 61*(3), 537–553.

Kadavil, S., & Chattopadhayay, S. (2007). *CHAI TIME: sustainable livelihood for small tea growers through CSR*. Partners in Change, New Delhi.

Koshy, T., & Tiwary, M. (2011). *Enhancing the opportunities for women in India's tea sector a gender assessment of certified tea gardens*. Prakruthi, Bangalore

Lama, S. D. (2019). *Tea industry and its workers in Darjeeling: An analysis of health, economy and state policies*. Unpublished doctoral thesis submitted to Centre for Social Medicine and Community Health, Jawaharlal Nehru University, New Delhi.

Loewenson, R. (1992). *Modern plantation agriculture: Corporate wealth and labour squalor*. Zed Books.

Makita, R. (2012). Fair trade certification: The case of tea plantation workers in India. *Development Policy Review., 30*(1), 87–107.

McKeown, T., Brown, R. G., & Record, R. G. (1972). An interpretation of the modern rise of population in Europe. In *Population studies* (pp. 345–382).

Minimum wages across years and industries in West Bengal. https://wblc.gov.in/min-wages-act

Minimum Wages Act. (1948). http://pblabour.gov.in/pdf/acts_rules/minimum_wages_act_1948.pdf

Neilson, J., & Pritchard, B. (2010). Fairness and ethicality in their place: the regional dynamics of fair trade and ethical sourcing agendas in the plantation districts of South India. *Environment and Planning, 42*, 1833–1851

PTI. (2020, April 4). First flush Darjeeling tea almost lost due to lockdown, say Bengal planters. *The New Indian Express*. https://www.newindianexpress.com/nation/2020/apr/04/first-flush-darjeeling-tea-almost-lost-due-to-lockdown-say-bengal-planters-2125819.html

Rajbangshi, P. R., & Nambiar, D. (2020). "Who will stand up for us?" The social determinants of health of women tea plantation workers in India. *International Journal for Equity in Health, 19*, 29.

Rasaily, R. (2003). *Labour and health in tea plantations: A case study of Phuguri Tea Estate*. Unpublished Ph.D. thesis submitted to Centre for Social Medicine and Community Health, Jawaharlal Nehru University, New Delhi.

Sarkar, K. (2016). Wages, mobility and labour market institutions in tea plantations. In *Globalisation, development and plantation labour in India* (p. 27).

Selvaraj, M. S., & Gopalakrishnan, S. (2016). Nightmares of an agricultural capitalist economy. *Economic and Political Weekly, 51*(18), 107–113.

Sen, D. (2018). *Everyday sustainability: Gender justice and fair trade tea in Darjeeling*. Women Unlimited.

Van Der Wal, S. (2008, June). Sustainability issues in the tea sector: A comparative analysis of six leading producing countries. *Stichting Onderzoek Multinationale Ondernemingen*. Retrieved June 23, 2015, from https://www.somo.nl/sustainability-issues-in-the-tea-sector/

Zahan. S. A. (2020, April 9). Assam, West Bengal tea gardens staring at 22% revenue loss. *Times of India.* https://timesofindia.indiatimes.com/city/guwahati/assam-west-bengal-tea-gardens-sta ring-at-22-revenue-loss/articleshow/75060322.cms

Chapter 18
Socioeconomic Disparities in Access and Utilization of Health Care Services in Nepal

Bamdev Subedi

Abstract Nepal has made impressive progress in some health indices in the last few decades. Despite this progress and policy intent of equitable access to quality health care services, disparities remain wide. Drawing from a field study conducted in a village in south-west Nepal, this paper looks into the disparity in access and utilization of health care services among three major caste/ethnic communities—Brahmin/Chhetri, Adivasi/Janajati and Dalits. While the field data suggest that Dalits are increasingly utilizing health post services, the local outlet of government health care services, they are the ones whom the official health care system serves the worst. They fall ill more frequently, rely more on local health traditions and resort (unwillingly) to government health facilities. In many conditions, they experience treatment failures, and incur a high expense per episode of illness, when they seek medical help from private health facilities. The paper discusses the issues of access and utilization of health care services among the marginalized caste/ethnic groups in the context of medical pluralism and the importance of enhancing local health knowledge and practices with reference to COVID-19. The paper concludes with a note that the inequality in health cannot be addressed merely by the policy rhetoric of equal access to quality health services unless the equity concern is seriously articulated into the health care delivery system, the quality of traditional medicine is improved, the health knowledge of marginalized communities is enhanced, and related social determinants addressed.

Keywords Health disparity · Caste/Ethnicity · Dalits · Herbs and healers · Nepal

Introduction

Despite prolonged political instability, Nepal has made impressive progress in some health indices in the last few decades. Significant progress has been made in achieving

B. Subedi (✉)
Medical Anthropologist and Social Activist, Kathmandu, Nepal

targets around maternal, infant and child health, which has been acknowledged internationally (NPC & UNDP, 2013). Between 1996 and 2016, maternal mortality ratio declined from 539 to 239 per 100,000 live births, infant mortality declined from 78 to 32, and under-5 mortality declined from 118 to 39 deaths per 1000 live births (NDHS, 2017). Similarly, life expectancy at birth increased from 54.2 to 66.6 years between 1991 and 2011 (CBS, 2014). The poverty headcount rate also declined from 41.8 during 1995–96 to 25.2 during 2010–11 (CBS, 2014) and overall HDI improved from 0.378 in 1990 to 0.558 in 2015 (UNDP, 2016).

While progress can be observed in overall health indices, the gap across socio-economic groups remains wide, and progress is more visible among certain sections of the population. Dalits are historically marginalized groups, and they are far below the national average in many indices related to health, education and poverty. For example, from 2006 to 2016, under-5 mortality declined from 76 to 31 deaths per 1000 live births among the Brahmin/Chhetri community compared to decline from 80 to 32 among Janajatis (except Newar) and from 90 to 51 among Dalits. Institutional deliveries increased from 24 to 68% among Brahmin/Chhetri, from 14 to 60 among Janajati and from 9 to 45 among Dalits (Bennett et al., 2008; Ghimire et al., 2019). Similar is the trend with deliveries attended by skilled birth attendants. The maternal mortality ratio for Dalits (273 deaths per 100,000 live births) is higher than Janajatis (207) and much higher than Brahmin/Chhetris (182) (Pradhan et al., 2010). On the contrary, life expectancy among Dalits is lower than Janajatis and much lower than Brahmin/Chhetris. People living below the poverty line declined to 25%, but the gap between Dalits (42%) and non-Dalits (23%) below poverty remains wide (CBS, 2011). In terms of human development, Brahmin/Chhetris have the highest HDI value (0.538), followed by Janajatis (0.482) and Dalits (0.434) (UNDP, 2016, p. 5). The disparity in these indicators signals the continued inequality in access to and utilization of health care services.

This paper draws from a field study conducted in a village in south-west Nepal and compares three major social groups in the access and utilization of health care services. According to the 2011 census, Brahmin/Chhetris constitute 28.8%, Janajatis constitute 35.8% and Dalits constitute 13.6% of the total population in Nepal (CBS, 2014). Though these groups are not homogenous and intragroup disparity exists among them (Subedi, 2016), comparison among them makes sense for socio-economic analysis.

Micro-level field data indicates that Dalits are increasingly utilizing primary health care services. However, their health-seeking behaviour and resort patterns suggest that they are the ones whom the official health care system serves poorly. They fall ill more frequently, rely more on local/folk health traditions, resort (unwillingly) to government health facilities, experience treatment failures in many conditions and incur a high expense per episode of illness when they seek private medical care. In this background, the paper discusses the issues of access and utilization of health care services among the marginalized caste/ethnic groups in the context of medical pluralism and the importance of enhancing local health knowledge with reference to COVID-19.

Caste and Ethnicity in Nepal

Nepal is home to approximately 26.5 million people with 125 caste and ethnic identities, 123 languages and 10 religions (CBS, 2012). Caste and ethnicity are important social categories to understand the inequality in Nepali society. Both caste and ethnicity refer to cultural identity or an ascribed status obtained by birth.

Muluki Ain, a national legal code proclaimed in 1854, had classified caste/ethnic groups into (i) *Tagadhari* (those castes who wear sacred thread) such as Brahmin, Chhetri, (ii) *Matawali* (those castes who consume alcohol such as indigenous people), and (iii) *Pani Nachalne* (Water unacceptable). *Matawali* were further divided into two groups: (a) Non-enslavable such as Magar, Gurung, and (b) Enslavable such as Gharti, Bhote, Tharu, and *Pani Nachalne* were further divided into two groups (a) *Sudra* (impure but touchable castes) such as Dhobi, Kasai, and (b) *Achhut* (impure and untouchable castes) such as Kami, Damai (Bhattachan et al., 2003; Subedi, 2010).

'Dalit' has become a widely accepted term among both Dalits and non-Dalits communities. According to Bharati (2002, p. 4339), 'Dalit is not a caste, it is a constructed identity. But at the macro-level analysis, Dalit is an appropriate term when one is studying caste phenomena'. Dalits are defined as 'those communities who, by virtue of atrocities of caste-based discrimination and untouchability, are the most backward in social, economic, educational, political and religious fields, and are deprived of human dignity and social justice' (Bhattachan et al., 2003, p. 3).

Similarly, the term Adivasi/Janajati is used to refer to indigenous communities. Adivasi/Janajati do not come under the caste system, even though many of them can be found following or to be influenced by the Hindu religion and practicing caste system, and many are even counted as the followers of the Hindu religion in the national censuses (Dahal, 2014). The National Foundation for Upliftment of Adivasi/Janjati Act, 2002 defines Adivasi/Janjati as 'a tribe or community as mentioned in the Schedule having its own mother language and traditional rites and customs, distinct cultural identity, distinct social structure and written or unwritten history'.

Caste/ethnicity, like poverty, has been recognized as one of the most important determinants of inequality in access and utilization of health care services (Acharya, 2010, p. 108). Acharya (2010, p. 1) asserts, 'Most poor are Dalits as well as most Dalits are poor'. The incidence of poverty is higher among Janajatis and the highest among the Dalit communities in Nepal. The poor health outcome of the Janajatis and Dalits communities affirms the fact that these groups are served poorly by the official health care system.

Studies conducted in various regions of the Indian subcontinent provide astonishing data about the caste/ethnic disparities and the gravity of discrimination and exploitation of these groups (Jodhka & Shah, 2010; Pyakurel, 2011; Bansod et al., this volume). It is the poor and Dalit who spend more (percentage of their income) than others for the treatment of both acute and chronic illnesses and fall into a debt trap (Sujatha, 2014). Dalit women and children suffer the most from the caste-based discrimination in access to health (Acharya, 2010; Thapa et al., 2021; Acharya, this volume).

Method and Material

This paper draws from a study which was conducted from November 2015 to December 2016 in a village (anonymized as *Anjaan Gaun*) of Dang district of mid-western Nepal, which lies approximately 450 kms South-west of Kathmandu and 700 km northeast of New Delhi. Field data was collected using qualitative measures from the village where 666 people (334 male and 332 female) with different caste and ethnic backgrounds, live in 126 households (50 households from Brahmin/Chhetri, 56 from Janajati and 20 from Dalit communities).

Village Setting

The village has three clusters inhabited mainly by Brahmin/Chhetri, Janajati and Dalit groups. These three groups represent the major caste/ethnic groups of Nepal. The village has fertile and irrigated land, making agriculture, along with animal husbandry the main occupation of the villagers. A sizable number of youths work as migrant workers and a small number of people are employed in service sectors.

When we walk through the village, we can see the growing crops in the surrounding lands, cowsheds and cattle, heaps of rice straw, traditional Nepali house (Namaste shaped rooftops), greenery of agricultural fields and people engaged in the agricultural activities, chirping of birds and sounds of morning roosters, smoke of dung cake and firewood, and the smell of dusty/muddy soil, perfectly giving a flavour of village life.

Semi-structured interviews were conducted with the heads or the elders of the households through repeated visits which helped increase familiarity and build trust. This also encouraged participants to share about private illnesses (like tuberculosis, reproductive health issues, mental illness) which are often surrounded by stigma and discrimination. Participatory methods like social mapping and well-being ranking were also utilized to triangulate the data. At the end of the field-stay, a clearer under-standing of socio-economic backgrounds, village power structures, common health issues and treatments sought was obtained.

Wellbeing Ranking

Five government school teachers, who were from Brahmin/Chhetri and Janajati community and from the same or adjoining village, participated in the well-being ranking. After briefing the process, the participants were given 126 cards on which the names of household heads were written. They were instructed to arrange the cards based on their well-being status. This order was based on the size of land-holding, amount of agricultural production, type of house, level of education, type of employment and income, possession of household assets (such as motorcycle, water pump and sanitation, biogas, agricultural equipment), number and types of domestic animals, social prestige, political involvement and health condition of the family members. At last, these cards were divided into three groups characterized as *sampanna* (well-off), *samannya* (average) and *bipanna* (poor).

The word *sampanna* means well-off, prosperous or accomplished. The *sampanna* households hold relatively large plots of irrigated land, have a good well-equipped house, usually connected to the main road and often have a housing plot in the nearest city of Ghorahi. These households give their land for sharecropping, and have enough wealth to hire labour for their fields, give loans to other villagers and buy shares in cooperative banks or boarding schools. Such households usually have someone in the family holding a government or private job or getting pension, and can afford to send their children to boarding schools and private colleges in distant cities, and have the access to go to cities like Nepalgunj, Butwal, Kathmandu and Lucknow (India) for treatment. Members of *sampanna* households hold a position of respect in the village and are sought for the resolution of local disputes.

The *samannya* (average) households hold smaller agricultural land and a good house. They have enough wealth and resources to provide for the family, cultivate their lands, send their children to school and afford basic health care services. These households have at least a few family members working outside the village, and some who have gone abroad, especially to Gulf countries for contractual work.

The *bipanna* (poor) households own significantly less land (often unregistered), and have thatched/tinned roof and mud-brick wall houses on the periphery of the village, with little to no assets. They mostly work as labour in other farms, or go to Indian cities to work as domestic or factory workers. Their children attend government schools and often have to drop out to work and contribute to the household income. Families are forced to borrow money from local money lenders frequently and live in a cycle of debt. *Bipanna* households are mostly shunned by the others and have little say in any decision-making.

Findings

Identity and Well-Being

In the well-being ranking, 56% of households from the Brahmin/Chhetri communities and 25% from Janajatis ranked sampanna, whereas not a single Dalit household qualified. Among the Brahmin/Chhetris, only 12% households came under the *bipanna* category, while 34% Janajati and 85% Dalit households ranked as poor

(Table 18.1). This reveals the remarkable difference in the socio-economic status of the three groups.

Brahmin/Chhetris hold more agricultural lands—23 *Kattha* on average (one *Kattha* is equal to 338.6 square metres) than Janajatis (12 *Kattha* on average) and much more than Dalits (5 *Kattha* on average). The possession of household assets such as motorcycles, television, solar panel and a biogas plant is positively associated with the people's socio-economic status. For example, among the Brahmin/Chhetris, 46% of the households have motorcycles, whereas only 16% of Janajatis and 10% of Dalits households possess motorcycles. Similar is the trend with other household assets. A point to be noted here is that poverty, and not caste/ethnicity, had a role to play in the lack of household assets. Only three per cent of the households ranked as poor had motorcycles, whereas two-thirds of households ranked as well-off had possessed all these items.

The place of residence in the village also shows the disparity among the three groups. Brahmin/Chhetris are concentrated at the centre of the village connected by the main road, which is the prime location in the village; Janajatis are concentrated on one side connected by secondary road, and Dalits on another side connected by tertiary road or foot trails (Fig. 18.1).

The total percentage of people without any education is the highest among Dalits, whereas the percentage of those with a School Leaving Certificate (SLC) and higher education is highest among the Brahmin/Chhetris (36%).

During the fieldwork period of 14 months, 15 children were born, and of them, six were born at home (one among the Brahmin/Chhetris, three among Janajatis and two among Dalits) with the assistance of traditional midwives. Among them, one was from a *sampanna* household, one from *samannya* and four were from *bipanna* families. Of the nine children born in hospitals, four were from Brahmin/Chhetris, three were from Janajatis and two were from Dalits. And among them, three were from *sampanna* households, five were from *samannya* households and one was from *bipanna* households. This indicates the differences between socio-economic groups in the use of maternity care services.

One of the most striking differences was noted while observing access to healthcare. On one hand, a Brahmin/Chhetri man from a *sampanna* household, diagnosed with diabetes 18 years ago, was living 'a disciplined life' in his eighties; on the other, a Dalit woman from a *bipanna* household, diagnosed with diabetes three years ago, died in her sixties. A woman of her age from Brahmin/Chhetri households who

Table 18.1 Wellbeing status of households by caste/ethnicity

Caste/Ethnicity	Total households	Well-off (*Sampanna*)	Average (*Samannya*)	Poor (*Bipanna*)
Brahmin/Chhetri	50 (100%)	28 (56%)	16 (32%)	6 (12%)
Janajati	56 (100%)	14 (25%)	23 (41%)	19 (34%)
Dalits	20 (100%)	0	3 (15%)	17 (85%)
Number of HH	126	42	42	42

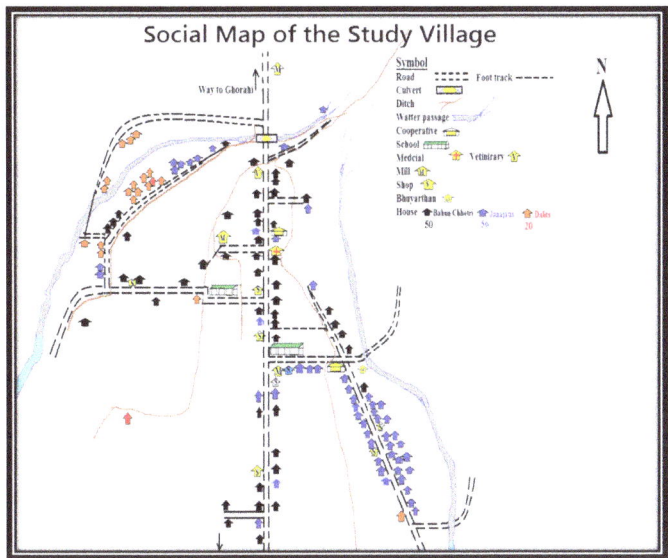

Fig. 18.1 Social map of the study village. *Source* Subedi (2018)

was diagnosed with diabetes 13 years ago was living fine with regular medication. The woman who died had to postpone her plan to visit the health facility because of the peak agricultural season. She would have survived had she belonged to a *sampanna* Brahmin/Chhetri family because they can afford regular tests and the cost of medicine. Moreover, they have better connections with the people in the health facilities and can avail free medicines which are meant for the poor and helpless. Half a dozen patients with asthma had been living fine with medication but among them one who was from *samannya* Brahmin/Chhetri family died. Many people with hypertension were on regular medication and living healthy but among them a person who was from a poor Janajati family died all of a sudden.

The persons who had experienced illness which were explained as *mansik rog* (mental illness), had experienced success or were living fine with regular medication or trying their best in search of better care, but among them, two families lost hope and were left with no choice. They could not afford the cost of care and stopped to seek any further treatment. And those were also from Dalit and Janajati families. Some people with diabetes were diagnosed because they suspected the early signs and symptoms, while others were diagnosed in seeking treatment for other problems without any suspicion of diabetes. Similarly, some were diagnosed with hypertension while doing regular check-ups, but some were diagnosed when seeking care for some other problems. Those who were diagnosed early were relatively better off, while the others who were relatively poor were diagnosed late. Among the six people who died during the course of fieldwork, one was from the well-off, three from average and two from poor families. The death data of a small village cannot be representative but can be taken as indicative that the poor diagnosed late, experience treatment failure, and for them, death comes sooner than those of socio-economically well-off.

Utilization of Health Post Services Based on Caste/Ethnicity

A network of health posts and primary health care centres has been expanded nation-wide, but they function poorly because of absenteeism of medical staff and shortage of supply. In each Village Development Committee (VDC), which is divided into nine wards, there is a health post to provide primary health care services to the local population. The health post data of Amuk VDC (pseudonymized) shows that more people were served from those wards closer to it than the ones farther off. For instance, from the ward where the health post was located, 903 people were served whereas only 48 people from one of the peripheral wards were served. This shows that the distance and geographical location of the health facilities influence the utilization of health care services. Another reason is the location of the health post. While the distance to go to the health post and Ghorahi is roughly equal, the health post is not located at the centre but almost at one corner of the VDC (Fig. 18.2).

Some participants also expressed fear of coming back without getting the help they needed at the cost of a whole day's work because there is no certainty that the medical staff or prescribed medication would be available. Some complained about the short and unsuitable opening hours and unwelcoming environment. Others expressed their doubt over drugs dispensed by the health post saying that 'they distribute whatever they have leftover in their stock'. Sometimes, local residents do not feel the need to

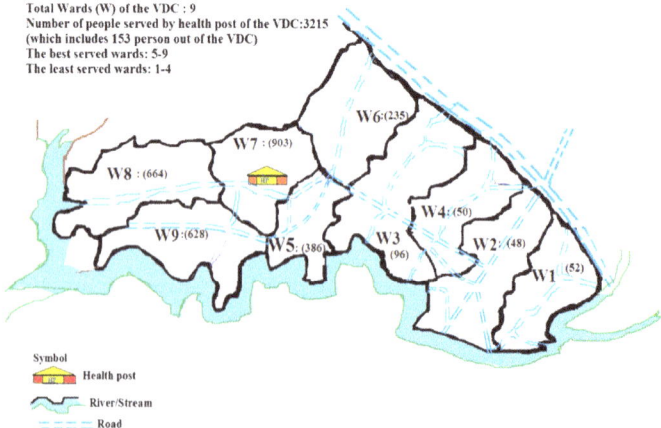

Fig. 18.2 Number of patients of Amuk VDC served by the local health post. *Source* Health Post of the Amuk VDC 2015, Subedi (2018)

Table 18.2 Caste/Ethnic composition of patients served at local health post

Caste/Ethnicity	Composition of population in VDC (%) Source Census data, 2011	Composition of patients served at health post (%) Source Health post annual data, 2016–17
Brahmin/Chhetris	31.3	26
Janajatis	60.3	57
Dalits	4.5	9.2
Others	3.9	7.8

Subedi (2018)

go to the health post in case of minor illnesses such as common cold, short headache and short-term fever, or if the illness is an indigenous one which can be treated with traditional/home remedies.

When comparing the composition of caste/ethnic populations with the composition of patients served by the health post in Amuk VDC, it was found that the patients' caste/ethnic breakdown is in line with their population size, highest being the Janajatis, followed by Brahmin/Chhetri and Dalits both in terms of population and number of patients served by the health post (Table 18.2).

The census data (2011) and health post's Annual Report (2016–17) were of different periods; however, since the VDC level caste/ethnic composition has not changed much since 2001 in terms of percentage of the caste/ethnicity, the comparison makes sense (According to 2001 census, the population of Brahmin/Chhetri was 30.7%, 60.2% Janajati, 3.8% Dalit and 4.3% others).

Dalits make up 4.5% of the VDC population, but 9.2% of the total people served by health post were from Dalits communities. This could largely be due to the propensity to pay, rather than proximity to the health post. This data reiterates that the Dalits who are mostly poor, prefer to use the public sector services and therefore appear to be better served by the local health posts. Analysis of the caste/ethnic composition of the population living in the proximity of the health posts suggest that of the total Brahmin/Chhetri population in the Amuk VDC, 38% live in closer wards (W5-W9) and 62% live in peripheral wards (W1-W4). This is similar to the Dalit population— i.e. 38% live in closer wards and 62% in peripheral wards. Also, there is a possibility that the households from well-off sections including the well-off Dalits and Janajati go to the private clinics or directly to the hospital in Ghorahi.

The health post had served 3215 persons, of which 153 (4.7%) were from outside of the VDC area, and among the 153 people, the Dalits per cent might be high. This does not hold a greater possibility but can be a third reason to increase the Dalits percentage. The frequent visit of the same Dalit patient for health post services may be the fourth reason, and this supports that the poor and Dalits fell ill more frequently or were not treated at the first recourse. Here, it is imperative to note that the poor and Dalits seek no treatment for minor illnesses many times; they also visit local healers more than other groups. Despite this fact, they visit health posts more, possibly supporting that they fall ill more or had recourse more than the other groups.

The high utilization of health post services by Dalits rather than Brahmin/Chhetri may not be true for other health posts. However, a study conducted in the Mid-Western hill district of Nepal also shows that Dalits and Janajatis had significantly more access to government health facility than the Brahmin/Chhetris, and the study also points to the possibility of Dalits being sick more often than those of Brahmin/Chhetri, and they are less likely to use private health facilities (Paudel et al., 2012) due to poor economic propensity. This indicates that using government health facilities by the poor and Dalits is because they cannot afford the healthcare from private facilities. But it is also evident from the data that the better-off and Brahmin/Chhetri utilize the public sector free health care services more than the poor, Dalits and Janajatis.

Among the medical staff in health facilities, from health posts to hospitals, in the study district, most of them are from Brahmin/Chhetri communities. They constitute the two-thirds majority of all the medical staff and hold most of the powerful positions. Janajati, Dalits and the poor are better represented as support staff such as nursing, paramedical and sanitation staff. Across the country the medical profession remains to be dominated by well-off, upper caste and men (Cameron, 2009; MoHP, 2013).

The local health post has six staffs: four staff from Brahmin/Chhetri and two from Janajati communities but not a single staff is from Dalit community. There are two FCHVs in the village, one each from Brahmin/Chhetri and Janajati communities, both from *sampanna* family and both of the private medical stores in the village are run by Brahmin/Chhetris. There are two healers from Dalit, four from Janajati and two from Brahmin/Chhetri communities in the village, and all of them are from *samannya* or *bipanna* households. Though caste-based discrimination and untouchability exists in the village, healers are consulted by all the caste/ethnic groups, often indiscriminately. However, it does not mean the non-existence of caste preference in seeking care.

One of the reasons why local healers (herbalists, shaman and midwives etc.) are consulted more by Dalits and Janajatis may be because the size of Dalit healers is much larger than the Dalits medical practitioners. Besides, Dalits as healers are more accepted but Dalits as medical practitioners, may not be accepted that much or may be discriminated (Cameron, 2009). The higher reliance of Dalits and Indigenous ethnic communities on local healers can be partly because of the size of their healers in the VDC.

The Use of Herbs and Healers

The use of medicinal herbs and healers is a prominent part of the community health tradition in Nepal. The importance of Nepalese Himalayan herbs has always been highlighted. Even politicians do not miss to mention the richness of Nepal in medicinal herbs. Home-based herbal healing serves is an option when people are optionless. For instance, in the beginning of COVID-19 pandemic, the use of home-based herbal practices increased significantly. The present state of home-based practices needs attention because these practices are associated with the treatment of many illness conditions. Besides, the responsibility of caring primarily falls upon the family members. Hence, herbal literacy and general health awareness among the family members contribute to good health.

There are eight local healers (faith healers, herbal healers and traditional midwives) in the village who provide shamanic or faith healing, herbal healing, massage and midwifery services. The shaman or faith healers handle illnesses such as *jhaskine* (startling), *daraune* (frightening), coping with nightmares, and attacks by unknown forces, the illnesses of emotional, spiritual, and mental conditions and those which are locally understood and explained.

The use of herbal healers has always been an integral part of community health practices and traditional midwives, who assist in childbirth and postpartum care and massage, have always been an important source of help. These indigenous traditional healers follow distinct healing methods, use healing mantras, herbal medicines and massage therapies (Subedi, 2019). These healers are often consulted first before visiting official health facilities and for some conditions such as jaundice, sprain, fracture, snake bites, people frequently visit them because of their expertise. However, it is notable that the people have become selective in their choice, and some of them express doubt over healing herbs because of a lack of scientific study and evidence (Subedi & Joshi, 2018).

They use various types of home-based herbs, food items and spices to deal with minor illnesses, but these constitute a major share of the number of illnesses they encounter. In managing chronic illnesses such as diabetes and hypertension, people also follow yoga exercise, brisk walking and dietary regimen. Based on the illness and severity, they try home-based practices first. They then move to local healers or medical practitioners, and to the health posts and hospitals, first within the district and then outside the district, sometimes across the border in India. The use of local herbs and healers is higher than the official traditional medicine such as Ayurveda, Homeopathy, Unani and Naturopathy. However, there has been a steady rise in the use of traditional medicine products and services. The expansion of private medical stores and health clinics has also contributed to the increased use of biomedicine, as private facilities outnumber public facilities.

There are several reasons why residents of the village were found to be relying on traditional healers more than the official systems, some of which have been discussed in the previous sections. On the one hand, sometimes people find no other option, and on the other, the cost comes as a barrier. Health care facilities are not at an accessible distance, nor are the health care services free. There are no special provisions to increase access and utilization of health care services to the poor. The private sector facilities charge high for medical examinations and surgical treatments. They fear that they will have to sell their assets when they go to a private hospital, pushing them deeper into the cycle of debt they are already caught in. A man from a poor family of the Brahmin/Chhetri community sought a bonesetter's service when he broke his hand after falling from a tree. When asked why he didn't go to the hospital, he replied, 'The amount of money which I had was not sufficient even to buy a plaster'. While some healers such as bonesetters, snake bite healers, reputed shamans with particular therapeutic skills, and traditional midwives have started to charge, people still find them more affordable than public facilities.

They also resort to folk healers because they have experienced successful treatment. A woman from a poor family of the Janajati community shared, 'I had gastric problems. I took medicine from the village medical store. That did not help. I took medicine from Ghorahi hospitals. That did not help either. It was the crude herbal medicine given by the healer who lives in the next village which truly helped me'.

Disparity in Health-Seeking and the Use of Medicine

The question 'What would you do if a doctor comes with free medicine in the village?' revealed how a large number of people were living with untreated illnesses due to a lack of access and resources.

During the course of the fieldwork, it was found that patients from Brahmin/Chhetri communities sought treatment sooner compared to Dalits and Janajatis. The number of patients who had not sought treatment among the Dalits was by far the highest. More Dalits and Janajatis than Brahmin/Chhetris were found not seeking treatment despite the need. While home-based treatment was a major source of treatment for all three groups, Dalits and the poor were found relying more on home remedies exclusively in many illnesses. Brahmin/Chhetris mostly used home remedies combined with official medicine. Similarly, more Dalits and Janajatis than Brahmin/Chhetris were found using traditional healers. More Brahmin/Chhetris were found visiting hospitals and private clinics located in faraway cities and even across the border in India. On the rare occasion the poor went to hospitals, it cost them far more than they could afford.

Based on Table 18.3, it can be noted that a higher percentage of Dalits sought treatment outside the district as compared to Janajatis. This can be attributed to the fact that many of them have family members working in Delhi, Haryana and Punjab. This reliance on family members, friends and acquaintances was observed across the three socio-economic groups.

As expected, Brahmin/Chhetris were found to have a more robust network outside the district whom they could rely on for support. They are more likely to find someone who at least knows budget hotels (or *dharamsala*) and public or charitable hospitals. The poor and Dalits lack such connections in the cities. For example, only one Dalit who was relatively better than others had gone to Kathmandu because he knew someone working there. However, among the well-off and Brahmin/Chhetris, there were many family members/friends/acquaintances in Kathmandu either working or studying. The socio-economically well-off also knew where to go for what kind of illness, which hospital provides affordable and quality care, and where to stay to save money.

Table 18.3 Reported treatment sites by caste ethnicity

Types/Place of treatment	Brahmin/Chhetris (N = 238)	Janajatis (N = 319)	Dalits (N = 109)
No treatment	0.4	1.3	3.7
Home treatment	8.4	5.9	10.1
Use of local folk healers	7.1	10	12.8
Official traditional medicine	2.1	1.6	0
Village medical stores	3.8	5.9	1.3
Within the district facilities	18.5	11.6	12.8
Outside the district facilities	15.9	7.5	8.2

This is another indication of how people with a poor socio-economic background often have to compromise in their treatment choices and experience treatment failures. The well-off sections have a relatively better chance to get the right care at the right time from the right practitioners. This is possible not only because they can afford the cost but also because they are more educated and can better use kinship and social networks. Most Dalits lack such networks, and they are likely to take additional recourse, thereby incurring additional costs. Moreover, Dalits suffer from stigma and discrimination. A woman from Dalit family said, '*Haamilai nahepne ko hola?* (Who doesn't look down on us?) All, even the doctors do'.

Discussion

Family and Folk Sector of Health

While explaining the structure of health care systems worldwide, Kleinman (1980) presented three overlapping sectors: the popular sector, folk sector and professional sector. The most important observation he made was that the popular sector plays a very important role in health maintenance and treatment of illnesses. In his study in Taiwan, he found that the popular sector treated almost 70–90% of the people. The popular sector, which includes the family, friends and social network's health care activities, constitutes a major share in the management of illness. This forms a major part of what has been termed as local health tradition in India, followed by the folk and professional sectors.

The family sector of healthcare often gets less attention. The family remains a primary source of care that supports sick members through self-medication, home remedies, home-based care and support. In a way, the professional practitioners' role is to help families in their effort to make sick members well. For instance, during the COVID-19 pandemic the role of the family increased in managing home isolation and providing care and support to the infected or sick members. The enhanced knowledge and skills of the family help evaluate and assess the condition of the sick person, seek required therapeutic services in time, and provide better home care and support. The better the family sector of care, the better the family can collaborate with professional practitioners. It is far more cost-effective and sustainable in many illness conditions to encourage home care than to increase the number of hospital beds and extended bed occupancy. The COVID-19 pandemic also helped realize the importance of the popular sector of care. The popular and folk sectors work as the base of the rural communities. Further effort needs to be made to strengthen this base. For instance, the contribution of FCHVs has been laudable in Nepal. Based on this experience, traditional healers hold a possibility to contribute to primary health care services and revitalize local health traditions.

Policy Rhetoric and Reality

There is an emphasis on equity in policy documents. The National Health Policy 2019 also emphasizes equitable access to quality health care services. The policy states one of its guiding principles as special health care services targeted to the marginalized Dalit and indigenous communities (MoHP, 2019). Such an affirmative policy initiative is vital to minimize the disparity on account of caste/ethnicity.

Constitutionally, everyone has the right to get free basic health care services from the state, and every citizen shall have equal access to health services. The directive policy of the state, as stipulated in the Constitution of Nepal 2015, is 'to arrange for access to medical treatment while ensuring citizen's health insurance' and 'to ensure easy, convenient and equal access of all to quality health to make people healthy by enhancing the public investment and making private health sector investment in health service-oriented by regulating and managing such investments'. Article 40 of the Constitution of Nepal stipulated various Rights of Dalits, and one of them is to make special provisions by law in order to provide health and social security to the Dalit community (Constituent Assembly Secretariat, 2015).

The local communities, particularly Dalit and Janajati, have better control over folk medicine and local health knowledge. However, a process has already begun to disregard and denigrate local health knowledge and make local communities resourceless, whereby neither will they have control over their indigenous health resources or have access to official resources. The number of traditional healers in Nepal is very large and better represents the Dalit and Janajati communities. However, traditional healers have not been included in the national official health care system, despite the Alma Ata recommendations for integrating and utilizing them as valuable resources. Traditional healers are not recognized or organized as health practitioners, and lack the political support to advocate for their rights and recognition. They are resourceless and fall below the power pyramid of health care practitioners. They also lack international support and funding to be trained, organized and integrated with the formal health care system.

If access to official health care facilities is to be enhanced, there should be a connection between traditional healers, whom the people visit first, and the local health facilities. Better health services cannot be ensured without the linkages between popular and professional sectors. For instance, the FCHV, who work as a grassroots structure in linking the community with the official health facilities, have shown the importance of such health workers. The linkages between the popular and professional sectors cannot be achieved without considering a role for traditional healers. They have been contributing as traditional health volunteers without any state support, and with recognition and some incentives, they can contribute to traditional medicine no less than FCHV to biomedicine. The continued utilization of traditional healers by rural communities shows their importance.

Even though targeted to the poor and Dalits in policy papers, the health care services have not and will not benefit much without enhancing their socio-economic conditions. The poor sections will remain deprived without social security and the measures to improve their livelihood conditions. From the perspective of equity and justice, the poor and Dalits need special attention. It is not enough to provide targeted incentives for utilizing official health care services; what they are using must not be of inferior quality, whether that is the food they eat, the condition in which they work, the environment in which they live or the medicine they use. This must include the quality concern of indigenous traditional medicine. The challenge is to provide quality health care services from the official service outlets, regulate the informal private sector and link indigenous traditional healers with the official traditional medicine service delivery system. The traditional knowledge system must not be broken down, and there should not be the Braminization of biomedical practitioners and Dalitization of folk practitioners.

Policy rhetoric is that all people should have access to safe, effective and quality health care services. They should not be exposed to financial hardship while using health care services. This is what is explained as universal health coverage. The logic is that biomedicine is the best, and they should also have access to the best. The policy intentions are seen directed to this end, increasing and expanding public and private health care facilities based on biomedicine. The kind of official health care services, in which they have some access (to be provided by the health post and primary health care services) are often of inferior quality, and to those facilities that provide better quality services, they do not have access, physically and financially. Many households are being pushed below the poverty line because of expensive health care services. When catastrophic health expenditure surpassed other issues, the agenda of universal health coverage got prominence. However, insurance-based universal health coverage is not free from problems both in terms of coverage (as many will be left uninsured) and the cost of the care (as the cost containment will be the new challenge). With national health insurance programmes, government expenditure on health will certainly increase, but it remains uncertain that the Dalits and poor will be better served. There are shreds of evidence that the countries on the path of health insurance have been struggling with cost containment. Some of the insurance models might work as the next level of privatization (Dao & Mulligan, 2016; Mukhopadhyay, 2013; Reddy & Mary, 2013). Besides, without strengthening the local health facilities, which are supposed to provide quality health care services to the local population, health insurance may cover but not improve patient experience significantly in access and utilization of health care services.

COVID-19 and Inequality

As highlighted above, caste/ethnic disparities exist and Dalits are the most marginalized groups. COVID-19 pandemic serves as an example which has exposed and exacerbated the disparity, and Dalits and marginalized Janajati and the poor suffered the most from the pandemic. Most of them who were informal sector workers, manual labourers, daily wage workers and contractual migrant workers lost their jobs. Many Dalits are landless or hold a minimal size of agricultural land and live below the poverty line. As historically oppressed and excluded groups, Dalits suffered even more from the pandemic. The nationwide lockdown, which was imposed to control the outbreak of the virus, severely affected the poor and Dalits. It was heart-rending when the poor and Dalits migrant workers who returned from India during the first wave of the pandemic were barred from entering Nepal. Some of the deaths were reported in the news due to starvation and extreme poverty. Many Dalits and marginalized people starved, and they were not provided with enough relief materials in time. The nationwide lockdown period of almost six months hugely affected them. Instances of caste-based discrimination and psychosocial sufferings abound. The pandemic also exposed the poor access to media among Dalit and marginalized communities. As in other South Asian countries, Dalits and ethnic communities suffered far more than other communities.

The disparity in health outcomes is not solely resulted from the disparity in access and utilization of health care services. Merely aiming to reduce health inequalities by providing equitable and affordable biomedical health care services would not bring the desired outcomes unless their social determinants are addressed. Factors such as living and working conditions, education and occupation, social securities and social network and social relations also have a greater role in health equities. What was more visible during the pandemic was that the poor and Dalits felt insecure because they did not have means of production, such as land. It is often said that disease does not discriminate. All people, irrespective of class, caste, gender, are equally affected by the disease. Against the epidemiological understanding of distribution and determinants of disease, such narrative was once again emphasized during the pandemic. However, studies have shown a strong association between socio-economic status and COVID-19 morbidities and mortalities (Mishra et al., 2021; Patel et al., 2020). Diseases do not affect all sections of the population in a uniform way. People are not equally affected by the COVID-19 and being Dalit and living in poverty itself is a risk factor for the disease and deaths.

The Use of Herbs During COVID-19 Pandemic

The use of various herbs increased exponentially during COVID-19 pandemic (Khadka et al., 2021). People used various types of herbs to boost their immune systems. Some medicinal herbs such as *Gurjo* (Tinospora cordifolia), *Tulsi* (Ocimum tenuiflorum) and *Besar* (Curcuma longa) were much publicized in (social) media. The widely held perception is that herbs are harmless, safe and free from side effects. People in the villages used whatever the knowledgeable persons or traditional healers suggested. Though traditional food items and herbs can help increase the body's ability to fight disease by improving the immune system, it is undeniable that use of unproven herbs or overuse of herbs can be harmful. There are suggestions that the *Gurjo* has side effects if used excessively. There are many benefits of using medicinal herbs if used in the right quantity but can adversely affect too, if used indiscriminately.

Prime Minister K. P. Sharma Oli also encouraged the use of herbs and home remedies even though he was criticized for downplaying COVID-19 and propagating unproven medical practices. People used various herbs to boost their immune system. The Department of Ayurveda and Alternative Medicine (DoAA) also recommended some herbs such as *Sutho* (dry ginger), *Besar* (turmeric powder), *Tulasi* (holy basil), *Asuro* (Justicia Adhatoda), *Marich* (black pepper), *Pipla* (long pepper), *Tejpaat* (Cinnamon) *and Daalchini* (Bay Leaf). What was lacking was the community connection of DoAA. The Department could not communicate effectively in time. The traditional herbal healers found in almost every village could have helped DoAA to be connected directly to the community had they been linked with the DoAA in the health care delivery system.

Conclusion

Whatever the political rhetoric be, the state has failed to benefit the Dalits and marginalized ethnic communities. Improving access and utilization of health care services among poor, Dalits and marginalized ethnic communities requires an improvement in the provisioning and service delivery. Ensuring access (financial, physical and cultural) to official health care services and enhancing local health knowledge and practices can help improve the health outcomes among the poor and Dalits. The local health post on which they have access must be strengthened, and traditional healing practices on which they rely must be improved. The accepted principle is that the kind of medicine they want and need must be of sufficient quality. This is important from the equity perspective. Inequality in health cannot be addressed merely by the policy rhetoric of equitable access to quality health care services unless the equity concern is articulated thoughtfully in the health care delivery system, the quality of traditional medicine on which they rely is improved, their traditional health knowledge enhanced and the social determinants addressed. Improving access and utilization of health care services is vital, but disparities based on class, caste and ethnicity cannot be reduced without dealing with the socio-economic issues. The socio-economic disparity in health requires a strong emphasis on the social determinants of health. Efforts should be directed towards developing policies and programmes to address the root cause of health inequality.

References

Acharya, S. S. (2010). *Access to health care and patterns of discrimination: A study of Dalit children in selected villages of Gujarat and Rajasthan* (Vol. 1, No. 2; Children, Social Exclusion and Development). Indian Institute of Dalit Studies and UNICEF.

Bennett, L., Dahal, D. R., & Govindaswamy, P. (2008). *Caste, ethnic and regional identity in Nepal: Further analysis of the 2006 Nepal demographic and health survey.* Macro International Inc. Retrieved October 7, 2014, from https://dhsprogram.com/publications/publication-fa58-further-analysis.cfm

Bharati, S. R. (2002). 'Dalit': A term asserting unity. *Economic & Political Weekly, XXXVII*(42), 4339–4340.

Bhattachan, K. B., Sunar, T. B., & Bhattachan, Y. K. (2003). *Caste-based discrimination in Nepal* (Vol. 3, No. 8; Working Paper Series). Indian Institute of Dalit Studies. Retrieved January 10, 2014, from http://idsn.org/fileadmin/user_folder/pdf/New_files/Nepal/Caste-based_Discrimination_in_Nepal.pdf

Cameron, M. M. (2009). Untouchable healing: A Dalit ayurvedic doctor from Nepal suffers his country's ills. *Medical Anthropology: Cross- Cultural Studies in Health and Illness, 28*(3), 235–267. https://doi.org/10.1080/01459740903070865

CBS. (2011). *Poverty in Nepal: Based on Nepal living standard survey III (2010–2011).* Central Bureau of Statistics, Government of Nepal.

CBS. (2012). *Volume 01, NPHC 2011: National population and housing census 2011 (national report).* Central Bureau of Statistics, Government of Nepal.

CBS. (2014). *National population and housing census 2011 social characteristics tables (caste/ethnicity, mother tongue and second language)* (Vol. 05, Part II).

Constituent Assembly Secretariat. (2015). *Constitution of Nepal 2015.* Constituent Assembly Secretariat.

Dahal, D. R. (2014). Social composition of the population: Caste/ethnicity and religion in Nepal. In *Population monograph of Nepal, Vol II (social demography).* Central Bureau of Statistics, Government of Nepal.

Dao, A., & Mulligan, J. (2016). Toward an anthropology of insurance and health reform: An introduction to the special issue. *Medical Anthropology Quarterly.* https://doi.org/10.1111/maq.12271a?

Ghimire, U., Manandhar, J., Gautam, A., Tuladhar, S., Prasai, Y., & Gebreselassie, T. (2019). *Inequalities in health outcomes and access to services by caste/ethnicity, province, and wealth quintile in Nepal. DHS further analysis reports no. 117.* ICF.

Jodhka, S. S., & Shah, G. (2010). Comparative contexts of discrimination: Caste and untouchability in South Asia *Economic and Political Weekly, 45*(48), 99–106.

Khadka, D., Dhamala, M. K., Li, F., Aryal, P. C., Magar, P. R., Bhatta, S., Thakur, M. S., Basnet, A., Cui, D., & Shi, S. (2021). The use of medicinal plants to prevent COVID-19 in Nepal. *Journal of Ethnobiology and Ethnomedicine, 17*(1), 26.

Kleinman, A. (1980). *Patients and healers in the context of culture: An exploration of the borderland between anthropology.* University of California Press.

Mishra, V., Seyedzenouzi, G., Almohtadi, A., Chowdhury, T., Khashkhusha, A., Axiaq, A., Wong, W. Y. E., & Harky, A. (2021). Health inequalities during COVID-19 and their effects on morbidity and mortality. *Journal of Healthcare Leadership, 13*, 19–26. PubMed. https://doi.org/10.2147/JHL.S270175

MoHP. (2013). *Human resources for health Nepal country profile*. Ministry of Health and Population (MoHP). Retrieved June 24, 2021, from http://www.nhssp.org.np/NHSSP_Archives/human_resources/HRH_Nepal_profile_august2013.pdf

MoHP. (2019). *Rashtriya Swasthya Niti 2076 (National Health Policy 2019)*. Ministry of Health and Population, Government of Nepal.

Mukhopadhyay, I. (2013). Universal health coverage: The new face of neoliberalism. *Social Change, 43*(2), 177–190. https://doi.org/10.1177/0049085713492281

NDHS. (2017). *Nepal Demographic and Health Survey 2016*. Ministry of Health and Population (MoHP). Retrieved December 27, 2017, from https://www.dhsprogram.com/pubs/pdf/FR336/FR336.pdf

NPC & UNDP. (2013). *Nepal millennium development goals progress report 2013*. Government of Nepal, National Planning Commission/United Nations Country Team of Nepal.

Paudel, R., Upadhayay, T., & Pahari, D. (2012). People's perspective on access to health care services in a rural district of Nepal. *Journal of Nepal Medical Association, 52*(185), 20–24. https://doi.org/10.31729/jnma.49

Patel, T. Y., Bedi, H. S., Deitte, L. A., Lewis, P. J., Marx, M. V., & Jordan, S. G. (2020). Brave new world:challenges and opportunities in the COVID-19 virtual interview season. *Academic Radiology, 27*(10), 1456–1460. CINAHL. https://doi.org/10.1016/j.acra.2020.07.001

Pradhan, A., Suvedi, B. K., Barnett, S., Sharma, S. K., Puri, M., Paudel, P., Chitrakar, S. R., Naresh Pratap, K. C., & Hulton, L. (2010). *Nepal maternal mortality and morbidity study 2008/2009*. Family Health Division, Department of Health Services, Ministry of Health and Population, Government of Nepal.

Pyakurel, U. P. (2011). A debate on Dalits and affirmative action in Nepal. *Economic & Political Weekly, Xlvi*(40), 71–78.

Reddy, S., & Mary, I. (2013). Rajiv Aarogyasri community health insurance scheme in Andhra Pradesh, India: A comprehensive analytic view of private public partnership model. *Indian Journal of Public Health, 54*(4), 254–259.

Subedi, M. (2010). Caste system: Theories and practices in Nepal. *Himalayan Journal of Sociology & Anthropology, IV*, 134–159.

Subedi, M. (2016). Caste/ethnic dimensions of change and inequality: Implications for inclusive and affirmative agendas in Nepal. *Nepali Journal of Contemporary Studies, 16*(1–2), 1–16.

Subedi, B. (2018). *Medical pluralism: Perceptions, practices and patterns of resort in dang, Nepal*. Ph.D. Thesis, Jawaharlal Nehru University.

Subedi, B. (2019). Medical pluralism among the Tharus of Nepal: Legitimacy, hierarchy and state policy. *Dhaulagiri Journal of Sociology and Anthropology, 13*, 58–66.

Subedi, B., & Joshi, L. R. (2018). (Un) popular traditional medicine: Community perceptions, changing practices, and state policy in Nepal. *eSocial Science and Humanities, 1*(2), 157–167. Retrieved September 9, 2018, from http://www.esocialsciences.org/eSSH_Journal/Repository/12N_(Un)%20popular%20Traditional%20Medicine_Subedi.pdf

Sujatha, V. (2014). *Sociology of health and medicine: A new perspective*. Oxford University Press.

Thapa, R., Van Teijlingen, E., Regmi, P. R., & Heaslip, V. (2021). Caste exclusion and health discrimination in South Asia: A systematic review. *Asia Pacific Journal of Public Health*. https://doi.org/10.1177/10105395211014648

UNDP. (2016). *Human Development Report 2016: Human Development for Everyone*. United Nations Development Programme.

Chapter 19
Social Epidemiology of Chronic Kidney Disease with Uncertain Etiology (CKDu) in Sri Lanka: Persistent Inequalities Among Agricultural Communities in a Dry Zone

Chandani Liyanage

Abstract Chronic kidney disease of uncertain etiology (CKDu) has become a critical health hazard in dry zone areas in Sri Lanka since the 1990s, devastating agricultural communities in affected villages. The disease was identified by local health care providers by accident after investigating patients who visited their institutions seeking treatment for various symptoms. Social scientific investigations indicate that structural violence and political economy of agricultural modernization as causal factors for this emerging disease. The present paper is based on ethnographic exploration carried out in two highly prevalent areas in a dry zone by adopting qualitative methodology. The paper explores how CKDu reinforces persistent inequalities among agricultural communities in the dry zone region and analyzes the State response to the emerging health hazard, the lived experience of affected communities with reference to psychosocial implications, issues related to healthcare-seeking behaviour, drawbacks in essential services provision and deficiency in the process of determining the uncertain etiology of disease. Findings reveal that CKDu is associated with stigma and communities being labelled as 'CKDu hot spots' carry adverse effects on victims reinforcing intergroup inequalities. Family vulnerability increases due to illness, pushing farmers into a new type of poverty. Significant gaps have been identified in service delivery points and the lack of cultural competency from local health care providers. In conclusion, disadvantaged socio-economic circumstances contribute in reinforcing persistent inequalities among agricultural communities through health hazards and widening disparities in health outcomes.

Keywords CKDu · Agricultural communities · Lived experience · Intergroup inequalities

C. Liyanage (✉)
Department of Sociology, Faculty of Arts, University of Colombo, Colombo, Sri Lanka
e-mail: chandaniliyanage@soc.cmb.ac.lk

© The Author(s), under exclusive license to Springer Nature Singapore Pte Ltd. 2022
S. S. Acharya and S. Christopher (eds.), *Caste, COVID-19, and Inequalities of Care*,
People, Cultures and Societies: Exploring and Documenting Diversities,
https://doi.org/10.1007/978-981-16-6917-0_19

Introduction

Over the past few decades, a growing epidemic of chronic kidney disease of uncertain etiology (CKDu) has appeared as a health hazard in the dry-zone region of Sri Lanka. The disease was identified in the 1990s by local health care providers in Anuradhapura district in the North Central Province when patients started visiting them seeking treatment for symptoms such as back pain, muscle pain, swollen body, urine infections and continuing fever for an extensive period. The number of patients with similar symptoms visiting those health care institutions gradually increased. After thorough medical investigation of those patients, the health care professionals confirmed that the patients were suffering from chronic kidney disease without presenting conventional causative factors such as diabetes, hypertension etc. which contribute in damaging human kidneys (Abeysekera et al., 1996; Bandara et al., 2008; Athuraliya et al., 2011; WHO & Ministry of Health, 2016b; Rajapakse et al., 2016; Herath et al., 2018 Ranasinghe et al., 2019). Therefore, the newly detected disease was indicated as 'chronic kidney disease of unknown etiology' that subsequently altered as 'uncertain etiology' after finding some susceptible causative factors through scientific investigation (Jayatilake et al., 2013). The latest information available at the Epidemiology Unit in the Ministry of Health reveals that 13 districts in the dry-zone region and surrounding areas have been affected by CKDu. The estimates indicate that incidents of CKDu in Sri Lanka have been doubling in every four to five years, the number of people affected are around 150,000 and nearly 3% of affected people die annually (Wimalawansa, 2015).

The empirical evidence clearly shows that underserved agricultural communities in dry zone areas involved in rice production have become more vulnerable to CKDu (De Silva et al., 2017; Jayasekara, et al., 2015; Jayasekara, et al., 2013; Gooneratne, et al., 2008). The number of those affected and dying has shown a progressive increase, threatening the existence of whole communities living in those areas, and repeatedly, the North Central Province has recorded the highest number of deaths due to chronic renal failure in Sri Lanka (Ministry of Health, 2017).

During the past few decades, a several scientific investigations have been carried out to determine the causative factors of the newly detected disease that goes beyond the conventional explanatory model with regard to chronic kidney disease (Jayatilake et al., 2013; Dharma-wardana, 2014; Jayasekara, et al., 2013; Jayasekara et al., 2015; Jayasumana et al., Jayasumana, Gunatilake, et al., 2015, Jayasumana, Paranagama, et al., 2015; Chandrajith et al., 2010, 2011; Bandara et al., 2008). However, findings of those studies resulted in only a large number of contradictory hypotheses without concrete conclusions with regard to uncertain/unknown etiology of chronic kidney disease that remain yet to be confirmed (Rajapakse, 2016; Ranasinghe et al., 2019). Though CKDu has attracted significant levels of medical, environmental and scientific investigations, only few studies are available from a social science perspective which have attempted to illuminate contextual relationships between CKDu and poverty, chemically-intensive agriculture, experiences of structural violence and burden of illness on affected families (De Silva et al., 2017; Bandarage, 2013; Silva,

2021; Liyanage, 2019). Findings of the study on structural violence of CKDu clearly demonstrate how conditions of structural inequalities have contributed in emergence of CKDu as a hazard in the dry zone districts in Sri Lanka (De Silva et al., 2017). Studies from the politico-economic perspective further reveal how the agricultural modernization processes have been associated with CKDu, and its impact on poor farmers who live in those areas resulting in a heavy burden on families (Bandarage, 2013; Liyanage, 2019; Silva, 2021). The present paper, based on an extensive ethnographic exploration in two agricultural communities in the North Central Province, explores the ways in which CKDu plays a dominant role in reinforcing persistent socio-structural inequalities and widening intergroup health discrepancies among marginalized agricultural communities in a dry-zone region in Sri Lanka. It critically reviews the strengths and shortcomings of state responses with regard to growing health hazards, analyses lay discourse on CKDu and lived experience of affected communities which are being labelled as 'CKDu hot spots'. Our involvement in the inclusion of sociological/anthropological perspectives into CKDu research aims to illuminate lived experience and wider impacts of CKDu on affected communities, significance of the transformation of 'CKDu hotspots' into sites of humanitarian concerns, local dynamics of healthcare-seeking behaviour and ascertaining gaps in fair distribution of health care services for the marginalized social groups. The following section describes the setting and methodology of the study.

Setting

Our ethnographic study focused on investigating socio-epidemiological aspects of CKDu that were carried out in two District Secretariat Divisions (DS Divisions)— Medawachchiya and Padaviya DS Divisions in Anuradhapura district in the North Central Province. The North Central Province is recorded as having the highest number of CKDu patients in Sri Lanka. Within the province itself, Medawachchiya and Padaviya DS Divisions have been reported as high prevalence areas of CKDu where it was originally detected in 1990s and continue to report a large number of cases till date (Jayatilaka et. al., 2013; Ministry of Health, 2017; Ranasinghe et al., 2019). Apart from being a CKDu prevalent area, the Anuradhapura district has a historical significance as the first ever ancient capital of the country (Nissan, 1989). Even today it is a place of archaeological and religious importance for Sri Lankans. Anuradhapura is one of the largest districts among the 25 districts in the country. The total area of the district is 9,741 km^2 which covers 68.5% of the whole province. Sri Lanka's hydraulic civilization was based in Anuradhapura and even today, the district has 2600 large, medium and small tanks irrigating large tracts of cultivable lands. Irrigation facilities are necessary as the district comes within the dry zone with little rain during certain months of the year. The annual rainfall for the district ranges from 1000 to 1500 mm per year (Abeywardana et al., 2018; Panabokke, 2009).

The above mentioned two DS Divisions were purposely selected for this study by considering high prevalence of CKDu and also the specific characteristics of each division for a comparative perspective in the analysis. Patients in these two DS Divisions have nearly three decades of lived experience with regard to impacts of CKDu at individual, family and community levels. At the same time, the two divisions have quite different social structures that are significant to take into account while assessing the level of vulnerability and coping strategies for resilience. Medawachchiya is predominantly based on a traditional village structure that has a comparatively easy access to both material resources and social capital from its social support networks. Padaviya comprises state-led resettlement schemes which were established in the 1950s after independence. People from different parts of the country have migrated into these areas and settled down as paddy farmers. Originally, each migrant family was given five acres of paddy land and two acres of high land. However, the second and third generations of migrant families living in those settlements at present face a lot of difficulties due to limited access to land as the original land has been divided among siblings of the extended family. Therefore, the inhabitants have limited access to cultivation and also inadequate social capital due to lack of integration among the inhabitants who came to the settlement from various parts of the country. Thus, the resettlements have been established without providing basic requirements for survival. The structural differences in the two divisions will be taken into account in analyzing repercussions of CKDu on relevant communities.

Methodology

The author has one decade of experience in interacting with CKDu patients, their family members and concerned communities which began in 2011 when the government declared CKDu as a disaster in the North Central Province. Since then, the author has been involved in a number of studies with reference to different aspects of CKDu that included as sociological study on the behaviour related to the prevalence of CKDu in Anuradhapura District in 2011 with the assistance of the Disaster Management Center and a community-based study on economic, and psychosocial impacts of CKDu in the North Central Province and interventions to support the affected households carried out as a part of National Research programme on CKDu initiated by the Ministry of Health in collaboration with WHO in 2012. The present study on social epidemiology of CKDu has been designed based on previous research experiences, focusing on the gaps identified through the aforementioned studies. This qualitative study adopted an ethnographic methodology in order to comprehend structural issues faced by victims of CKDu in their everyday lives from their own perspectives. The study population included 200 households with CKDu patients, 100 households from each division, elderly people who have a life-long experience of living in these areas, community leaders, local health care providers and other service providers in both localities. In addition, 13 households in Medawachchiya, and 9 households in Padaviya DS Divisions were included in the study where death was reported due to CKDu in order to get a comprehensive understanding of illness burden for the family and their coping strategies from the beginning to the end. The ethnographic investigation in two settings was carried out during a period of twelve months from 2017 to 2018 and continued with several follow-up visits till the end of April 2019.

A mixed method approach has been used for data collection which included in-depth and semi-structured interviews, focus group discussions, interviews with key informants and observation. Secondary data sources have also been used in the analysis. In-depth interviews with patients and their family members were conducted in their local language at their residential places and times convenient to them to minimize the negative impact of recalling past events. We allowed them to speak up in their own way, by using their own vocabulary and gathered necessary information by using phenomenological perspective. This convenient approach made them express their own interpretations regarding the illness experience in their everyday life. Supplementary to the illness narratives of patients, a number of focus group interviews were conducted with the villagers and a number of key informant interviews were conducted with elderly people in the agricultural resettlement, and with community leaders and service providers. An interpretive thematic analysis has been conducted by using procedures of qualitative data analysis where the transcripts and observational notes were utilized to identify patterns in data which are presented under relevant themes in the form of percentages, quotes, narrations and summary statements.

Socioeconomic Backgrounds of CKDu Patients

Socioeconomic background plays a key role in determining the health status of people and to locate patients in their social context to assess impacts of health hazards like CKDu. In both study locations, 90% of the population are Sinhala Buddhist. The purposive sample of CKDu patients included 65 male and 35 female patients in Medawachchiya and 66 male and 34 female patients in Padaviya. The country statistics of CKDu patients reveal that the prevalence rate among male patients is higher than that of females. Age distribution of patients reveals that 70% of CKDu patients in both DS divisions belong to the 41–60 age category, 25% of them above 60 and only a few patients below 40 years old. The age distribution of patients indicates a negative impact on the labour force as the greater majority of patients are in the productive age and their illness led to the loss of the main income to the family especially when farming communities lack a formal social protection system. The second implication is the lack of access to social security schemes for old age as only 25% of patients came under elderly category. Looking at the marital status of the patients, there is an important gender difference. While a majority of male patients are married, a significant number of female patients were widows. This could indicate that women can be more vulnerable by not having the care of a spouse and having to depend on children. However, division wise there was no considerable difference except that the number of female widows in Padaviya was higher than Medawachchiya. A majority of the male patients in both DS divisions were heads of households, their illness making the whole household vulnerable both economically and socially.

The education level of patients in Medawachchiya shows that 40% of them have completed secondary level education and 36% of patients completed primary education. In Padaviya, 54% of patients have studied only till the primary level. It is also important to note that 7% of patients in Medawachchiya and 4% of patients in Padaviya have not received any formal education.

The majority of patients have mentioned that they are unable to actively engage in economic activities due to their illness. However, more than 50% of patients in both locations point out that they are involved in agricultural activities and fulfilling their responsibilities though their capacity is limited due to illness. In both Medawachchiya and Padaviya, a majority of patients are engaged in paddy cultivation. This is more obvious in Padaviya as it is an irrigated settlement area where cultivation is the main economic activity for the majority. Paddy farming is mainly dependent on water supplied by tanks through channels distributed among paddy fields. However, due to a lack of the required water supply, farmers often face difficulty in obtaining the maximum output and are thereby unable to repay their debts obtained from various sources for farming activities. There are some occasions where the paddy farmers have been unable to cultivate both seasons, the *maha* and *yala kanna* (major and minor seasons of cultivation) due to severe drought in the dry zone. Geographical features in Padaviya further fuel the uncertainty of villagers, due to its close proximity to marginal forested areas which exposes them to the risk of snake bites and wild-elephant attacks. To add to this, there have been boarder villages in war zones during armed conflict over the last 30 years, endangering their lives even more. CKDu has added further uncertainties into the lives of people in endemic areas with more suffering.

Looking at the residential status, there is a difference in the two DS divisions. Medawachchiya has a traditional village structure, the economic status of patients is comparatively stable and their social networks are strong. Padaviya being a settlement, a majority had migrated to the area receiving state land who have now been living in the area for more than 30 years. Agriculture is the main livelihood of the majority. However, access to land is limited due to the original being divided among siblings of the original migrant family. The loss of productivity from illness, the costs of care and preventive action have taken a toll on the lives of those people who are surviving in a subsistence economy. The youth population in both locations slowly moved away from agriculture while joining both the civil and armed forces and migrating to urban areas seeking employment opportunities.

CKDu Local Discourses

Multiple methods were employed in collecting information from patients, family members, fellow villagers and leaders of the two communities to grasp insight of local perception on causative factors of CKDu and illness experience of the common people who live in communities which have been labelled as 'CKDu hotspots' for the past few decades. Narratives were collected through in-depth interviews with patients, the caretakers and family members while conducting a number of focus group discussions with diverse groups in the two communities. Key informant interviews were conducted with the elderly people and leaders of concerned communities. Participant observation was also used as a technique while attending healing rituals, harvesting ceremonies, funeral rites and diverse activities within the community itself during the period of our ethnographic investigation.

As mentioned earlier, a majority of patients were diagnosed with CKDu at an acute stage when they were at a productive age. Both Medawachchiya and Padaviya DS Divisions were labelled as CKDu hotspots by health care providers due to the highest number of patients reported from these areas. The empirical evidence reveals that the locals have constructed a popular discourse on CKDu based on their lived experiences, the knowledge received from outsiders and beliefs in traditional culture. This includes their interpretations with regard to the origin, etiology and prevalence of CKDu in their locality. The two communities perceive the disease as a 'struggle between life and the death' in their everyday lives. It is obvious that the calamity has resulted in deteriorating the well-being of patients, family members and also the entire community over the past three decades. As one of the female patients at Medawachchiya pointed out, CKDu articulates in the local social context not simply as a 'life threatening' and 'incurable' disease but also an illness that is associated with huge injustice (*asadharana ledak—an illness with injustice*). The emerging discourse on CKDu in these communities raises several critiques with regard to its prevalence in their locality. The community members who contributed in our focus group discussions, key informant and in-depth interviews have raised a number of questions: Why are only these particular geographical locations vulnerable to CKDu but not Colombo or other areas of the country? Why has CKDu become a problem at present but was not in the past? And why are only some members of the family/community affected while others are safe?

The villagers have different interpretations regarding etiology of CKDu which is based on their own experience as well as explanations given by various specialists who investigated the etiology of CKDu. It's a dilemma within the community discourse itself as to whether CKDu is a recent phenomenon in their locality or if it was prevailing in the past as well. Most of the patients believe that the tragedy is a recent phenomenon due to adverse effects of socio-economic and cultural transformations which have been happening over the past few decades. They also attribute it to misconduct that took place after the agricultural modernization process began in their locality after the introduction of open economic policies in Sri Lanka in 1977. They strongly believe that CKDu is a man-made disaster that the previous generations never experienced as they were capable of maintaining a harmonic balance between the natural environment, socio-economic activities and cultural practices. They gave numerous examples of good practices from the past aimed to protect the natural environment and water sources, along with healthy food practices.

However, recalling their experience during our qualitative interviews, the elders of the village explained that they have witnessed a similar type of disease with symptoms such as disfigured face, swollen body and breathing difficulties that are locally known as '*pittapanduwa*' (a condition of anemia). They believe that those symptoms were caused due to lack of blood in the body and therefore, patients were treated with foods which were considered as most nutritious including meats, milk, curd and certain types of locally available vegetables and leaves.

Within the discourse, there are many possible causes for CKDu including poor quality of drinking water, heavy usage of pesticides and chemical fertilizers, dehydration due to hot weather in the dry zone region, snake bites, genetic factors, hypertension, diabetes, heavy use of alcohol, prolonged usage of medicines and hard work that associated with their livelihood activities. Even though the villagers have identified many possible causes for CKDu, they consider the heavy usage of agrochemicals and the poor quality of locally available drinking water as the main causes. As a result, they are in search of potable water from suitable sources, even agreeing to bear out-of-pocket expenditure. All the patients have changed their drinking water source/s from ground wells to the Reverse Osmosis (RO) system. There is a community-based system to operate and maintain the RO watershed in the village that has been subsidized for the families who have CKDu patients (Kafle et al., 2019).

The identified patients have been categorized into stages while considering the severity or the progress of disease and level of kidney function by health care providers based on their biomedical model of renal failure. Even though the community discourse on CKDu is overlapping and interrelated to a certain extent with the above biomedical explanatory model, the locals also have their own culture specific interpretations in this regard. Accordingly, both communities in Medawachchiya and Padaviya have recognized three categories of CKDu which are based on their illness experience over the past few decades. The categorization has an impact on their treatment seeking behaviour.

The three categories of CKDu locally identified are *Vakugadu ekilenawa* (the kidneys shrink, or the shrinking of kidneys); *Vakugadu diyawenawa* (the kidneys dissolve, or the dissolving of kidneys) and *Vakugadu idimenawa* (the kidneys swell, or the swelling of kidneys). As verified by the villagers in both communities, each category can be identified based on its symptoms. The cause/s of illness may vary depending upon the illness category. According to village narratives, the physical appearance of people who suffer from 'shrinking of kidneys' looks like they are very healthy and no visible symptoms are generally found except for passing protein with urine that is identified by the health care providers through a screening process. However, people believe that western medicine is not required for this condition and use some herbal medicine locally available. According to their experience, urine infections are very common in their locality due to dry climatic conditions. They believe that this type of illness can be controlled by increasing daily water consumption. Most patients were diagnosed with CKDu due to screening tests conducted at grassroots level. However, they were not given any medication and instructed to go for a check-up at the clinics once in six months.

The villagers believe that kidneys can gradually dissolve due to various reasons and associate breathing difficulties, back pain and headache as some of the symptoms. They also believe that it is impossible to recover completely even though such symptoms can be controlled by taking medicine. On the other hand, swelling of kidneys is considered as the worst category of CKDu by the villagers. According to their narratives 'it is a matter of life and death' and is indicated by as swollen body, severe breathing difficulties, loss of appetite. The villagers inevitably put any patient-recommended dialysis under this category. The empirical evidence suggests that there is a fear among the villagers to go through dialysis as it symbolically suggests the imminent, and painful death of the patient by the third time. The narratives indicate that there is an emerging trend of avoiding dialysis as a treatment for CKDu by the concerned communities. There are some cases where patients have completely stopped visiting the clinic when they are prescribed dialysis and have been found searching for alternative treatment methods. There is a popular belief that this condition is a result of karma, and any patient suffering from it is stigmatized. This was further verified from a case study of a 40-year-old woman who died due to swelling of kidney in Medawachchiya during our investigation period. The relatives of the patient and villagers strongly believed that the death was due to bad karma in the previous as well as present birth.

Economic Impact of CKDu on Affected Communities

CKDu has adverse effects on the economic conditions of patients and their families due to low productivity of the ill member/s while bearing additional expenditure that is required for health care and preventive measures. As mentioned earlier, a majority of households being considered are often poor even prior to diagnosis. The livelihoods are predominantly agricultural, with uncertain and low incomes. The male rate of CKDu patients is higher than that of the female and most male patients in our sample were also heads of their households, in the age group of 41–60 years. In an agricultural setting, the men play a crucial role in the process of land preparation, cultivation and harvesting while the women play a dual role in assisting the agricultural process while bearing the caregiving responsibility. The evidence also reveals that there is a large dependent population, so the loss of income and labour has a major adverse impact on the household expenditure as well as in providing care to the patient. The study found the families to be largely nuclear: with the modal family size being four in Medawachchiya and five in Padaviya. The economic impact of CKDu incurs out-of-pocket expenses for the patients and their families in accessing healthcare which includes transport, expenses during hospital stay, out-patient visits, special diet for patients, expenditure for medical care using complementary systems such as indigenous medicine, religious, ritual and other healing systems, and preventive measures such as obtaining or purchasing water from different sources, etc. This additional economic burden often ends up pushing families into poverty.

Psychosocial Impact of CKDu

The empirical evidence clearly suggests that there is fear and stigma associated with CKDu. More and more people are hiding the illness from the neighbourhood and even their close relatives to avoid stigma and associated discrimination. On one hand, the patient who wishes to keep CKDu as a secret attempt to hide it from fellow villagers by saying that they attend another clinic (hypertension or diabetic) and not the CKDu clinic at the hospital. On the other hand, there is a trend of labelling people as CKDu patients if they attend other clinics at the nearest hospital. The empirical evidence also shows that there is a trend among patients to avoid the nearest health care facility and visit faraway places even with lots of difficulties just to maintain the confidentiality of their disease within the community.

It is very clear that CKDu has contributed to the deteriorating overall mental well-being of patients, family members and members of concerned communities. The patients' narratives reveal that fear, anxiety, anger and sleeping disorders are common symptoms among all CKDu patients. However, the service delivery system is not yet ready to provide the required psychosocial counseling for the patients and family members to cope.

The psychological dimension of CKDu has been extremely neglected in the clinical setting where patients go for regular treatment. The evidence reveals that there are a number of gaps in the process of diagnosis and treatment including communication gaps, internal arrangements/organizational structure of the clinic, long waiting times and problems related to infrastructure facilities contribute to further deteriorating the mental well-being of CKDu patients. Issues related to communication gaps between the patient and the health care providers is identified as one of the factors that should be given priority in this context. The patient is treated as a passive object where they receive only instructions to follow but hardly get any explanation with regard to their ill-health and relevant treatment which adds to the patient's anxiety and fear. The evidence further highlights the importance of integrating clinical social workers into the local health care delivery system urgently in order to minimize and overcome the above limitations. Such clinical social workers can work in collaboration with health care providers to address the emotional well-being of patients.

While it is important to identify individual patients when evaluating mental well-being, evidence of this study stresses on the importance of considering family as a unit when examining the psychological/emotional impact of ill-health related to CKDu. As Dwyer correctly pointed out, the western conceptions of self and emotional stress that the human subject is held to be singular and unique. However, in the Asian context, the individual is not an autonomous independent agent where it would be impossible to evaluate mental well-being of an individual by investigating them from the western notion of authority. As evident from this study, the family can be identified as a collective unit of suffering even though the individual patients have responded quite differently to similar situations based on their internal capacity.

The whole family needs to be strengthened with necessary interventions throughout the process to enhance its capacity to face this long-term challenge. While each person's experience with CKDu is unique and depends on individual internal and external factors, there are some common feelings and concerns. CKDu has become a social issue, and the entire community has been gradually deteriorating due to illness. There is hardly any significant distinction between different social categories based on age, gender, social class, level of income, ethnicity, etc. The findings clearly suggest that the entire community needs to be considered as a vulnerable group in this context when designing interventions with regard to mitigating adverse effects of CKDu. There are a number of occasions where the community has expressed their tension and dissatisfaction when interventions have been targeted only for CKDu patients but not the entire community. The empirical evidence further suggests that there is a need for organizing and strengthening the community in order to mobilize its resources to face the challenge of stigma and discrimination. Integrating social workers who are capable of organizing such communities to mobilize their various resources at different levels can play a crucial role.

Social Impact of CKDu

Besides emotional damage, CKDu has many adverse effects on other aspects of the everyday life of a patient and their families. The illness has brought about drastic changes within the family in terms of resource allocation, consumption patterns, setting priorities and maintaining social relationships. Finally, the entire community has been affected due to CKDu in the form of deteriorating social capital and material resources available in these communities.

The findings of the study suggest that the everyday life of patients has been disturbed to a great extent not only due to physical discomfort and emotional damage caused by the illness but also due to issues related to the treatment process and the negative image that comes with being labelled as a CKDu patient. The impact of CKDu on a patient's everyday life can be elaborated in relation to their participation in livelihood activities, domestic tasks including duties and responsibilities associated with social roles, personal activities and social activities at the community level. The narratives reveal that there is a general pattern with regard to everyday life of CKDu patients. Most patients struggle to continue with the same lifestyle with little adjustments even after their diagnosis as CKDu until they become inactive or incapable of movement. It is quite important to take into account that besides medical explanation, patients have their own criteria to evaluate their personal health condition where physical fitness and the ability to work are crucial for the villagers in evaluating their health condition. The evidence suggests that most of the patients are compelled to continue with the same lifestyle if they feel physically comfortable even though their productivity gradually deteriorates due to illness. Some of the patients in the sample have been diagnosed as CKDu when they were at a critical condition where the lifestyle of those patients had been changed within a short period of time after the diagnosis. It is of vital importance to note that there are some exceptional cases where a patient's everyday life has become more active than in the past after diagnosis and expedited certain tasks in order to fulfill their social responsibilities with regard to the family before their health becomes critical. It's a common feature that most of the patients have considerably increased the amount of time set aside to engage in religious and ritual activities due to illness, it can be seen as the main strategy adopted by them for restoring and enhancing mental well-being.

Impact of CKDu on Livelihood

The empirical evidence of this study strongly suggests that CKDu has had an adverse effect on productivity. As mentioned earlier, most of the patients are farmers and they are compelled to continue with the same livelihood activities even after being diagnosed as CKDu patients until they become physically inactive. The illness has some adverse effects on the contribution of patients in domestic tasks including duties and responsibilities that are associated with various social roles. This narrative further suggests that most patients voluntarily become silent within the family by disengaging themselves from important activities while accepting the sick role when they start experiencing physical discomfort as a result of the progression of the illness. There is some evidence to prove that patients have taken immediate actions to fulfill some of the responsibilities with regard to children's matters before the sickness becomes critical.

Impact of CKDu on Patients' Families

Family is one of the most important social institutions that helps society in organizing most social roles for its smooth functioning. Thus, the family is responsible for activities related to both production and reproduction while mutually sharing its resources, fulfilling emotional needs of its members and providing care to members within. The findings of this study show that the family has been greatly affected by CKDu in various ways. As discussed earlier, the family is viewed as a unit of suffering that has been affected in three ways. Firstly, the family has been affected by the low productivity of the ill member; secondly, by allocating its resources, both human and material, to manage the health of that particular member and thirdly, the emotional and social cost of illness on the family.

On the one hand, the patient's family members have to take up the added workload that was previously done by the patient. On the other hand, the family members have to accept the additional workload of caregiving. In some families, the members had to find new income generating activities in order to cope with additional expenses incurred due to illness. By contrast, there are some families where the members have had to reduce or completely stop their livelihood activities in order to provide necessary care for the patient. It was observed that comparatively, family members have to suffer more when the patient functions as the head of the family. The spouses have faced a lot of difficulties while trying to deal with duties and responsibilities that are attached to the family unit. The children have also been affected badly because of an ill parent. As evident from this study, most family members have adjusted to the situation by adopting different strategies through limited engagement in leisure activities, and sacrificing on future endeavours.

The education of children has been affected as some of them have had to drop out of school due to sickness of one member in the family. In some cases, the academic performance of children decreased after a family member had been diagnosed with CKDu, while some faced difficulties in attending extra classes for tuition due to financial problems within the family. When the patient is the head of the family, schooling becomes irregular for some children who have to take up work to help the family in generating lost income or to take care of the ailing family member.

As revealed by empirical evidence, the impact of CKDu on marriage can be seen in two ways. In some cases, parents have had to arrange early marriages for their children due to the illness of a mother or father. In some cases, marriages of children have been delayed and one parent has had to take the whole responsibility for it. For several families, it was also found that finding suitable partners for the children of CKDu patients has become problematic due to many reasons. Some of the geographical locations in the area have been labelled as high-risk areas for CKDu, this has also had a negative impact on the image of the people living in these areas. It becomes further problematic because of the stigma associated with the disease and the popular notion among locals that genetic factors are also a cause for illness as there are a number of incidents where several members in same families have been affected from CKDu. However, scientific investigation is required to verify this factor. Development activities related to family have been another aspect impacted by CKDu in many ways. Most of the construction work has been delayed, but there are a few exceptional cases where the family has taken immediate action to complete construction of house and other arrangements before the patient's condition becomes critical. However, most of the evidence suggests that people have had to sell some of their lands, livestock, vehicles or equipment related to agriculture due to meet the increased expenses linked with the disease, or had to delay purchasing land, equipment, etc. as they have given their main priority to managing CKDu.

As far as food and water are concerned, consumption patterns change greatly in a family after the disease is diagnosed. In most families, a separate meal is prepared for the patient while others eat whatever is available. It should be highlighted that there are drastic changes with regard to water consumption by patients after diagnosing them as CKDu for which they have to bear extra expenses. Most of them hardly use water from their own wells and spend money to buy filtered water from Rivers Osmosis system, use bottled water and drive distant places searching for potable water from spring wells.

The study has also found that CKDu has had a positive as well as negative effect on social relationships. Emotional bonds within families have been seen to be stronger, children who live in distant places have come to see their sick family members, even those who weren't always close with their family. However, as mentioned earlier, the general pattern is that family ties with relatives and neighbours become strengthened at the initial stage of diagnosis of a family member as CKDu and they are weakened in the middle stage and re-strengthen at the end stage. In addition to the above pattern there are some occasions where the family networks become weakened throughout the process and as against some networks continuing while mobilizing their resources throughout the process to manage the patient's care.

Through the course of the study, it was observed that while some challenges remain common for most families, the experience may differ from one to the other depending on available resources, access to social networks and specific characteristics of an individual. This further suggests that each family needs to be considered as a unique unit when designing interventions for mitigating the adverse effect of CKDu on the family. This could be done by using family social workers who could draw up individualized care plans for patients and their families.

Impact of CKDu on the Community

Communities become more vulnerable when there are a large number of CKDu patients as they are unable to help each other. The other issue that remains is the stigma. In Padaviya it was reported that one family had left the village in order to escape from being labelled a 'CKDu family'. Although this is just one case, in the time to come, if the problem is not addressed there can be more families moving out of these areas. The study locations are comparatively more vulnerable to many hazards such as drought, wild-elephant attacks, etc. where CKDu has added further uncertainty to make the situation worse. There are hardly any signs of addressing relevant issues at the community level even though there are some existing Community Based Organizations contributing in indirect ways to provide necessary resources only when matters become critical.

Healthcare-Seeking Behaviour

A social behaviour perspective was adopted to scrutinize the healthcare-seeking behaviour of patients in the two DS Divisions. It was observed that despite registering at the nearest CKDu clinic, nearly 50% of patients utilize Ayurvedic or traditional medicine simultaneously. Every patient acknowledged that they were diagnosed clinically by a biomedical clinic in the area. Only a few patients have visited private hospitals in urban areas to get confirmation of the diagnosis made at the clinic. Based on narratives shared by patients, it is clear that there is a lot of confusion around the treatment procedures since all of them were given similar medication, irrespective of the different stages of the disease. All the patients also maintained that they were not properly educated about the illness by the physicians. Based on three decades of experience, the community has concluded that CKDu is an incurable deadly disease. They are aware that the medications given by the clinic only halt the progression of the disease. The patients pointed out that their quality of life never improved, even though they had been taking medication for months, some for years. Most patients added that they had never experienced any physical comfort. This is most likely why patients in the area have selected Ayurveda/traditional medication to replace biomedicine. They seek Ayurveda/traditional medicine from local as well as far-off practitioners. Social networks and lay referrals play a crucial role in searching for multiple therapeutic options. In comparison with western medicine, the patients highlighted some of the improvements in their health condition with the use of Ayurveda/traditional medicine. According to patients, the functional capacity of their everyday life has improved to a great extent with reduced sleeping disorders, improved appetite and added hope for life. The evidence suggests that patients see the different medical systems as complementary to each other. However, from a provider perspective the different types of practitioners never collaborate with each other to address critical health hazards like CKDu.

The government has initiated providing a monthly cash subsidy for CKDu patients to cover their expenses. The patients who utilize Ayurveda, simultaneously attend the CKDu clinic just to maintain a good record of attendance to fulfil the eligibility criteria for the monthly allowance and to preserve the choice to utilize the hospital in case of an emergency. Many feel a sense of guilt for discarding the free medication provided by the government, and also do not share their experience of using Ayurvedic medicine with health care providers out of fear of judgement. The patients' narratives suggest that there is a huge gap in doctor–patient interactions. However, patients seem very silent in the clinical setting, but they are very dynamic in other spheres of their lives.

State Response

CKDu is one health issue that has been thoroughly investigated by experts from various disciplines to determine its unknown/uncertain etiology. The government also initiated the National Research Programme with the collaboration of World Health Organization (WHO) including a multidisciplinary team of experts to investigate diverse aspects of CKDu. However, while a large number of studies have been carried out during the past few decades to discover the etiology of the disease, it is yet to be determined (Rajapakse, 2016). Our empirical evidence reveals that the common people were marginalized throughout the process of the scientific investigations by minimizing their involvement and using water samples, food items, soil samples etc. instead. However, the citizens have their own discourse with regard to CKDu based on their local knowledge and lived experience as discussed earlier. They critique contradictory explanations with regard to the etiology of CKDu expressed by experts.

The state in Sri Lanka has given high priority to address CKDu and established a specific Presidential Taskforce to design and implement required interventions. It has also taken immediate actions to provide renal care services in concerned areas by strengthening the public health care delivery system. Simultaneously, regular clinics have been established in local health care institutions for health management. In addition, a special unit has been established under the Ministry of Health in Anuradhapura for CKDu to implement possible interventions for prevention. A surveillance system has been established to understand the burden of disease and to assess its geographical distribution. The health care providers noticed that patients were visiting the health care institutions at a late stage of disease progression as CKDu symptoms appear very slowly. As a result, community level screening programmes have been implemented in high-risk areas and a large number of people have been detected as CKDu patients. The patients who were at early stages were recommended to visit the clinic once in six months for check-ups, the patients at middle stages of disease progression were asked to visit the clinic once in three months and the patients who were at critical stages were requested to visit monthly. Dominant attention was given for early detection and management of CKDu and gradually, facilities for dialysis in the late stages have been expanded (Ministry of Health, 2017).

The public health care delivery system plays a crucial role in disease management with regard to CKDu. However, the health services are burdened by the illness. Most of the services were strictly inadequate in the beginning to provide essential service for a rapidly growing demand and there were indications that there was an implicit rationing of some of the services. For example, older persons with chronic kidney disease were not being provided with dialysis and kidney transplantation was recommended only for those who can afford out-of-pocket expenditure, etc. The situation slowly started changing with state intervention to improve the facilities for dialysis and kidney transplantation. However, our empirical evidence reveals a number of limitations in those interventions. The patients are reluctant to go for dialysis mainly due to misconceptions that they developed through their experience. As mentioned earlier, a facility for dialysis was initially given only for the patients who were at the end stage due to lack of facilities. Most people were not aware about the rationality behind rationing of services and rejected the same when the facility was given assuming that a rapid death can occur if they go for dialysis. The patients' narratives also reveal drug shortages in public health care institutions; they are regularly requested to buy medicine and get laboratory tests from the private sector.

CKDu is one health issue that has been thoroughly investigated by experts from various disciplines to determine its unknown/uncertain etiology. The government also initiated the National Research Programme with the collaboration of World Health Organization (WHO) including a multidisciplinary team of experts to investigate diverse aspects of CKDu. However, while a large number of studies have been carried out during the past few decades to discover the etiology of the disease, it is yet to be determined (Rajapakse, 2016). Our empirical evidence reveals that the common people were marginalized throughout the process of the scientific investigations by minimizing their involvement. However, the citizens have their own discourse with regard to CKDu based on their local knowledge and lived experience. They critique contradictory explanations with regard to the etiology of CKDu expressed by experts.

   The state interventions have strengths as well as some limitations as most of the interventions have been implemented in an ad hoc manner rather than properly planning them in advance. The local knowledge and experience of affected communities and their perspectives have not been taken into account in designing interventions and implementation processes. Three decades of lived experience of CKDu patients and concerned communities highlight a number of gaps in state interventions and issues with regard to the scientific investigation process of etiology of CKDu in local social context.

Discussion and Conclusion

Sociological and Anthropological studies clearly show interconnections between structural violence and poor health outcomes among marginalized social groups in different societies (De Silva et al., 2017; Farmer, 2004; Bourguignon & Farmer, 2004; Scheper-Hughes, 1993). In analyzing structural violence of CKDu, de Silva shows the factors and forces that have contributed to the emergence of CKDu among paddy farmers and agricultural labourers in Medawachchiya DS Division (De Silva et al., 2017). Silva (2021) shows how globalization processes have contributed to the emerging CKDu in the local context through the agricultural modernization process. Bandarage suggests the significance of taking the political economy of epidemic kidney disease in Sri Lanka into account in determining uncertain etiology of CKDu (Bandarage, 2013). The findings of the present study indicate that the affected communities have been marginalized throughout the process of discovering unknown/uncertain etiology and the decision-making process on health management. The biomedical system plays a dominant role in health management and currently faces a number of limitations. Findings of present study illuminate the ways in which CKDu contributes in reinforcing persistent inequalities among geographically underserved, marginalized agricultural communities in the North Central Province in Sri Lanka.

   The country has a well-established public–private mixed health care delivery system. The public health care delivery system plays a dominant role in providing free renal care services in the endemic areas though the patients have to bear some out-of-pocket expenditure. The government has paid dominant attention during the past few years to improve renal care services and cater to the growing demand and minimize the burden on patients. However, huge gaps can be seen in service delivery points and the country lacks sufficient social protection systems to support marginalized social groups who are involved in the informal economy of the country. The burden of CKDu has resulted in severe psychosocial and economic challenges for affected families/communities and an emerging trend of a new type of poverty that reinforces intergroup inequalities among disadvantaged social groups. Thus, the affected communities only have minimal access to social protection and support services. It is significant to incorporate knowledge about health-seeking behaviour into health service delivery strategies which are sensitive to the local dynamics of the community. Empirical evidence reveals an emerging discourse on efficacy of complementary medicine that demands an integrated approach for health care delivery systems. However, policy alternatives are required to incorporate collaborative strategies into the health care delivery system in Sri Lanka. A conceptual transformation is also required with ethno-medical perspective to address CKDu related issues in a culture sensitive manner (Kleinman, 1981). Integration of social workers into the local context is crucial to deal with humanitarian issues while improving communication skills among health care providers. The health care delivery system requires a biopsychosocial approach to address emerging issues that are associated with contemporary health hazards and for fair distribution of health care services among marginalized social groups.

Acknowledgements I acknowledge with thanks all respondents who shared their lived experience of CKDu with me to develop this paper. I thank Nishantha Wickramanayake, and Sumithra Rajapaksha for their assistance in conducting field work and Thiran Liyanage for technical assistance. I acknowledge the University of Colombo for providing a Small Research Grant to carry out this research.

References

Abeysekera, D. T. D. J., Kaiyoom, S. A. A., & Dissanayake, S. U. (1996). Place of peritoneal dialysis in the management of renal failure patients admitted to General Hospital Kandy. In *Kandy society of medicine 18th annual academic conference*.

Abeywardana, N., Bebermeier, W., & Schütt, B. (2018). Ancient water management and governance in the dry zone of Sri Lanka until abandonment, and the influence of colonial politics during reclamation. *Water, 10*(12), 1746. https://doi.org/10.3390/w10121746

Athuraliya, N., Abeysekera, T., Amerasinghe, P., Kumarasiri, R., Bandara, P., Karunaratne, U., et al. (2011). Uncertain etiologies of proteinuric-chronic kidney disease in rural Sri Lanka. *Kidney International, 80*(11), 1212–1221. https://doi.org/10.1038/ki.2011.258

Bandara, J., Senevirathna, D., Dasanayake, D., Herath, V., Bandara, J., Abeysekara, T., & Rajapaksha, K. (2008). Chronic renal failure among farm families in cascade irrigation systems in Sri Lanka is associated with elevated dietary cadmium levels in rice and freshwater fish (Tilapia). *Environmental Geochemistry and Health, 30*(5), 465–478.

Bandarage, A., (2013). Political economy of epidemic kidney disease in Sri Lanka. Sage Open, *3*(4). https://doi.org/10.1177/2158244013511827.

Bourguignon, E., & Farmer, P. (2004). Pathologies of power: Health, human rights and the new war on the poor. *The Antioch Review, 62*(1), 175. https://doi.org/10.2307/4614627

Chandrajith, R., Nanayakkara, S., Itai, K., Aturaliya, T., Dissanayake, C., Abeysekera, T., Harada, K., Watanabe, T., & Koizumi, A. (2010). Chronic kidney diseases of uncertain etiology (CKDue) in Sri Lanka: Geographic distribution and environmental implications. *Environmental Geochemistry and Health, 33*(3), 267–278.

Chandrajith, R., Dissanayake, C., Ariyarathna, T., Herath, H., & Padmasiri, J. (2011). Dose-dependent Na and Ca in fluoride-rich drinking water—Another major cause of chronic renal failure in tropical arid regions. *Science of the Total Environment, 409*(4), 671–675.

De Silva, M. W. A., Albert, S., & Jayasekara, J. (2017). Structural violence and chronic kidney disease of unknown etiology in Sri Lanka. *Social Science & Medicine, 178*, 184–195.

Dharma-wardana, M., Amarasiri, S., Dharmawardene, N., & Panabokke, C. (2014). Chronic kidney disease of unknown aetiology and ground-water ionicity: Study based on Sri Lanka. *Environmental Geochemistry and Health, 37*(2), 221–231.

Farmer, P. (2004). An anthropology of structural violence. *Current Anthropology, 45*(3), 305–325. https://doi.org/10.1086/382250

Gooneratne, I., Ranaweera, A., Liyanarachchi, N., Gunawardane, N., & Lanerolle, R. (2008). Epidemiology of chronic kidney disease in a Sri Lankan population. *International Journal of Diabetes in Developing Countries, 28*(2), 60. https://doi.org/10.4103/0973-3930.43101

Herath, C., Jayasumana, C., De Silva, P., De Silva, P., Siribaddana, S., & De Broe, M. (2018). Kidney diseases in agricultural communities: A case against heat-stress nephropathy. *Kidney International Reports, 3*(2), 271–280. https://doi.org/10.1016/j.ekir.2017.10.006

Jayasekara, J., Dissanayake, D., Adhikari, S., & Bandara, P. (2013). Geographical distribution of chronic kidney disease of unknown origin in North Central Region of Sri Lanka. *Ceylon Medical Journal, 58*(1), 6.

Jayasekara, K., Dissanayake, D., Sivakanesan, R., Ranasinghe, A., Karunarathna, R., & Priyantha Kumara, G. (2015). Epidemiology of chronic kidney disease, with special emphasis on chronic kidney disease of uncertain etiology, in the North Central Region of Sri Lanka. *Journal of Epidemiology, 25*(4), 275–280.

Jayasumana, C., Gunatilake, S., & Siribaddana, S. (2015a). Simultaneous exposure to multiple heavy metals and glyphosate may contribute to Sri Lankan agricultural nephropathy. *BMC Nephrology, 16*(1).

Jayasumana, C., Paranagama, P., Agampodi, S., Wijewardane, C., Gunatilake, S., & Siribaddana, S. (2015b). Drinking well water and occupational exposure to Herbicides is associated with chronic kidney disease, in Padavi-Sripura, Sri Lanka. *Environmental Health, 14*(1).

Jayatilake, N., Mendis, S., Maheepala, P., & Mehta, F. (2013). Chronic kidney disease of uncertain etiology: prevalence and causative factors in a developing country. *BMC Nephrology, 14*(1).

Kafle, K., Balasubramanya, S., & Horbulyk, T. (2019). Prevalence of chronic kidney disease in Sri Lanka: A profile of affected districts reliant on groundwater. *Science of the Total Environment, 694*(2019), 133767, ELSEVVIER.

Kleinman, A. (1981). Patients and healers in the context of culture. *An exploration of the borderland between anthropology, medicine, and psychiatry*. University of California Press.

Liyanage, C. (2019). Burden of chronic kidney disease of uncertain etiology on families of patients and their coping behaviour in two farming communities in Sri Lanka. *Journal of Social Sciences and Humanities Review, 4*(1), 27. https://doi.org/10.4038/jsshr.v4i1.26

Ministry of Health, Nutrition & Indigenous Medicine in Sri Lanka. (2017). *Weekly epidemiological report*, epidemiology unit, Vol. 44 (7). 11–17 February 2017.

Nissan, E. (1989). History in the making: Anuradhapura and the Sinhala Buddhist nation. *Social Analysis: The International Journal of Social and Cultural Practice*, (25), 64–77. Retrieved June 4, 2021, from http://www.jstor.org/stable/23163052.

Panabokke, C. R. (2009). *Small village tank systems of Sri Lanka: Their evolution, setting, distribution, and essential functions*. Hector Kobbekaduwa Agrarian Research and Training Institute.

Rajapakse, S., Shivanthan, M., & Selvarajah, M. (2016). Chronic kidney disease of unknown etiology in Sri Lanka. *International Journal of Occupational and Environmental Health, 22*(3), 259–264. https://doi.org/10.1080/10773525.2016.1203097

Ranasinghe, A., Kumara, G., Karunarathna, R., De Silva, A., Sachintani, K., & Gunawardena, J. et al. (2019). The incidence, prevalence and trends of chronic kidney disease and chronic kidney disease of uncertain aetiology (CKDu) in the North Central Province of Sri Lanka: An analysis of 30,566 patients. *BMC Nephrology, 20*(1). https://doi.org/10.1186/s12882-019-1501-0.

Scheper-Hughes, N., (1993). *Death without weeping: The violence of everyday life in Brazil*. University of California Press.

Silva, K. T. (2021). Globalization as a trigger for emerging new diseases? Contestations on chronic kidney disease of unknown etiology in Sri Lanka. *Current Research Journal of Social Sciences, 03*(1), 63–72.

Wimalawansa, S. J., (2015). Agrochemicals and chronic kidney disease of multi-factorial origin: Environmentally induced occupational exposure and occupational exposure disease. *International Journal of Nephrology and Kidney Failure (ISSN 2380–5498), 1*(3). https://doi.org/10.16966/2380-5498.111.

World Health Organization and National Science Foundation (NSF), Sri Lanka., (2016a). *Designing a step-wise approach to estimate the Burden and to understand the Etiology of CKDu in Sri Lanka*

World Health Organization., (2016b), *International expert consultation on chronic kidney disease of unknown etiology held in Colombo.* 27–29 April 2016.

Ingram Content Group UK Ltd.
Milton Keynes UK
UKHW022225160323
418671UK00002B/6